The Tufts University Guide to
TOTAL NUTRITION

The Tufts University Guide to
TOTAL NUTRITION

STANLEY GERSHOFF, PH.D.
Dean of the Tufts University School of Nutrition

**with Catherine Whitney and the Editorial Advisory Board
of the *Tufts University Diet & Nutrition Letter***

Foreword by Dr. Jean Mayer
President, Tufts University

1817

HARPER & ROW, PUBLISHERS, New York
Grand Rapids, Philadelphia, St. Louis, San Francisco
London, Singapore, Sydney, Tokyo, Toronto

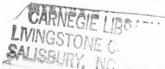

FIRST EDITION

Designed by Alma Orenstein

Library of Congress Cataloging-in-Publication Data

Gershoff, Stanley W.
    The Tufts University guide to total nutrition / Stanley Gershoff, with Catherine Whitney, and the editorial advisory board of the Tufts University diet & nutrition letter ; forward by Jean Mayer. — 1st ed.
      p. cm.
    ISBN 0-06-015918-9
    1. Nutrition. 2. Food. 3. Diet. I. Whitney, Catherine (Catherine A.)
II. Tufts University. III. Tufts University diet & nutrition letter. IV. Title.
    [DNLM: 1. Nutrition.]
TX353.G4 1990
613.2—dc20
DNLM
for Library of Congress   89-46124

---

90 91 92 93 94 DT/RRD 10 9 8 7 6 5 4 3 2 1

Dedicated to William H. White, whose vision made this book possible; and to the scientists and researchers whose work has led to a greater understanding of human nutrition in our time.

Contents

Acknowledgments

The development of this book depended on the efforts of many people. I would like to thank, in particular, my literary agent, Jane Dystel, who was instrumental in the book's conception, and who gave many long hours to assure its smooth development; Carol Cohen, a talented and enthusiastic editor, whose instincts about appealing to the popular market have always been on target; and Catherine Whitney, the writer who transformed the scientific information into practical, readable advice for consumers.

The staff of the *Tufts Diet & Nutrition Letter* have supported this work in countless ways. The late Bill White fought to make the book a reality and contributed considerable time to defining its direction and contents. Deborah White has used her experience with popular media and her strong marketing skills to assure the book a wide reading. The newsletter staff has been most generous in allowing me access to the excellent material they have gathered and has helped keep the book up-to-date during its development. In partic-ular, I am grateful for the assistance of Lawrence Lindner, Gail Zyla, Viola Roth, Marie Johnson, and the members of the newsletter's editorial board. I have appreciated the support and input of Marilyn Crim, M.D., Ph.D., assistant professor for nutrition, and Robert Nicolosi, Ph.D., visiting professor of nutrition.

Jean Mayer, the president of Tufts University, has distinguished himself as a leader in the nutrition and medical communities. His guidance and support have been essential to the work we have done at the School of Nutrition. I would also like to thank others at Tufts.

I am grateful for the work of Maureen Callahan, the nutritionist who consulted on this book. In particular, Maureen's contribution in developing practical food plans and appealing menus was critical. I would also like to thank others who contributed to portions of this book, including art designer, John Schuler, who developed some of the charts and art.

Tables, Charts, Illustrations

Nutrition Quizzes

Foreword

It is a pleasure to write this foreword for the first edition of *The Tufts University Guide to Total Nutrition*. You will find that this book is both readable and reliable. *Total Nutrition* is based on the research and knowledge of the Tufts University School of Nutrition and the *Tufts University Diet & Nutrition Letter,* which is edited by Dr. Stanley Gershoff, dean of the Tufts University School of Nutrition, a man whose name guarantees thoroughness and accuracy in the nutrition field.

Not only will readers be able to trust the information in this book, they will also be able to understand it. And that, when I think back, is a compliment I could not have paid the American public twenty years ago. At the time of the 1969 White House Conference on Food, Nutrition and Health, which I organized and chaired, I characterized Americans as "nutritional illiterates," a description fully deserved at the time but one that is no longer true.

The conference had many positive outcomes. The large federal food programs were expanded to the point that ten years later hunger (but not poverty) had largely disappeared from the United States. For consumers, a full review of the GRAS (Generally Recognized as Safe) list of food additives was initiated. This resulted not only in the removal of several potentially dangerous additives from foods, but also in unit pricing, open dating, ingredient labeling, the concept of standard packaging, and, most important, nutrition labeling on foods. Another consequence of the conference was the expansion of research on the role of diet in health and disease.

The interest of the American public in nutrition was permanently stimulated. One result of this growing awareness and knowledge about diet is the evidence of changes in food buying patterns over the last decade. Consumption of meats and dairy products (which are high in fat) and eggs (with their high cholesterol levels) has been cut back. There has been a rise in the consumption of polyunsaturated oils and fats, low-fat animal foods such as chicken and fish, fruits, vegetables, grains, and legumes. Salt consumption has also declined. People have not suddenly started to dislike those foods; they are simply eating less of them because they know it is better for their health. In response, food producers are beginning to alter the composition of foods. Although dietary changes may not account for the over one-third decline in cardiovascular mortality since 1970, they certainly play an important role. And in the case of the degenerative diseases of middle age, prevention, at this point, has proved easier than finding cures.

The increased interest in and knowledge of nutrition is attested to by the marked decrease of fad books on the market. Twenty years ago, not a week passed without the appearance of a "dieting" book which denied the basic laws of nutrition and made its author a millionaire on the basis of erroneous claims. For example, at a time when obesity and drunken driving represented two of the greatest threats to the survival and health of Americans, the virtues of the high-calorie, high-fat "Drinking Man's Diet" were extolled.

True, we still have the occasional book or article announcing that you don't have to worry about your blood cholesterol, for example, but these episodes are getting mercifully rarer and are questioned when they do take place. All in all, present-day Americans have had much more exposure to nutrition facts and have developed much greater critical abilities toward diet claims than they had twenty years ago.

The introduction to this book goes into the ways you can identify trustworthy nutrition information. The book itself is, I believe, an excellent source of such information and enjoyable to boot.

Good health and good reading.

Dr. Jean Mayer
President
Tufts University

Introduction

Nutrition has been a human preoccupation since the beginning of time. Our prehistoric ancestors served as the "laboratory subjects" for many of the foods we eat today, testing the viability of everything that grew or moved on the earth's surface. Over time, the human diet in different parts of the world settled into relatively stable, safe consumption patterns.

It was not until the eighteenth century that scientists began to draw more specific links between food and function. And it wasn't until the twentieth century that vitamins were discovered as essential elements in the human diet. Given the state of our nutritional understanding today it is hard to believe that only 100 years ago rickets was the most common disease among American young people, scurvy afflicted large numbers of sailors, iron deficiencies were common even among the wealthy, and dental cavities were a fact of life for children. Two hundred years ago, the average human life expectancy was 35 years. One hundred years ago, it was only 40 years. But as a result of medical advances and improved nutritional understanding, a child born today in the United States has an average life expectancy of 75 years.

In some respects, the rapid growth of nutrition-related discoveries, the elimination of common deficiencies, and the breakthroughs in the prevention and management of diseases have fostered a population of people with very high expectations for scientific research. People today expect positive discoveries to be made overnight; they are impatient with the slow, grinding process of research. They are better informed than ever, bolstered by a wealth of books, magazines, newspapers, and television programs that focus attention on nutrition. Yet in some ways they are less well informed than ever, lost in a sea of what appear to be constantly conflicting "expert" opinions. There seem to be so many scientific controversies that they don't know who to believe.

Thus, it may surprise you to know that, when it comes to most facets of nutrition, there is hardly any controversy within the scientific community. Nutritional authorities in this country and around the world have reached a clear consensus on many important aspects of nutrition—indeed, the recommendations of the 1988 Surgeon General's Report on Nutrition and Health were born of that consensus. The only major controversy is the debate that is constantly waged between the scientific community and the nonscientific community.

The media is always ready to give full play to the "discovery" of a new magic potion. For example, although the scientific community is in complete agreement that laetrile is not a vitamin and does not cure cancer, it continues to be promoted as a cure, and cancer victims continue to spend precious time and money traveling to Mexico to receive treatments.

In one sense, the scientific community is at a disadvantage when unsupported or false claims are made. Few scientists are willing to spend their limited research time and resources to prove to public satisfaction that a quack remedy will not cure cancer or a variety of other ailments. The more meaningful task is in the discovery of medical or nutritional links that might work.

Consumers are easily persuaded by false claims because they grow so impatient with the slow process of research. (Of course, research isn't *that* slow when you consider that most of the essential discoveries have been made in the last century.) The human body is a complex organism with thousands of possible interactions. Every time scientists discover a previously unknown contribution of one nutrient, their discovery has the potential for illuminating the metabolic roles of other nutrients. Before making a recommendation concerning food or nutrient therapy, however, scientists must not only rule out potentially detrimental interactions, they must also examine factors such as age, sex, environment, hereditary patterns, and potentially harmful practices, such as smoking. These factors are examined by studies on animals and human beings. Sometimes they take place over a period of many years, since long-term effects must be taken into account.

People who are confused about what to believe can use the following guidelines to judge the validity of a nutritional claim. A statement should probably be considered questionable if:

The claim sounds too good to be true. Consumers should take a skeptical view of diets, herbs, vitamins, minerals, enzymes, or "special foods" promoted as simple "cures" for, or "dramatic relief" from, a host of ills. Most scientists speak in terms of treating or reducing the risk of a disease rather than curing it. Furthermore, while dietary factors such as fat can play a role in the development of heart disease, cancer, and

other disorders, anyone who suggests that diet alone is to blame for most ailments and that nutritional supplements offer a remedy is leading you astray.

A promoter repeatedly refers to unproven remedies as "alternatives" to medically proven treatments and/or belittles established medicine. Physicians in the medical community generally welcome new treatment options, provided they are supported by solid research. If an "alternative" has not been accepted by legitimate health-care providers, it's because sufficient research is lacking or, even worse, the treatment has proved to be dangerous.

Anecdotes and testimonials alone are used to support a claim. Scientists rely on carefully controlled experiments to measure the effectiveness of treatments, not random comments from consumers who use them before they're rigorously tested. Often claims are made based on the personal experience of the author—hardly a reliable way to make pronouncements for the general population. It takes a good deal of time and careful study to determine if the seeming effects of a food or drug actually are what they're said to be.

The recommendation limits variety. Human beings need protein, carbohydrate, fat, and a number of essential vitamins and minerals to grow and develop. Diet prescriptions that are based on excluding essential foods or that focus on one or several "special" foods are not valid. In effect, these dietary theories take us back to the "dark ages" of nutritional understanding, when deficiencies were rampant. Likewise, the "more is better" philosophy is fallacious. Vitamin and mineral megadoses can often lead to toxicity and negatively influence the absorption of other nutrients. Overdoing the use of a positive substance, such as fiber, will lead to problems.

It contradicts consensus. At times, it becomes fashionable to mistrust the scientific and health establishment—as though there were an establishment in the sense that we all got together in a room and formulated proclamations. In fact, there is no formal establishment in the field of nutrition. Rather, the things we know about food and its functions have emerged over time as the consensus of scientists and other experts. It is absurd to heed the advice of self-proclaimed outsiders, many of whom have no training whatsoever in the disciplines they are evaluating. It can be frustrating for those of us who work in this field to see consumers listening to people who preach misinformation when there is so much that we *know*. Granted, some erroneous recommendations seem to be benign; while they won't help you, they probably won't hurt you either. But others are not so harmless and can lead to health problems that might easily have been avoided.

It is our hope that this book will provide the public with a reliable, commonsense guide to nutrition. It contains hundreds of different suggestions for better eating; it includes data on the most current scientific research underway, both here at Tufts and elsewhere; and it offers advice for people who are "average" as well as for people who have special concerns and needs.

We also hope that, in the process of reading and using this book, you will begin to experience some of the excitement about the possibilities that exist for human nutrition as we move toward the end of the twentieth century. Good nutritional practices can improve the lives of many millions of Americans, and we look forward to the time when they are available to every person in the world, as well. It will be a different planet indeed when that dream is realized.

PART ONE

The Fundamentals of Good Food

When you sit down to the dinner table, you probably don't look at the food and exclaim, "That protein smells delicious!" or "Please pass the vitamin C." Rather, what you see is food that has been prepared in a certain way. The aroma and presentation influence your reaction, as do the setting of the meal, the people with whom you share it, and a variety of other factors, including your food preferences, how hungry you are, and the way you live. These factors are, in their own ways, fundamental to the practice of good nutrition, since all of them influence what foods you consume and how you consume them.

In the course of our busy lives, most of us don't stop to consider the incredible logic of nature. Nutrition may seem an abstract concept to us. We're not sure exactly why it's so; we only know that if we follow certain guidelines, we'll probably lead healthier, longer, lives. But nutrition is not abstract at all.

The saying "You are what you eat" was originally coined as an admonition to those who might feast on fatty foods or ingest empty calories. But it is not exactly true that we are what we eat. A more accurate way to state the principle is: In order to reach our greatest potential for growth and development and to maintain good health, we must consume nutritious foods.

To better understand the role of nutrition in life functions, it is important to grasp the fundamental design of food and the role it plays in nourishing your body. Once you grasp the basic science of nutrition, you'll find that your options for developing a healthier diet will increase.

The simplest way to define food is to say that it is the plant and animal products we ingest that enables our bodies to operate. It accomplishes this function in three ways: by supplying energy, by providing the building blocks to support growth and tissue repair, and by delivering the nutrients necessary to keep our metabolic systems running smoothly.

Food which supplies calories primarily consists of three elements: *carbon, oxygen,*

1

and *hydrogen*. Carbohydrates and fat are essentially composed of these compounds. Protein is composed of these three plus *nitrogen* and *sulfur*, which sets it apart from other nutrients in the role it plays.

When we eat food, we are not actually consuming nutrients. But once we start chewing, our bodies' food-conversion mechanisms kick into action in a remarkable way. The diagram demonstrates, for example, how the body might process a peanut butter and jelly sandwich. First, the protein, carbohydrate, fat, vitamins, and minerals must become separated by the process of digestion. The pipeline for food processing is called the *gastrointestinal (GI) tract*. The GI tract is composed of somewhat elastic muscles that

How Food Moves Through the GI Tract

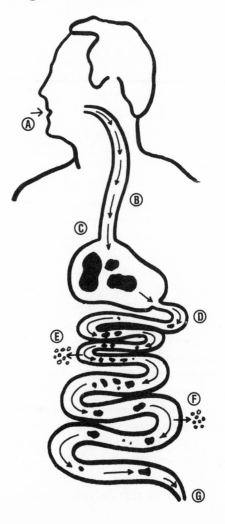

(A) Mouth: Chewing and saliva reduces food to a soft wad. Breakdown of carbohydrate begins.

(B) Esophagus: Muscles propel saliva-lubricated food down to stomach.

(C) Stomach: Stomach has about a 2-quart capacity. Food is churned into liquid mass. About every 20 seconds, some of this mass is released into the small intestine.

(D) Small intestine: Chemical activity breaks down protein, fat, carbohydrate.

(E) Nutrients now pass into the bloodstream to feed and fuel cells.

(F) Large Intestine: Beginning with the colon, water and salts pass into the bloodstream, leaving undigested waste for excretion.

(G) Anus: Exit for fecal waste. The entire process takes 1 to 2 days.

in an adult would measure about 26 feet in length if stretched completely straight. But the GI tract is not straight; it is a twisted pipeline made up of pouches and tubes, including the mouth, esophagus, stomach, small intestine, and large intestine. Through the process of *peristalsis* (contractions) and digestion, food moves through the pipeline and is pulverized and lubricated so that it becomes finely divided and suspended in a watery, mushy solution. At various points in the digestive tract, hydrochloric acid, bile from the liver, and enzymes from the mouth, stomach, pancreas, and intestines are added.

The walls of parts of the GI tract are permeable, allowing nutrients to pass through them into the bloodstream. These nutrients consist of amino acids from protein, fatty acids from fats and oils, simple sugars from carbohydrates, and vitamins and minerals. As nutrients are absorbed, the bloodstream and lymphatic system transport them to the cells. But not all the material in food is absorbed. The nutrients the body needs pass through the walls of the small intestines, and the waste material is passed on to the large intestine for excretion.

Each of the various food compounds has specific roles to play in our bodies. Once the various nutrients enter the cells, they go to work performing their unique functions, which are described in the following sections.

1

Protein: The Body Builder

Our need for dietary protein stems from its function in providing and replenishing the protein that is the structural core of the human body. Protein might easily be called "the stuff of life," as it is at work in every cell of the body. In fact, about one-fifth of our total weight is protein—one-half of it in muscle, a fifth in bone and cartilage, a tenth in skin, and the rest in other tissues and body fluids.

Protein performs the most important jobs in the body, including all three of the functions of nutrients:

▶ Protein is essential for growth and the repair and formation of new tissues.

▶ Protein is the regulatory agent for our important body processes, since all enzymes and many hormones are proteins. They are useful in transporting nutrients and oxygen through the body. Since antibodies and other components of our immune system are proteins, they play a major role in fighting diseases.

▶ Protein is a source of energy.

The Makeup of Protein

Protein consists of a variety of nitrogen-containing compounds, called *amino acids,* which are linked together in different, genetically controlled sequences. There are 22 separate amino acids, and the sequence in which they appear in a protein defines its biological activity. For example, even though liver proteins are made of the same amino acids as muscle proteins, the different ways they are linked allows them to perform separate functions. The nitrogen (and in some cases sulfur) in amino acids makes proteins different from fat and carbohydrate, even though all three contain carbon, oxygen, and hydrogen.

Chemically, amino acids are absorbed into the body and rebuilt into various proteins through what is called a *peptide linkage*. When you eat protein foods, the digestive enzymes in the intestines, some of which come from the pancreas, break the proteins down, first into *peptides* (small groups of amino acids) and finally into amino acids. The amino acids are absorbed through the intestines, and the body then builds them up again in the various sequences that define the functions they will serve.

Thirteen of the amino acids can be manufactured in the body. But nine of the amino acids needed to make up the body's protein cannot be manufactured in the body. We must eat protein to supply these nine *essential amino acids*. If we don't our bodies cannot function. Dietary protein is not optional.

The essential amino acids are histidine, isoleu-

5

cine, leucine, lysine, methionine, phenylalanine, threonine, tryptophan, and valine. The term "essential" is somewhat misleading. All of the amino acids are necessary for good health. But since the body doesn't produce these nine, they must be consumed in the foods we eat; they are an essential part of the human diet. If your diet lacks even one of these amino acids, you can't produce enough new protein, and you will suffer muscle and other tissue loss.

In addition, many of the amino acids support other body functions. For example, *tryptophan* is converted into the B vitamin niacin and into the neurotransmitter *serotonin,* which influences alertness and mood. Likewise, *histidine* is converted into *histamine,* a compound associated with allergic reactions. *Methionine* is involved in the synthesis of substances which affect transport of fats from the liver. One of the nonessential amino acids, *tyrosine,* can be converted to the hormone *thyroxine.*

Anyone who is even vaguely familiar with nutrition can list a wide variety of foods that are significant sources of protein. But not all protein food sources are equal when it comes to supplying the nine essential amino acids. Since we must have adequate amounts of all nine of them, it is important to know the difference between complete proteins and incomplete proteins.

Complete proteins contain all nine essential amino acids in sufficient quantities. Incomplete proteins lack or have limited amounts of one or more of the essential amino acids; by themselves, they cannot support the body's growth and maintenance.

In general, animal proteins are more complete than plant proteins. While the proteins in meat and other animal products are not exactly the same as the proteins in the human body, they are similar enough in composition that they're likely to provide essential amino acids in the ratios needed. However, don't assume that this is always the case. Gelatin, for example, is a particularly poor protein source; it lacks or has inadequate amounts of several amino acids.

Proteins from vegetable sources (which include grains and legumes) are usually incomplete. By itself, a vegetable food that lacks or has insufficient quantities of one or more of the nine essential amino acids cannot adequately support the body's growth. However, it is possible to combine incomplete proteins to make up a complete protein. Some incomplete proteins are "complementary," making up for each other's deficiencies by forming a complete protein when eaten together.

Unfortunately, in many parts of the world, single grains that contain incomplete proteins are the primary protein source for the population. In some Third World countries, 70 percent of the protein consumed is derived from incomplete sources like wheat. However, it is rare that people eat only a single source of protein; if there is adequate food, different grains can be combined with vegetables, legumes, and small amounts of animal products to create complete protein patterns. One good example is a meal pattern that has evolved in Latin America, where two complementary protein sources, rice and beans, are eaten together.

Protein deficiencies are rarely a problem for North Americans, since we tend to consume such a wide variety of foods. However, people who go on fad diets that emphasize one or two foods with incomplete proteins (such as rice) are putting themselves in danger.

Good Sources of Complete Protein

Animal products, which contain complete proteins, provide a major part of the nine essential amino acids in the American food supply. These include meat, fish, poultry, eggs, milk, and cheese. Of course, these foods are not simply "pure" protein; they are rich sources of vitamins and minerals and may also contain fat and cholesterol. You can benefit from the protein without consuming excessive amounts of fat and cholesterol, or too many calories, if you follow some of the practical guidelines that are discussed in other sections of this book.

Combining Incomplete Protein Sources

But what if you want to restrict your consumption of animal products? Does this necessarily mean that you will suffer protein deficiencies? Not necessarily, but such a diet requires planning. If the complementary foods are eaten together, your body treats them as if they were one food. An incomplete protein source like corn, for example, is low in the amino acids tryptophan and lysine. Beans are high in tryptophan and lysine, but low in methionine, which corn has in sufficient amounts. Therefore, if you eat corn and beans together, you will have eaten a meal that contains all the essential amino acids.

On the other hand, soybeans and many nuts contain all the essential amino acids, but they don't have enough of one or more of them to make them effective in completely meeting protein needs. Soybeans are limited in methionine, so if they are combined with wheat, which has high levels of that amino acid, the result is a complete protein source.

You can also create a high-quality protein meal by adding a very small quantity of an animal food to an incomplete protein. For example, cereal with milk or spaghetti with a little ground beef or grated cheese will supply the essential amino acids in the necessary quantities.

(Note that fresh, dry, or sprouted kidney, navy, pinto, and soy beans contain substances that can interfere with the digestion of proteins. To be on the safe side, make sure that these and other dried beans are thoroughly cooked, since heat deactivates the inhibitors.)

How Much Protein Do We Need?

Anyone who has access to and consumes a variety of foods shouldn't have a protein problem. And,

---

Protein Combinations to Make a Meal "Complete"

lentil soup with corn bread
rice and kidney bean casserole
peanut butter on whole-wheat bread
corn tortillas with pinto beans
vegetable-tofu stir fry over rice
navy bean–potato soup with rye bread
peanut–sesame seed snack mix
rice cakes with peanut butter
chile with a side of whole wheat bread
chick peas or black-eyed peas with corn
   bread

or use small amounts of animal protein:

spaghetti with tomato–meat sauce

shredded chicken or pork with stir-fried vegetables
cereal with low-fat milk
spinach salad sprinkled lightly with bacon
   and hard-cooked egg
vegetable–clam chowder
bean tortillas with shredded cheese
   topping
meatless chile bean soup, topped with shredded cheese
baked potato with low-fat yogurt and chives
potato–egg salad
macaroni casserole with tuna or grated
   cheese
split pea soup with diced ham

► NUTRITION QUIZ ◄

Do You Know the Truth About Protein?

Most people know that protein is essential, but there are many misconceptions about how much the body needs and what are the best sources. Take this true-or-false quiz to see if you know the facts.

1. Most Americans eat more than enough protein.
   True _____ False _____

2. Proteins that come from animals contain all the essential amino acids the body needs.
   True _____ False _____

3. As adults age, they require less protein.
   True _____ False _____

4. High-protein diets are not recommended for the obese.
   True _____ False _____

5. Red meats are better protein sources than poultry or fish.
   True _____ False _____

6. Athletes need significantly more protein than nonathletes.
   True _____ False _____

ANSWERS

1. (True). Most Americans consume double their requirement for protein. For example, the RDA for a 130-pound woman is easily met by eating three ounces of lean meat, one slice of bread, one-half cup of cottage cheese, and 1 cup of milk.

2. (True). Animal proteins are considered "complete," meaning that they contain the needed amounts of the nine essential amino acids your body must get from food. Vegetables are not complete sources of protein; they lack essential amino acids or do not contain them in sufficient quantities to meet your body's needs. Only by combining complementary vegetables on the same day (e.g., rice and beans) can you receive a complete protein source.

3. (False). Current thinking is that the RDA for protein remains the same on a weight basis throughout adulthood. Some investigators think that because of changes in the body's efficiency in using protein, the elderly might require more. However, since calorie needs decrease as we age, it is wise for the elderly to select low-fat sources of protein.

4. **(False).** High-protein, low-carbohydrate, very low-calorie diets can be effective for weight loss in obese people (those who are approximately 25 percent or more above their normal weight range). After an initial water loss, significant amounts of fat are also lost. However, these diets can be hazardous and are recommended only for people whose obesity places them at high risk for heart disease or adult-onset diabetes. And they should always be undertaken with medical supervision.

5. **(False).** Red meats tend to be higher in fat, so the percentage of protein on an ounce-for-ounce basis is lower than in fish or poultry.

6. **(False).** Although an athlete may need slightly more protein during the initial stages of training or competition, that need is not very great. Since most Americans already consume more than enough protein, chances are the increased need has already been met by a normal diet.

although it has been suggested that North Americans consume too much protein, few people suffer from too much protein. The exceptions are people who deliberately choose a diet very high in protein, or those who, because of kidney and liver problems, should restrict the amount of protein that they eat. In fact, since our bodies store very limited amounts of protein, we need to eat it every day to prevent muscle breakdown and a lapse in other bodily functions.

On the other hand, many Americans have inflated views of how much protein they need. From time to time, high-protein diets (often based on misconceptions) are advertised as providing special benefits. For example, one currently popular diet theory proposes that the amino acid tryptophan converts to an alertness-related neurotransmitter and, thus, that animal protein should be eaten in abundance when we need to stay alert. Another popular notion is that, because protein is needed for the development of muscle, a high-protein diet will make a person muscular. These ideas are unproven, or at the very least gross oversimplifications that can lead to trouble when people take them literally. As eagerly as we might seek "magical" effects from food, the simple, if dull, fact remains that only by eating a balanced variety of foods can we get all

the nutrients we need in the amounts we need them.

In fact, consuming an overabundance of protein can be expensive and inefficient. Our bodies are not able to store the amino acids they can't use, so the excess is used either for energy or to build fat. Consider, too, that the waste products from excess protein metabolism are lost in the urine. Overconsumption can place a strain on the kidneys. Furthermore, the cholesterol and fat content of many high-protein foods can place you at risk for heart disease if you eat too much of them.

The amount of protein most people need is approximately 8 or 9 percent of their total calories, with needs being highest during periods of growth, such as childhood. For women who are pregnant or lactating, they are even higher. Americans consume an average of 12 to 14 percent of their calories in protein, yet we could eat even more—say, 20 percent—and still be healthy.

As we've pointed out, most Americans, if they have access to a variety of foods, don't have to worry about not getting enough protein. However, if you are concerned, it is easy to calculate your individual protein requirement by weight. If you look at the breakdowns of Recommended Dietary Allowances (RDAs) in chapter 7, you will find guidelines that cover 18 standard profiles.

These guidelines aren't meant to be taken as rules. But they're useful in determining the general range of nutrients appropriate for a person of your age or special circumstances.

If you want to develop an even more personal version of your daily protein requirement, here's how: The current recommendation for adults over the age of 19 is a little over a gram of protein per kilogram of body weight. (A kilogram is equal to 2.2 pounds.) By making the following calculations, a 130-pound adult woman can determine her daily protein requirement:

$$130 \text{ pounds} \div 2.2 = 59 \text{ kilograms}$$

$$59 \text{ kilograms} \times 0.8 \text{ grams} = 47 \text{ grams of protein}$$

$$\begin{aligned} 47 \text{ grams} \times 4 \text{ (calories} \\ \text{per gram)} \end{aligned} = 188 \text{ calories}$$

Note that this is only a few grams different from the RDA. It can easily be met within the structure of a a normal diet. But counting protein grams isn't a simple matter of weighing high-protein foods, since they contain other components as well. Get in the habit of reading labels to familiarize yourself with the protein content of common foods. And be aware that few foods are perfect sources of the nutrients they provide. For example, a 3-ounce lean round cut of beef, broiled, has 179 calories, with 26 grams or 104 calories contributed by protein. Most of the remainder is fat, plus a variety of vitamins and minerals.

We provide the following breakdowns for those who are interested or who need, for specific health reasons, to calculate their intake more precisely. But we stress that, for most people, a general awareness of the content of various foods will provide the tools they need to formulate a well-balanced diet. It is hardly our suggestion that you carry a pocket calculator to count your grams of protein each day. As a matter of fact, not consuming your requirement on occasion for a day or two will not have a long-term effect on your health. However, the greater the deviation and the longer it occurs, the greater the chance you'll suffer from a deficiency.

THE PROTEIN CONTENT OF COMMON FOODS

Serving of Food	Grams of Protein
Meats	
ground beef, 3 oz. broiled	21
beef round bottom, 3 oz., broiled	25
beef tenderloin, 3 oz., broiled	22
ham, 3 oz., roasted	18
veal, 3 oz., round, broiled	23
Poultry	
chicken, 3.5 oz., roasted	27
turkey, 3.5 oz., roasted	28
capon, 3.5 oz., roasted	29
Seafood	
salmon, 3.5 oz., baked/broiled	27
halibut, 3.5 oz., broiled	21
mackerel, 3.5 oz., broiled	22
flounder, 3.5 oz., baked	30
bluefish, 3.5 oz., baked/broiled	26
tuna, 3.5 oz., canned in water	28
swordfish, 3.5 oz., broiled	28
scallops, 3.5 oz., steamed	18
Processed Meats	
beef bologna, 1 oz.	3
chicken roll, 1 oz.	6
beef frankfurter, 1	6
ham, sliced, 1 oz.	5
turkey bologna, 1 oz.	4
Dairy Products	
milk, 1 cup, whole/low-fat/skim	8
buttermilk	8
yogurt, 8 oz., low-fat, plain	12
yogurt, 8 oz., low-fat, fruit	9
cheese, 1 oz., cheddar	7
cream cheese, 1 oz.	2
cottage cheese, ½ cup, low-fat	15.5
eggs, 1 large, boiled	6

Source: U.S. Department of Agriculture (figures are approximate)

2

Carbohydrates:
Our Nutrient Staple

Many Americans born after World War II grew up believing that protein was the equivalent of dietary manna, while carbohydrates contributed little to health. In fact, for some time, carbohydrate foods were widely believed to be leading culprits in excess weight gain. Fortunately, as consumer education about nutrition has grown, Americans have opened their eyes to the benefits of many foods high in complex carbohydrates.

The Complex Carbohydrate Story

Carbohydrates are organic compounds composed of carbon, oxygen, and hydrogen. All carbohydrates are constructed from multiple units of simple sugars connected to each other. The most basic form of carbohydrate is that of the *simple sugars,* the most important of which are *glucose, fructose,* and *galactose.* Simple sugars are small compounds that have six carbons. In the same way that amino acids are the builiding blocks of protein, simple sugars are the building blocks of the *complex carbohydrates* (the starches).

Each simple sugar is called a *monosaccharide.* When it is chemically combined with another simple sugar, the result is a *disaccharide.* The most common disaccharide is ordinary table sugar, or

sucrose, which is composed of one unit of glucose and one unit of fructose. Another disaccharide, *maltose,* is composed of two units of glucose. And *lactose,* the disaccharide found in milk, is composed of one part glucose and one part galactose.

When more than two glucose molecules are joined together, they form a more complex carbohydrate called a *polysaccharide.* When they occur in plants, polysaccharides are known as starches; in animals, they are called glycogens. Polysaccharides are in the form in which plants and animals store carbohydrate energy. They contain anywhere from 300 to 1,000 glucose units linked together, and it is the nature of the links that determines whether a polysaccharide is starch or glycogen.

The Dietary Role of Carbohydrates

From a nutritional standpoint, plant starch is the most important source of complex carbohydrates. There is very little glycogen in animals, but there's a great deal of starch in plants.

When we eat complex carbohydrates, the digestive enzymes in the mouth and intestines break down the polysaccharides into disaccharides and, ultimately, into glucose. It is glucose that is absorbed into the system and converted into energy.

If complex carbohydrates are broken down and absorbed as sugar, why are we so concerned about the importance of eating starch? Why not just eat glucose? There are two important reasons.

First, if you gave one person starch and another an equal amount of glucose, you would achieve entirely different results because the simple sugars are released from starch more slowly into the bloodstream. The rate of release has a number of consequences, one being that it affects the way *insulin* is secreted. This factor is particularly important for diabetics. It's not that diabetics can't eat sugar. While they can't tolerate a big dose of sugar all at once, they can handle the slow release of sugar that takes place in their systems through the breakdown of starch.

Second, starch differs from simple sugars in a very important way. When we eat simple sugars —in sweets or table sugar—these literally are "empty calories," because there's nothing else in the sugar. It doesn't carry other nutrients. If you eat a pound of hard candy, all you've eaten is sucrose. There are no vitamins or minerals. (Honey and brown sugar are not more healthful; those sources of sugar do not really add significant nutrients.) There's a big difference between eating a bowl of sugar and a bowl of rice, because when you eat rice you're also getting protein, minerals, and vitamins.

To illustrate, let's compare a small baked potato with an ounce of gum drops. Both contain about 100 calories, but they come in very different packages. The potato, rich in glucose in the form of starch, provides about one-half of the RDA for vitamin C, along with small amounts of protein, B vitamins, about six minerals, and fiber. The gum drops, whose glucose is contributed as the simple sugar sucrose, supplies the same amount of energy but no other nutrients in significant amounts.

What about fruit, which contains the sweetest-tasting sugar, fructose? Fruit does not contain a substantial amount of starch, but that does not make it nutritionally undesireable. Since fruit is mostly water (91 percent of the edible part of a watermelon is water), its fructose concentration is relatively low and therefore does not drive up the number of calories or make it taste overly sweet. And the fruit has fiber. Moreover, like starchy foods, many fruits come packed with vitamins A and C, and some contain minerals.

Are Starchy Foods Fattening?

It used to be that if you wanted to lose a few pounds, you cut out bread, pasta, rice, and potatoes. But today these very foods (without the rich toppings) are considered to be the best foods to include in a weight-loss diet. Starch has no more calories than protein—just four per gram. And, unlike some high-protein foods such as meat and dairy products, most starchy foods are almost fat free.

But there's another reason why starch is good for weight control. It appears that the process of metabolizing carbohydrate uses more energy (calories) than metabolizing fat. Some studies have shown that as many as 25 percent of the excess calories we take in as carbohydrate are used to convert the carbohydrate to body fat. This means that only about 75 percent of the extra carbohydrate calories are "added on" as body weight. By contrast, only 3 percent of excess fat calories are needed to convert dietary fat to body fat, and a full 97 percent of extra fat calories wind up "on the body."

Does Sugar Cause Problems?

There is some evidence that humans are born with a "sweet tooth." In tests conducted with newborn babies, researchers sought to discover what their automatic, untrained response might be to various substances. When a drop of water was placed on the babies' tongues, they showed no response. A drop of sour substance caused them to scrunch up their faces. Salt made them cry. And when a drop of sugar was placed on the babies' tongues, their faces relaxed into a contented expression.

Sugar has been called the culprit for everything from heart disease to cancer to diabetes to hyperactivity. But recently, a panel of scientists at the Food and Drug Administration, known as the Sugar Task Force, concluded that sugar does not directly contribute to any health problems other than dental cavities.

The main concern we have about sugar is that its overconsumption can potentially lead to other problems, such as obesity, and that it supplies no nutrients. A teaspoon of sugar used to sweeten a cup of coffee or tea contains only 16 calories and is relatively harmless. But when it is one of the main ingredients in a product such as soft drink, candy, sugar-coated cereal, or ice cream, the picture changes. A 12-ounce can of sugar-sweetened soda, for instance, contains about 10 teaspoons of sugar, or 160 calories' worth. Sugar also contributes more than a fourth of the calories in a small slice of chocolate cake. Similarly, it takes about four teaspoons of sugar—totaling 64 calories—just to sweeten one ounce of chocolate, which is naturally bitter in taste. In other words, sugar can add a substantial number of calories to food. And these calories are "empty"—they supply nothing in the way of vitamins or minerals.

But that's not all. Many of the foods people like because of their sweet taste are also loaded with fat. For example, a number of popular candy bars are about 25 percent fat by weight.

A report by the Center for Science in the Public Interest constructed the following analysis of where Americans get their sugar. Their report listed the sources of sugar consumption as follow:

Soft drinks: 25 percent

Sweets (table sugar, jams, syrups, etc.): 18 percent

Baked goods (cookies, cakes, pies): 13 percent

Ice cream and other dairy products: 10 percent

Bread and grain products: 6 percent

Breakfast cereals: 5 percent

Candy: 2 percent

Other minor sources add up to 21 percent. These include various packaged foods, dressings, cured meats, etc.

How Much Carbohydrate Should We Eat?

Carbohydrates are abundant in our food supply. The many nutritional benefits of foods that contain them lead most health professionals to recommend that 50 to 60 percent of our calorie intake be contributed by carbohydrates, and that about 80 percent of those be complex carbohydrates.

It wasn't very long ago that complex carbohydrates accounted for this amount of our daily diet. At the beginning of this century, Americans consumed 40 to 50 percent of their calories this way. But today complex carbohydrates comprise only 20 to 25 percent of the average American's diet. The decrease is largely the result of the fact that as we have become more affluent, we have turned to relatively expensive animal foods, such as meat and poultry, for our protein and away from the less expensive carbohydrate-containing grains and legumes that once played a greater role in meeting our protein needs.

Good sources of complex carbohydrates include all vegetables, cereal, rice, bread, pasta, nuts and seeds, grains, and legumes. It is best to consume a variety of high-carbohydrate foods to insure that you get adequate amounts of the vitamins and minerals you need.

Have a High-Carbohydrate Day

Statistics show that the average American consumes only 20 to 25 percent of his or her daily calories in the form of complex carbohydrates, only half the amount most health professionals recommend. This one-day menu adds up to about 1,800 calories, with 53 percent of them from complex carbohydrates, 30 percent from fat, and 17 percent from protein.

Food	Carbohydrate (grams)	Food	Carbohydrate (grams)
Breakfast:		**Dinner:**	
1 cup cornflakes	21.7	3½ oz baked, skinless	
1 cup 2% milk	11.7	chicken breast	0
½ banana	13.4	2 pieces 4″ corn on the	
1 slice whole-wheat toast	11.4	cob	44.6
1 tsp. polyunsaturated		½ cup cooked green	
margarine	0	beans	4.9
½ cup orange juice	12.9	2 tsp. polyunsaturated	
		margarine	0
Lunch:		tossed salad, with	
roast beef sandwich,		1 cup lettuce, and ¼	
with		cup each of carrots,	
2 oz. lean roast beef	0	mushrooms, tomato,	
2 slices rye bread	24.0	celery	7.2
lettuce	0	1 tbsp. French salad	
¼ medium tomato	1.8	dressing	2.7
1 tbsp. mayonnaise	0.4		
1 cup black bean soup	19.8	**After-dinner snack:**	
½ cup grapes	7.9	2 oatmeal raisin cookies	17.8
		1 cup 2% milk	11.7
Midafternoon snack:			
1 medium apple	21.1		

3

Fiber:
A Dietary Bonus from Plants

It may surprise you to know that fiber is not a substance with nutritive value. The word "fiber" is used to describe a variety of substances in plant foods that may have no relationship to one another except for the fact that they are not digested. Fiber is not necessary for life and growth, but it does perform a useful role in the digestive process and may contribute other benefits.

Fiber comes in two forms. Water-insoluble fibers, which make up the structural parts of plant cell walls, include substances like cellulose, hemicellulose, and lignin that are found primarily in whole-wheat products, wheat bran, and fruit and vegetable skins. Water-soluble fibers come primarily from fruits, vegetables, beans, and oats, and include pectins and gum, some of which are extracted for use as food additives. All plant foods contain some combination of the various types of fiber. For example, fruits and vegetables contain cellulose as well as pectin; in general, fruits are higher in pectin, and vegetables have more cellulose.

Fiber's Problem-Solving Qualities

Fiber is clearly the new "darling" of the nutritional media. Many health claims have been made, some based on early scientific evidence, and others based on unproven theories.

Since fiber is not necessary to human nutrition, what true benefits can it really have? There is very good evidence that fiber serves a number of problem-solving functions in the body:

▶ Most experts agree that the chemical nature of fiber (especially the insoluble kind) enables it to pick up water, which adds bulk to the stool and enhances the transit time of undigested foods through the GI tract. There are several advantages to this. First, when you have soft, bulky stools, there is less trauma to the bowel. In the case of hemorrhoids (swollen distended veins in the rectal area), the larger, softer stools that result from eating foods high in water-insoluble fiber (such as wheat bran) may lead to less strain during defecation.

▶ There is also evidence that fiber protects against a common condition in the GI tract called diverticulosis. This disease is characterized by pouches that develop in weak areas of the large intestine. It is believed that a low-fiber intake might increase the likelihood of this problem developing because the muscles of the intestine become "out of shape" as a result of insufficient stimulation. Until recently, fiber was not recommended for people with diverticular disease. But now a high-fiber diet and sometimes coarse wheat bran are recommended to relieve the accompanying constipation. (However, a high-fiber diet is not advised for complicated cases in which there is intestinal bleeding, perforation, or abscess.)

► There is some evidence that certain types of fiber—namely those in fruits, vegetables, and oats—can decrease blood lipids and therefore reduce the risk of heart disease. Some studies have reported that the soluble fiber found in oat bran and dried beans is effective in lowering blood cholesterol. A recent study, which was given enormous unwarranted media coverage, questioned the value of oat bran in reducing cholesterol. We believe that oat fiber has a real anti-cholesterol effect, but it is a relatively small effect, and one would be foolish to think that oat bran or any other dietary component is the answer to cholesterol problems. Other studies have revealed that pectin and guar—a type of gum—can also reduce blood cholesterol.

Potential Benefits Still Being Researched

It appears that the health benefits of fiber may reach even further. However, these speculations are as yet based on limited data, and much more research must be done before scientific conclusions can be made. There are two areas of current speculation:

► *Diabetes aid.* Accumulating studies demonstrate that dietary fiber can improve the control of blood sugar and decrease insulin requirements for some diabetics. Some doctors have found that diets high in both fiber and complex carbohydrates can effectively lower blood sugar. This result can be achieved with many different fiber sources, including legumes, whole-grain products, fruits, and vegetables. Some people with adult-onset diabetes have been able to go off oral

medication and insulin injections altogether. However, not all doctors have had favorable results when they've tried high-fiber diets with diabetics. (Under no circumstances should a diabetic try such a diet without medical supervision.)

► *Cancer prevention.* Some studies suggest that cancer of the colon, which is one of the most common malignancies in the Western world, with a 50 percent mortality rate, may be related to a low intake of fiber. Cancer of this portion of the large intestine is virtually nonexistent in areas where the dietary fiber intake is high.

Fiber is thought to protect against colon cancer by increasing the bulk of stools, thereby diluting potential cancer-causing agents. Fiber may also bind some carcinogens so that they're less available to cause damage. In addition, since fiber can move waste material through the intestines more quickly, it may give carcinogens less time to work.

The fiber-cancer connection has received a great deal of attention, but the data are so scanty that it is premature to assume that there is a direct link. If and until there is valid scientific evidence, we believe it is unacceptable for the federal government to allow food manufacturers to advertise their high-fiber products as being related to cancer prevention.

Can Fiber Aid Weight Loss?

Fiber's weight-reducing properties were first promoted by companies that marketed supplements containing guar gum and cellulose. Fiber, they suggested, provides bulk that makes you feel full faster and slows down the rate at which your stomach empties. Another theory holds that since high-fiber foods usually require more chewing, you'll eat more slowly, and therefore less.

There is some evidence that slower eaters actually consume less in the long run. And high-fiber, low-calorie fruits and vegetables are good fillers, whose bulk may help you eat less of other foods. In these indirect ways, foods high in fiber may help some people who want to lose weight.

However, fiber supplements are another matter. Although researchers are studying the weight control effects of fiber supplements containing guar and other substances, the Food and Drug Administration has no evidence that guar is safe or effective for long-term weight loss. Keep in mind that aside from the harmless small amounts of guar gum used as thickeners in some processed foods, guar is not present to any substantial degree in foods. It is not known what, if any, potential problems might arise from using it as a regular dietary supplement.

Even if the FDA deems guar-containing supplements safe, do not be misled by the extravagant claims of some promoters about fiber's near-magical weight loss qualities. These supplements are just one more weight-loss gimmick. Rather than trying to "trick" yourself into not feeling hungry, you would be wiser to concentrate on creating a balanced diet of nutritious foods and enrolling in a regular program of exercise.

Too Much of a Good Thing

It seems to be characteristic of human nature to embrace a nutrition concept with such enthusiasm that we go overboard. But it is not necessarily true that if a substance is good for us, then more of it will be better. And this is the case with fiber.

Overconsumption of fiber-rich foods is hardly a problem for most Americans. But with the easy availability of fiber supplements, as well as packages of raw wheat and oat bran, you should be careful not to overdo it on these fiber products. Such profuse and concentrated doses may undercut the natural process of the GI tract and interfere with your body's absorption of important nutrients. Fiber has a binding effect on substances that pass into the intestines, and too much fiber may bind minerals such as calcium, iron, and zinc,

causing them to be lost in the stools rather than absorbed into the bloodstream.

Too much fiber can actually be harmful, especially when large doses are taken without adequate amounts of liquids. Your intestines can become blocked with indigestible matter.

Finally, there is concern that some people (especially growing children and those with poor appetites) may fill up too fast when they consume fiber supplements or concentrated sources of fiber and, as a result, may eat less than they need of nutrient-rich foods.

We suggest that you depend on a variety of fiber-rich foods for your daily intake. There is no Recommended Dietary Allowance for fiber, but you should strive for between 20 and 35 grams per day. (Americans currently average only 11 grams per day.) Some manufacturers have begun to include fiber grams on their labels, particularly for cereal, bread, and grain products.

Good Fiber Sources—Eat a Variety!

High-fiber foods include whole-grain breads, cereal, and pasta (including wheat, rye, and oat products); brown rice, fruits, and vegetables, dried beans (legumes), nuts, and seeds. Refined grain products are low in fiber since the fibrous grain husk is removed during processing.

Ounce-for-ounce, vegetables and fruits have less fiber than grains because of their high water content. And not all vegetables are high in fiber. Lettuce, for example, has very little fiber, while peas have a great deal. Following is a list of good fiber sources. We suggest you get your daily fiber from several of these sources. These foods are good sources of fiber and they should be part of a balanced approach to eating. When you plan your daily diet, you should consider the essential nutrients you need that may not be found in these foods.

During 1988 and 1989, the nation's leading health authorities, including the surgeon general, the American Medical Association, the National Cancer Institute, and the American Heart Association, publicly stressed the importance of consuming a diet rich in high-fiber foods. While the full implications of fiber's role in the prevention of disease are still being explored, it seems clear that it's a dietary course that can be beneficial nutritionally.

A WIDE VARIETY OF FIBER-RICH FOODS

Food	Serving	Fiber (grams)	Food	Serving	Fiber (grams)
Bread			Figs, dried	2	7.4
Bran muffin	1	4.0	Orange	1 medium	2.8
Cracked-wheat bread	2 slices	2.4	Pears	1 medium	4.0
Pumpernickel bread	2 slices	3.2	Raisins	5 tbsp.	3.0
Whole-wheat bagel	1	2.7	Raspberries	½ cup	9.2
Whole-wheat bread	2 slices	3.2			
			Vegetables/Legumes		
Grains			Broccoli, cooked	¾ cup	5.0
Barley, dry	1 oz.	2.1	Brussels sprouts, cooked	1 cup	5.0
Brown rice	⅔ cup	3.0	Corn, sweet, cooked	½ cup	4.7
Wheat bran	1 oz.	11.3	Green peas, cooked	½ cup	3.1
			Kidney beans, cooked	½ cup	9.7
Cereals			Lentil beans, cooked	1 cup	9.0
All-Bran	1 oz.	8.5	Lima beans, cooked	½ cup	7.4
Bran Buds	1 oz.	7.9	Green peas, cooked	½ cup	5.0
100% Bran	1 oz.	8.4	Pinto Beans, cooked	½ cup	8.9
Corn Bran	1 oz.	5.3	Spinach, cooked	½ cup	6.5
			String beans, raw	3½ oz.	3.4
Fruits					
Apple	1 medium	3.2	*Nuts*		
Banana	1 medium	3.0	Almonds	1 oz.	5.0
Blueberries	½ cup	3.0	Peanuts	1 oz.	2.5
Blackberries	½ cup	4.5	Pecans	1 oz.	2.0
Cranberries	½ cup	4.0			

4

Fat:
Good News and Bad News

For most people, the word "fat" is associated with a number of negatives, especially heart disease and obesity. But, in itself, fat is not bad. It's a fundamental part of the body's structure and operation, as are protein, starches, and sugars.

Actually, the word *fat* is a misnomer. The real term for body substances that won't dissolve in water, but will dissolve in organic solvents, is *lipids*. Technically, lipids are more than fats, although they are primarily fats. Lipids also include several hormones, sterols (one being cholesterol), waxes, and other substances.

Like carbohydrates, fats are composed of carbon, hydrogen, and oxygen, but their structure is different. One very important difference is that fats contain much less oxygen in their molecules. The lower amount of oxygen in relation to carbon results in fat being a more concentrated source of energy. In effect, when the body burns fat it produces more than twice the number of calories than when it burns the same amount of protein and carbohydrate. That is why one gram of fat is equivalent to nine calories, while one gram of carbohydrate or protein is equivalent to only four calories.

How Fats Are Constructed

The chemical structure of fats starts with a framework of linked carbon atoms. To this framework, called *glycerol,* three *fatty acids* are attached. This structure is called a *triglyceride*. In fat, each carbon atom forms bonds with another carbon atom and usually with hydrogen or oxygen atoms. Many of the atoms form bonds with two carbon and two hydrogen atoms.

▶ If no hydrogens are missing from the structure of a fatty acid, it is called *saturated*. Animal fats found in meat and dairy products are high in saturated fatty acids, as are plant oils such as coconut oil and palm oil.

▶ If one pair of hydrogens is missing from the structure of a fatty acid, it is called a *monounsaturated* fatty acid. Avocados and olive oils are mostly composed of these.

▶ If two or more pairs of hydrogens are missing from the structure of a fatty acid, it is called a *polyunsaturated* fatty acid. Most vegetable oils (including safflower and sunflower) and fish oils are composed of polyunsaturated fatty acids.

Our bodies have the capability to synthesize saturated fatty acids, but not certain important polyunsaturated fatty acids. For this reason, we must consume these polyunsaturated fatty acids in our diets. They are called *essential fatty acids* and should account for about 3 percent of our daily calories to avoid a deficiency disease. Three fatty acids have been found to be most essential: *linoleic, arachidonic,* and *linolenic.* Of these, linoleic is most important, since the other two can be made from it. Linoleic acid is present in high quantities in corn, safflower, and soybean oils.

Essential fatty acids are necessary for maintaining healthy cell walls, for normal cholesterol metabolism, and in the formation of each important cell regulators as *prostaglandins,* hormone-like compounds that are involved in a wide variety of functions, such as regulation of blood pressure and blood coagulation.

In our food supply, few fats and oils are completely composed of saturated, polyunsaturated, or monounsaturated fatty acids. Most contain all three in some ratio; it's the makeup of this ratio that makes a food "high in saturated fat" or "high in polyunsaturated fat." In the following table, common cooking oils are broken down to show the ratio of the fatty acids. Safflower oil is the least saturated; coconut oil is the most saturated. (Note that the totals do not add up to 100 percent, since these items also contain small amounts of other substances.)

FATTY ACID BREAKDOWN OF COMMON OILS

	Saturated (%)	Mono-unsaturated (%)	Poly-unsaturated (%)
Coconut	87	6	2
Corn	13	24	59
Cottonseed	26	18	52
Olive	13	74	8
Palm	49	37	9
Palm Kernel	81	11	2
Peanut	17	46	32
Safflower	9	12	75
Sesame	14	40	42
Soybean	14	23	58
Sunflower	10	20	66

The Role of Fat in a Healthy Diet

Every body cell contains some form of lipid, and lipids perform critical roles in the body. They store energy, support the cell walls, and store or circulate the fat-soluble vitamins: A, D, E, and K.

For this reason, we need some fat in our diets, especially the polyunsaturated kind that the body can't make on its own. Fat is a necessary source of energy, and it also helps to make the foods we eat palatable. But it is widely believed that Americans consume too much fat.

In a 1988 report, the surgeon general called for a reduction of all types of fat, especially saturated fat, in the American diet. Evidence supports the relationship between excessive fat intake and a number of chronic conditions:

▶ *Obesity.* Because fat sources usually contain little water and take up less volume, we can eat more fat without feeling full. And because of its chemical nature, fat contains more calories per gram than other foods. It also takes less energy to store excess fat calories as body fat than those that come from carbohydrates and protein. So it may be easier to get fat on a high-fat diet.

Obesity increases the risk for high blood pressure and consequently for stroke. It is also associated with an increase in blood cholesterol levels, which has been associated with heart disease. Obesity is a critical factor in adult-onset diabetes.

▶ *Cancer.* There is compelling evidence that certain kinds of cancer—specifically, colon, lung, and bladder cancer—are more prevalent in people who have high-fat diets. There is also evidence that breast and uterine cancer are more common in obese women.

▶ *Cholesterol.* There is an enormous amount of data to support the premise that a high intake of saturated fat raises blood cholesterol levels and increases the risk of heart disease. Saturated fat is highest in animal foods, and dietary cholesterol is

Recommended Daily Fat Intake

Daily Calories	Calories from Fat	Fat (grams)	Saturated Fat (grams)
1,000	300	33.3	11
1,200	360	40	13
1,500	450	50	17
1,800	540	60	20
2,000	600	66.6	22
2,500	750	83	28
3,000	900	100	33

found only in animal foods. Animal foods are the major source of fat in the American diet.

Many authorities now suggest that, for most people, the maximum percentage of daily calories from fat should be 30 percent, with the bulk of these calories coming from unsaturated fats and not more than 10 percent of total daily calories coming from saturated fats. We have broken down the ratios for average diets in the box above.

In general, the more liquid a fat is at room temperature, the less saturated it is. But what about nonliquid foods such as margarine, which are made from vegetable oils high in polyunsaturated fatty acids? Many prepared foods are hydrogenated, a process that, in effect, hardens a liquid oil. If margarine were not hydrogenated or partially hydrogenated, it would be a puddle of liquid at room temperature. Unfortunately, hydrogenating makes a fat more saturated. Your best compromise is to choose margarines and similar products that list a liquid oil as the first ingredient. They are somewhat less saturated than those that list a hydrogenated or partially hydrogenated fat as the first ingredient.

Trimmer Beef on the Way

In recent years, the warnings about highly saturated fat and cholesterol in beef have led to a steady decline in consumption—a fact that finally hit home for beef producers and retailers. A number of steps have been instituted within the beef industry to make beef a leaner choice for the American consumer.

The search for leanness starts on the ranch, where many ranchers are cross-breeding their stock with cattle that are naturally lean or are importing genetically lean breeds from Europe. In addition, many ranchers now leave their cattle in the feedlot for shorter periods of time, resulting in less fatty beef.

The efforts do not end on the ranch. At packing houses, supermarkets, and neighborhood meat stores, butchers are trimming away more of the "separable" fat—that is, the layer of fat surrounding the beef. The half inch or more of external fat that butchers once left on beef has been reduced to a quarter inch or less.

In 1987, the United States Department of Agriculture (USDA) developed new beef labeling standards that required that beef labeled "lean" or "low-fat" could not contain more than 10 percent fat by weight. "Leaner" or "light" meat, which once meant anything retailers wanted it to mean, now must contain less than 10 percent fat or be 25 percent lower than usual—the "usual" being an actual meat cut with which it can be compared. The exception to the grading system is ground beef. The USDA also changed the grade for leaner cuts from "good" to "select," hoping to give lean beef a classier name, especially since the fattiest cuts are graded "choice."

One new direction of research may permanently change the fat profile of our nation's meat supply. Biotechnology may enable meat producers to genetically alter the makeup of an animal to make it naturally leaner. The time is coming when, rather than being considered an impediment to a low-fat diet, beef might be one of the best sources of high-quality, low-fat protein.

5

The Two Faces of Cholesterol

Cholesterol is a lipid, present in every cell, that is used by your body to make some very important things happen. For example, cholesterol contributes to the formation of sex hormones (estrogen and testosterone), skin oils, digestive juices (bile), vitamin D, and the sheaths that protect nerve endings. It is also necessary for the development of each cell. Cholesterol differs from fat in its carbon and hydrogen configuration. There is a difference between blood cholesterol and the dietary cholesterol we consume in food.

We don't need to consume cholesterol, since our bodies are capable of manufacturing all we need; our livers produce it at the rate of one to two grams each day, using acetate, a product derived from the metabolism of glucose, amino acids, and fats.

Cholesterol travels back and forth from liver to cells by way of the bloodstream. But, since it cannot move through the bloodsteam on its own, it must be carried. The carriers of cholesterol are called *lipoproteins*. Lipoproteins, produced in the liver from protein products, are distinguished by their density. One might view high-density lipoproteins (HDLs) as strong carriers that remove cholesterol from each cell and deliver it safely to the liver for processing. Low-density lipoproteins (LDLs) can't "grab" as much cholesterol from the cells and, on the way to and from the liver, they

tend to have "accidents" and drop cholesterol along the way. This is what distinguishes "good" HDL cholesterol, the kind processed in your liver, from "bad" LDL cholesterol, which is left behind in the arteries.

The cholesterol deposited in the arteries contributes to *plaque* formation. As plaque builds up, it hardens and closes off the arterial pathway (in other words, it causes a type of hardening of the arteries), slowing the flow of blood. If too much plaque builds up, the flow of blood can stop completely. In an artery that supplies blood to the heart, this can cause a heart attack. In an artery that supplies blood to the brain, it can cause a stroke.

In addition to being more reliable transporters of cholesterol, HDLs can sometimes reduce the damage done by LDLs by sweeping some of the cholesterol deposits out of the arteries and carrying them to the liver.

What Happens to the Cholesterol We Eat?

Although we do not need to eat cholesterol, most of us do. Every food that comes from an animal contains some cholesterol, including eggs (one of

23

the highest), cheese, meat, milk, poultry, and fish. Plant foods and plant oils do not contain any cholesterol.

Some of the cholestrol we consume or synthesize is incorporated into cell structures, where it has essential functions. Some is converted into biologically important compounds such as sex hormones and vitamin D. Some is broken down metabolically or excreted in the bile through the intestines. And finally, cholesterol can be deposited in tissues, particularly in the arteries, where it represents a major health risk.

The High-Risk American Diet

Since Americans consume so much fat and cholesterol, there is much concern among medical professionals and nutritionists about the risks associated with high cholesterol levels in the blood. In fact, heart disease is the leading cause of death among Americans. The National Institutes of Health report that the average American currently consumes between 450 and 500 milligrams of cholesterol per day, a great deal higher than the 300 milligram maximum recommended by the Heart Association and other health agencies (see chapter 18). Cholesterol-rich foods that raise total cholesterol levels include eggs, organ meats (such as liver), whole milk, cheese, ice cream, butter, and fatty meats.

Cholesterol-containing foods are often high in fat, and fat is even more important in raising total cholesterol levels than dietary cholesterol. Among fat-rich foods, those containing saturated fats— the most damaging—include palm and coconut oils, and dairy fat. Saturated fats decrease the body's ability to break down cholesterol.

Polyunsaturated fats are believed to lower cholesterol by increasing its excretion and breakdown and decreasing its synthesis in the liver. Polyunsaturated fats are highest in vegetable oils like safflower, sunflower, corn, soybean, and cottonseed.

Monounsaturated fats are also believed to lower total cholesterol, but they are less effective. They also may cut down the risk of hardening of the arteries. The food that contributes the most monounsaturated fat to our diets is olive oil.

The Facts about Oats and Cholesterol

The excitement generated in the marketplace about the cholesterol-combatting effects of oat bran has sent consumers rushing out to stock up on sacks of the substance or to purchase the new wave of products that now contain oat bran.

Oats contain water-soluble fiber, long believed to be influential in lowering cholesterol. Soluble fiber forms a gel as it moves through the intestines and, in some way not yet fully understood, may interfere with the absorption or metabolism of cholesterol, more efficiently excreting it from the body.

Oat bran hit the news when research scientists at Northwestern University School of Medicine published the results of a study showing that just two ounces a day of either oatmeal or foods containing oat bran could lower cholesterol by almost 5 percent in a matter of weeks.

The researchers arrived at their conclusion via a two-step process. First, they placed 208 men and women, aged 30 to 65, on a "heart healthy" diet for six weeks, limiting fat calories to 30 percent of the total and cholesterol to 250 milligrams a day. After the six weeks, cholesterol levels had dropped from an average of 208 to 198 milligrans per deciliter (mg/dl).

In the second phase, all the participants were told to continue following the reduced fat, reduced cholesterol diet for six more weeks. But two-thirds of them were also instructed to eat two ounces of oat products every day, either in the form of hot oatmeal cereal or foods made with oat bran, such as muffins. The blood cholesterol levels of these people dropped even more—to

THE FAT AND CHOLESTEROL CONTENT OF COMMON FOODS

	Amount	Total Fat (grams)	Choles-terol (grams)		Amount	Total Fat (grams)	Choles-terol (grams)
Beef*				flounder fillet	3 oz./85 g	.68	41.0
well-marbled	3 oz./85 g	27.2	79.9	shrimp meat	3 oz./85 g	.65	127.5
lean cuts	3 oz./85 g	10.5	77.3	oysters	3 oz./85 g	.8	187.0
salami	1 slice	8.8	14.0	tuna in oil	3 oz./85 g	17.4	47.0
bologna	1 slice	6.5	13.0	tuna in water	3 oz./85 g	2.5	53.5
hot dog	1	16.8	22.0				
pot pie	8 oz./225 g	22.7	38.0	**Milk**			
				whole	1 cup/244 g	9.0	34.0
Pork				2% fat	1 cup/246 g	4.9	22.0
chop (without				1% fat	1 cup/246 g	2.5	15.0
bone)	3 oz./85 g	13.1	75.0	light cream	1 cup/240 g	49.4	158.0
ham	3 oz./85 g	22.6	48.0	whipped			
sausage	2 oz./53 g	25.0	39.0	cream	1 cup/60 g	22.0	51.0
Lamb				**Cheese**			
leg	3 oz./85 g	13.8	55.3	blue	1 oz./28 g	7.8	24.0
Chicken				cheddar	1 oz./28 g	9.0	28.0
breast with				Swiss	1 oz./28 g	7.8	28.0
skin	3 oz./90 g	4.5	74.0	American	1 oz./28 g	6.2	25.0
skinless				cottage, 1%			
breast	3 oz./80 g	2.0	53.0	fat	4 oz./112 g	10.8	92.0
leg and skin	2 oz/53 g	3.3	47.0	cottage, 2%			
pot pie	8 oz./225 g	25.9	29.0	fat	4 oz./112 g	42.8	192.0
Turkey				**Eggs**			
skinless light				white	1 large	0.0	0.0
meat	3 oz./85 g	1.2	51.0	yolk	1 large	30.6	213.0
skinless dark							
meat	3 oz./85 g	4.3	64.0	**Fats**			
Seafood				butter	1 tbsp./14 g	11.3	35.0
cod fillet	3 oz./85 g	.25	42.5	vegetable-oil			
pink salmon	3 oz./85 g	3.10	29.8	margarine	1 tbsp./14 g	12.2	0.0

* Meats are trimmed and cooked

about 190 mg/dl—while the cholesterol levels of those who did not include the oat products in their low-fat diets remained at approximately 198 mg/dl. It should be noted that the further reduction in cholesterol occurred even though many of the oat eaters only took in one ounce, not two ounces, of oat products per day.

The tests strongly suggest that oats have a beneficial effect on blood cholesterol. But since oatmeal contains only half the fiber of oat bran, why were two ounces of oatmeal as effective as two ounces of oat bran in reducing cholesterol? One explanation is that the oat bran muffins in the study were made with cholesterol-rich eggs, thereby increasing the cholesterol intake of anybody who chose them over oatmeal. By the time the study was completed, it was found that those who generally ate the oatmeal had reduced their daily cholesterol intake to an average of 206 milligrams. The muffin eaters, on the other hand, had increased their intake to 288 milligrams a day.

Good studies from the University of Kentucky support the hypothesis that oat fiber will lower blood cholesterol. A Harvard study questioned the mechanism by which the lowering of cholesterol is achieved, but that study has many critics.

The discovery that oats may contribute to lowering cholesterol has led to something of an oat fanaticism, but simply adding a lot of oats to your diet won't necessarily lead to low cholesterol. For one thing, the oat products in the study were shown to be helpful only when they were part of a moderate-fat, moderate-cholesterol diet. Whether they would work with a high-fat, high-cholesterol diet isn't known, but no one should count on oatmeal or oat bran to combat the effects of a diet filled with fatty foods. Nor has it been shown that more than two ounces of oat products a day are better. Overall, the tendency to go overboard on isolated foods is not a good nutritional habit. While oats may help lower cholesterol, they should only be eaten in combination with a variety of healthy, carbohydrate foods. Keep in mind, too, that oats are not the only form of water-soluble fiber. Although they were singled out because of the studies, other good sources of soluble fiber include fruits, legumes, and vegetables. For example, apples, which contain pectin, are a very good source. If soluble fiber has a beneficial effect in lowering cholesterol, many of these foods would accomplish it.

There is also early evidence that soluble fiber may not be the only fiber that has cholesterol-lowering benefits. Animal tests conducted by the USDA show that rice bran, the outer layer of brown rice, which is a source of insoluble fiber, might be just as effective in lowering blood cholesterol as oat bran. Although scientists are speculating that it might be the oil in rice bran, not its fiber content, that is the beneficial element, these tests should provide further proof that a varied diet, rich in many different nutritious foods, is the best course of action.

The Niacin Controversy

The B vitamin known as niacin, or nicotinic acid, has received a good bit of publicity for its ability to lower cholesterol. It is important to note that in the studies where niacin was shown to be effective it was used as a drug in medically supervised conditions, sometimes in combination with other drugs and therapies. Such use is a far cry from recommending that people purchase niacin supplements and self-treat themselves with high doses (a recommendation being made in at least one well-known cholesterol-lowering diet program). Niacin toxicity can have a number of troubling side effects. The most common is the so-called niacin flush—intense reddening and itching of the face and upper body. More severe side effects might include gastrointestinal problems, abnormal liver functioning, and elevated blood sugar levels.

Do Fish Oils Lower Cholesterol?

Research now being disputed suggests that fish oils, which contain omega-3 fatty acids, may lower blood cholesterol levels. This possibility was first studied when scientists found that Eskimos, who consume large quantities of fatty fish, tend not to suffer from heart disease.

The fat in fish is polyunsaturated (if it were saturated, it would harden in cold water), but fish oils are constructed differently than other polyunsaturated oils, their primary fatty acids being eicosapentaenoic acid (EPA) and docosahexaenoic acid (DHA), which have characteristics that are very different from plant oils.

Omega-3 fatty acids are believed by some to lower blood cholesterol levels more markedly than other polyunsaturated fatty acids by decreasing liver synthesis of cholesterol. Omega-3 fatty acids are also converted into a series of compounds that increase the time it takes blood to coagulate, so that the development of clots at the point of plaque buildup in the arteries may be avoided.

The caution to apply when considering the health benefits of fish oils is that their misuse can result in problems with excessive bleeding and anemia, and may increase the possibility of stroke. Eskimos have shown a tendency to bruise and, when cut, they bleed longer than other groups of people.

It is probably healthy to eat moderate amounts of fish high in omega-3 fatty acids. Even if omega-3 fatty acids turn out to be less instrumental in lowering blood cholesterol than some believe them to be, fish is still an excellent source of protein and much lower in fat than other cholesterol-containing foods.

Fish and other marine foods that are good sources of omega-3 fatty acids include the following:

Albacore tuna	Mussels
Anchovies	Pollock
Bluefish	Rainbow trout
Clams	Salmon
Cod*	Sardines**
Crab	Scallops
Halibut*	Shrimp
Herring**	Striped bass
Lake trout	Trout
Mackerel**	Whiting

* Although cod and halibut are good sources of omega-3 fatty acids, some people have assumed that consuming cod liver oil or halibut liver oil is a cheap and efficient way to get fish oils. But these products may contain high levels of vitamins A and D, which can be extremely toxic when consumed in large quantities.
** Often these fish are prepared in a manner that makes them high in sodium, saturated fat, and

calories. Pickled herring is high in sodium and, when it's accompanied by sour cream, also high in saturated fat and calories. Mackerel is often smoked and dried, making it high in sodium. And tuna and sardines are not always packed in fish oils; frequently, vegetable oils are used, increasing their fat and calorie content and, depending on the oil used, altering the ratios of unsaturated and saturated fatty acid.

Should You Take Fish Oil Capsules?

Millions of Americans have been swallowing fish oil capsules, eager to reap the alleged benefits of omega-3 fatty acids. But researchers have found that the capsules generally do not contain the levels of omega-3 fatty acids stated on their labels.

Researchers at Tufts, led by Ernest J. Shaefer, M.D., chief of the Lipid Metabolism Laboratory at the Human Nutrition Research Center, and head of the Lipid Clinic at the New England Medical Center, analyzed 10 major brands of fish oil supplements, including Pro-Mega and Proto-Chol, and found that the capsules, on average, had only 38 percent of the omega-3 fatty acid EPA and 85 percent of the omega-3 fatty acid DHA that the companies claim are present. In part, the reason is that the vitamin E used in the capsules to prevent oxidation (breakdown) of the fatty acids is not added in sufficient amounts. In addition, it is present in what is known as the acetate form, which is not the form that best protects against oxidation.

The American Heart Association (AHA) has strongly recommended that fish oil supplements should never be taken without medical supervision. The AHA has gone on record warning against their indiscriminate use. There is little evidence, they say, that the omega-3 fatty acids in fish oil supplements are useful for substantially reducing LDLs in the blood. They have, however, been shown to lower abnormally high triglyceride levels, which is a reason some doctors may prescribe them.

6

Vitamins and Minerals: Nature's Delicate Balance

Until the beginning of this century, most medical experts believed that the only things necessary for a good diet were protein, fat, carbohydrates, and minerals. But early in the 1890s, a series of studies suggested that there were other materials in food that were essential to health. The first to be identified was Vitamin B-1, whose chemical composition included an *amine*. Thus, in 1912, the word "vitamine" was coined, meaning "an amine necessary for life."

As the years went by, it became obvious that there were many of these substances, that some were fat-soluble (absorbed with and stored in body fat), that others were water-soluble, and that most of them were not amines. Thus, the "e" was dropped from the word and these substances came to be known as vitamins.

There are 13 known vitamins, 9 water-soluble and 4 fat-soluble. They are organic compounds composed almost entirely of carbon, oxygen, and hydrogen, and they are essential in minute amounts for the normal functioning of the body. Many people would be surprised to learn how little of the material in food is really vitamins. For example, if you were to remove the water from the diet of an average adult, he or she would consume about 600 grams of food each day. Of this amount, only about one-tenth of a gram (or 100 milligrams) would consist of vitamins. But

their lack of volume should not imply a lack of importance, as we could not survive without vitamins in our diet.

While some scientists at the turn of the century were busy discovering the biological activities of vitamins, others were concentrating on unraveling the mysteries of minerals. The role of minerals in the diet is a vastly complex matter, and even today there are many things that are not known. Early in the study of minerals it was determined that, since our bones are composed of calcium and phosphorus, those minerals needed to be in the diet. Similarly, there was early evidence of the need for minerals such as magnesium, sodium, and potassium. These became known as macrominerals. However, as investigators and their analytical equipment grew more sophisticated, it became clear that there were other minerals, such as iron and iodine, that were needed in very small amounts in the diet; these became known as trace minerals.

Scientists are continuing to learn about the role vitamins and minerals play in the diet, how they interact with one another, and the potential they may have for reducing the risk of chronic disease. The Recommended Dietary Allowances (see chapter 7) are based on what is currently known about our daily need for vitamins and minerals, in addition to protein.

28

Water-Soluble Vitamins

There are nine water-soluble vitamins—eight B vitamins and vitamin C. In the preparation of foods, some water-soluble vitamins can easily be washed away or destroyed by light and heat. In the body, most are not stored very well and need to be replenished frequently.

You might find the way the B vitamins are identified perplexing. Why is there B-1, B-2, B-6, and B-12, but no B vitamins with intermediate numbers? This resulted from the way the B vitamins were discovered. At various times during the first half of this century there were reports of materials that were given numbers like B-7 and B-8. But more careful study revealed that the substances either were not vitamins or that the researchers were looking at compounds that had already been identified and given a number or name. In recent years, there have been unscientific claims that substances like pangamic acid and laetrile were B vitamins. But neither of these materials are vitamins, nor are they medications with any demonstrable value.

Vitamin B-1 (Thiamin)

Thiamin is an essential dietary component. Because it is poorly stored in the body, deficiency symptoms will show up very quickly if it is not consumed.

The primary role of thiamin is to help convert carbohydrates into energy. It travels through the bloodstream to every part of the body, helping to burn carbohydrates for fuel. When thiamin is not present, the deficiency causes loss of energy, nerve damage, muscular weakness, and, in extreme cases, paralysis and heart failure. The severest form of thiamin deficiency, the disease beriberi, is rare in the United States except in chronic alcoholics.

One of the most important sources of thiamin is whole-wheat products, where the bran is retained. Pork, liver, and peas are also good sources. In addition, many flour and grain products in the United States are fortified with thiamin, along with other vitamins and minerals.

Food must be stored and prepared properly to maintain thiamin levels. It is sensitive to heat and, like some other water-soluble vitamins, is easily leached into cooking water.

Vitamin B-2 (Riboflavin)

Riboflavin is an essential nutrient that plays a role in a large number of enzyme interactions that are designed to convert the food we eat into energy. When it is absent from the diet, a variety of pathologic changes occur, causing dry, scaly skin, cracks on the lips and corners of the mouth, and extreme sensivity of the eyes to light. In many animal species, chronic riboflavin deficiency leads to cataract formation.

Riboflavin is abundantly available in the food supply, in meats, fish, whole-grain foods, milk products, vegetables, and legumes, as well as products fortified with B vitamins. Since it is rapidly destroyed with exposure to sunlight, these foods are best stored in a pantry, in bins, and, when perishable, in the refrigerator to avoid nutrient loss.

Niacin

The B vitamin called niacin is an essential nutrient that either must be present in the diet or formed in the body from the amino acid tryptophan, found in proteins. Like riboflavin, niacin helps living cells generate energy from food. Its nutritional value was first discovered in 1938 when it was found to eliminate the deficiency disease known as pellagra. In advanced cases, pellagra leads to severe mental impairment, hallucinations, and delirium. It also causes inflamed mucus membranes, with swelling in the tongue and mouth, and diarrhea. In the 1930s, approximately 200,000 Americans a year suffered from pellagra, and about 10,000 of them died from it. It was most often seen in poor people on corn-based diets which were lacking both niacin from food as well as tryptophan.

In addition to the niacin that is formed from tryptophan, niacin is present in foods such as whole-grains, milk products, and liver.

In supplement form, niacin is sometimes prescribed to lower blood cholesterol and, for reasons hard to support scientifically, it has gained popularity as an energy and strength booster. But megadoses of niacin (that is, excessive consumption above RDA levels) can be dangerous, leading to liver damage, ulcers, and high blood sugar. Commonly, large doses of niacin also cause rashes and stinging sensations in the skin. As concern with high blood cholesterol has mounted, many people have taken it upon themselves to self-prescribe megadoses of niacin supplements, not realizing that in large doses vitamins like niacin become drugs with potentially dangerous side effects.

Vitamin B-6

Also called pyridoxine, Vitamin B-6 is required by the body for protein metabolism, helping to break down and convert amino acids to energy. B-6 is also responsible for the synthesis of non-essential amino acids. It is important in many diverse roles, including the synthesis of muscle protein, hemoglobin, insulin, and the antibodies necessary to defend the body against infection. Acute vitamin B-6 deficiency, which rarely occurs in the United States, is accompanied by convulsions and severe anemia.

Vitamin B-6 is available in a wide variety of common foods, including meats, fish, nuts, beans, whole-wheat products, and some fruits and vegetables.

Traditionally, it was believed that there was no danger of toxicity from B-6 since it was a water-soluble vitamin whose excess would simply be excreted out of the body. But evidence in recent years shows that this is not the case. According to a report in the *New England Journal of Medicine,*

large doses of vitamin B-6 may cause severe nervous dysfunction. Dr. Herbert Schaumburg and colleagues from four prestigious medical centers described the symptoms of seven adults who had been taking large doses of vitamin B-6—from 2,000 to 6,000 milligrams—for periods ranging from 2 to 40 months. This amount exceeded the RDA for B-6 by 1,000 to 3,000 times. The symptoms that developed included unstable gait and numbness of the feet, which eventually became so severe that a cane had to be used for walking. With time, numbness in the hands also occurred, and there was an impairment in the sensations of touch, temperature, pinprick, vibration, and joint position. The afflictions were so severe that four of the patients were considered to be seriously handicapped. But when the B-6 supplements were stopped, the symptoms subsided.

It is not known at what levels toxicity begins. However, as early as 1964 it was reported that the ingestion of 200 milligrams of vitamin B-6 per day for 33 days by healthy young men resulted in metabolic and physiologic abnormalities. Further, the men in the experiment became dependent on the vitamin at this dosage level, thus increasing their requirement for it.

More recently, scientists have reported the development of problems associated with high doses taken by women to relieve premenstrual symptoms. Although there is no firm scientific evidence that vitamin B-6 relieves Premenstrual Syndrome (PMS), the treatment became popular during the 1980s. Only one out of four well-controlled studies suggested a positive effect, and this was at relatively low levels. In the mid-1980s, researchers from the University of California School of Medicine, San Franciso, reported that two women experienced severe nervous system problems after taking 500 milligrams of B-6 daily, one for eight months and the other for two years. One woman who consumed only 200 milligrams a day for three years had similar symptoms. Furthermore, thirteen other people who consumed at least 2,000 milligrams daily all experienced neurological changes.

Folacin

The B vitamin called folacin, or folic acid, is required for DNA metabolism and plays an important role in genetic functions such as cell division and tissue growth. Folacin is also involved in the formation of hemoglobin in red blood cells.

Folacin is available in abundance in many foods. Foods that are high in folacin include liver, kidneys, dark-green leafy vegetables, fruits, and beans and peas. However, since folacin is easily destroyed by oxidation, the vitamin may be lost in the cooking and processing of foods.

Pregnant women need to be particularly attentive to getting their RDA of folacin since it is needed to produce the genetic material of cells. Absence of folacin can lead to anemia in pregnancy, miscarriage, and infants born with deformities.

A further caution exists as a result of the symptomatic similarities of folacin deficiency to vitamin B-12 deficiency. There have been cases where people taking large amounts of folic acid in supplement form masked the blood symptoms of vitamin B-12 deficiency so they first became aware of the vitamin B-12 lack when they developed severe neurological damage.

Vitamin B-12

Vitamin B-12 is also known as a cobalamin because it contains cobalt. Like folacin, B-12 is important for DNA metabolism. It also assists in red blood cell formation and maintenance of the central nervous system.

There are no plant food sources for vitamin B-12. However, certain microorganisms can make the vitamin, and this factor has formed the basis for the commercial production of B-12. Some fermented foods, such as soy sauce, miso, and tempeh may have some vitamin B-12, resulting from the presence of microorganisms used in the fermentation process.

For certain people, consuming the required amounts of vitamin B-12 won't necessarily guarantee that they are absorbing enough of the vitamin. In order to absorb vitamin B-12, people need a substance, called intrinsic factor, that is produced by the lining of the stomach. Some people with congenital stomach abnormalities, or who have experienced stomach surgery, may not be able to produce intrinsic factor. It has also been discovered that elderly people sometimes produce less intrinsic factor and develop a bacterial growth in their gastrointestinal tracts that interferes with vitamin B-12 absorption. The result of vitamin B-12 deficiency is a disease called pernicious anemia, which is characterized by anemia followed by severe neurological abnormalities. It can be treated with periodic vitamin B-12 injections. (Other alleged benefits of vitamin B-12 injections as energy boosters are completely unsupported by scientific evidence.)

Vitamin B-12 is abundant in many animal foods that are common in our diets, such as milk and milk products, eggs, and fish. Vitamin B-12 is also found in liver, kidney, and muscle meats.

There have been no reported cases of people suffering from vitamin B-12 toxicity. But this fact does not in any way lend validity to its use by injection as an energy booster. The average adult needs only 3 micrograms of the vitamin daily to maintain the required level, and there is no evidence that normally healthy people will benefit from greater amounts.

Pantothenic Acid and Biotin

Requirements for the B vitamins pantothenic acid and biotin have not been determined, since deficiencies have never been observed except in experimental settings. Pantothenic acid, which is essential for synthesizing and metabolizing fats and the formation of hormones and cholesterol, is widely distributed in plant and animal foods. Safe and adequate ranges have been set for pantothenic acid at 4 to 7 milligrams, but there is little need to be concerned about deficiency if you're eating a relatively balanced diet.

Biotin aids in the formation of fatty acids and

Do You Know Your B's?

The B vitamins are essential to good health. Do you know how to maximize their potential? Take this test and find out.

1. The B vitamins are numbered up to twelve. But how many actually are there?
   (a) 5   (b) 8   (c) 12   (d) 20

2. True or false? Roasted, fried, and broiled meats retain more B vitamins than braised or stewed meats.

3. Which of the B vitamins is most readily destroyed in cooking?
   (a) B-6   (b) B-2   (c) pantothenic acid   (d) thiamin

4. Deficiency of which of the B vitamins causes anemia?
   (a) riboflavin and biotin   (b) niacin and pantothenic acid   (c) folacin, B-12, and B-6

5. One of the best sources of B vitamins is
   (a) organ meats   (b) citrus fruit   (c) yellow vegetables

6. True or false? Rice and flour are good sources of the B vitamins.

7. Women on oral contraceptives may need added
   (a) thiamin   (b) riboflavin   (c) B-6   (d) folacin

8. Strict vegetarians are likely to get too little
   (a) biotin   (b) B-12   (c) niacin   (d) thiamin

ANSWERS:

1. (b) The eight are thiamin (B-1), riboflavin (B-2), niacin, B-6, folacin, B-12, pantothenic acid, and biotin. Food faddists have dubbed laetrile as B-17 and pangamic acid as B-15, but they are not vitamins, and health claims made about them are false.

2. (True) Also, meats cooked rare lose fewer B vitamins.

3. (d) Thiamin is the most fragile, followed by B-6 and pantothenic acid.

4. (c) B-12 deficiency creates pernicious anemia; deficiencies of folacin and B-6 also lead to anemia.

5. (a) Organ meats are one of the best sources of the vitamins—particularly liver and kidney.

6. (True) But since milling and polishing remove so much of the vitamins, flour and rice in the United States are usually enriched with thiamin, riboflavin, and niacin.

7. (Possibly all) But there are data indicating a need for additional B-6 and folacin.

8. (b) There is no vitamin B-12 in plant foods.

carbohydrate metabolism. In addition to being present in many of the same foods from which we receive the other B vitamins, biotin is also manufactured by microorganisms in our intestinal tracts. Safe and adequate ranges have been set at 100 to 200 micrograms, but deficiency is very rare. There is an undigestable protein in egg white that binds biotin, making it unavailable, but unless one is consuming very large quantities of egg white, it is unlikely that its consumption will affect biotin needs.

Vitamin C: Ascorbic Acid

The function of vitamin C was first discovered in 1747 by British physician James Lind, who found that the bleeding gums, loose teeth, anemia, and skin hemorrhaging characteristic of scurvy could be cured by eating citrus fruits. Vitamin C was not actually extracted from fruits and vegetables until 1928; it was not synthesized in the laboratory until the 1930s. Only during the past twenty years, in the wake of a large number of health claims, has the market for vitamin C supplements emerged.

Scientists are not certain exactly how vitamin C works, but it is believed to be involved in the formation of collagen, a protein-based substance necessary for healthy bones, teeth, skin, and tendons.

Vitamin C also appears to play a role in the healing of wounds, resistance to infection, the metabolism of some amino acids and folic acid, and the body's ability to properly absorb iron.

Scurvy, the vitamin C deficiency disease, is rarely seen in the United States, except in infants who consume nothing but cow's milk, or in alcoholics and elderly people who are malnourished. All you need to prevent scurvy is a scant 10 milligrams of vitamin C a day. The remaining vitamin C consumed contributes to the body's stored reserve of approximately 1,500 milligrams.

A variety of factors may alter the need for vitamin C. Cigarette smokers have been discovered to have low blood levels of vitamin C. For them, the requirement may be as much as 50 percent greater than for nonsmokers. Age and sex may also alter vitamin C absorption. Women appear to break down and absorb the vitamin differently than men. In particular, women who take birth control pills may need more vitamin C, as well as more B-6 and folacin.

It has been shown that environmental stresses, such as work in a very hot climate, may increase vitamin C requirements. In one study, South Africans working in very hot mines needed considerably more than the RDA to maintain normal levels of the vitamin. But this is an extreme case —it does not imply that people need to increase vitamin C when the seasons change. In the United States, people usually consume more vitamin C-containing fruits, vegetables, and drinks during the summer months.

Vitamin C is concentrated in some foods, particularly fruits, vegetables, and some fortified foods such as fruit drinks. When you select foods for their vitamin C content, remember that their value can be greatly altered by the way they are processed, cooked, and stored. Vitamin C is vulnerable to air and heat, and because it is water-soluble, it leaches out of food into cooking water. The best way to lock in the vitamin is to cover containers of juice and cut fruits and vegetables with lids, foil, or plastic wrap. Avoid premature chopping or paring since the more surfaces that are exposed to air, and the longer they are exposed, the greater the loss of the vitamin. If possible, keep the skins intact on foods like potatoes and apples. And remember that the outer leaves of foods such as lettuce typically contain the most vitamin C.

There are some concerns associated with megadoses of vitamin C. Although the vitamin, at RDA levels, helps fight infection, high doses have been shown to interfere with the white blood cells' ability to kill bacteria. It can also interfere with the absorption of copper. Some people who megadose on the vitamin have suffered gastrointestinal side effects such as nausea and diarrhea.

Pregnant women who take vitamin C in excessive amounts may give birth to babies with unusu-

► NUTRITION QUIZ ◄

Are You Vitamin C Savvy?

Have you learned how to separate fact from fiction about one of our most important nutrients? Take this test and find out.

1. Vitamin C megadoses are helpful in preventing, but not curing, the common cold.
   True _____ False _____

2. Vitamin C helps to prevent cancer.
   True _____ False _____

3. Chemical vitamin C, made in a laboratory, is as effective as "natural" vitamin C, as extracted from rose hips.
   True _____ False _____

4. Exercise increases the body's need for vitamin C.
   True _____ False _____

5. It is harmless to take large doses of vitamin C because the body takes what it needs and excretes the rest.
   True _____ False _____

6. Potatoes are a good source of vitamin C.
   True _____ False _____

7. Vitamin C deficiency effects the ability of wounds to heal.
   True _____ False _____

8. Men need more vitamin C than women.
   True _____ False _____

ANSWERS

1. (False) Despite repeated attempts, carefully controlled studies have not been able to demonstrate that vitamin C megadoses have any significant effect either in preventing or curing the common cold. While some studies have reported that the vitamin has a slight effect on decreasing the severity of cold symptoms, over-the-counter pharmaceuticals do a better job.

2. (False) There is no firm evidence that vitamin C will prevent the development of cancer. Studies that suggest vitamin C might help block the formation of carcinogenic nitrosamines, formed from nitrates and nitrites that are present in some foods, are still unclear, although research continues in this area.

3. (True) Vitamin C that has been extracted from a plant has exactly the same chemical structure as vitamin C that is chemically synthesized in a laboratory. The body cannot tell the difference between the two forms.

4. (False) Exercise does not affect the body's requirement for vitamin C.

5. (False) There are enough reports of harmful effects of megadosing to suggest a need for caution in consuming very large amounts of vitamin C or any other nutrient.

6. (True) White potatoes, in particular, are a good source. One medium potato offers about one-third of the daily requirement for the vitamin. However, the more they are whipped, the more vitamin C is lost.

7. (True) The healing process involves many factors, one of them being proper nutrition, which includes vitamin C because it is necessary for the formation of collagen, a type of connective tissue. The need for vitamin C appears to increase significantly during recovery from surgery, injuries, and severe burns.

8. (False) The RDA is the same for both men and women, under normal circumstances. Pregnant and lactating women need more.

ally high vitamin C requirements, a condition known as "rebound scurvy." There have been incidents reported where women who took more than 400 milligrams per day during pregnancy had babies who developed scurvy when they were fed normal amounts of the vitamin.

Vitamin C megadoses can obscure the results of some medical tests. If people with diabetes take high doses, they may get false negative results when the Testape method is used for measuring sugar in the urine. On the other hand, too much vitamin C can yield false positive results when the Clinitest method is used. Finally, megadoses of vitamin C can interfere with the drugs heparin and coumadin, both used to keep blood from clotting.

Fat-Soluble Vitamins

Four vitamins—A, D, E, and K—are fat-soluble, meaning they are not soluble in water but will dissolve in organic solvents or liquid fats. They are stored in the body's fat and are transported to cells by blood, often attached to proteins. Unlike water-soluble vitamins, they are not excreted in the urine, but remain in the body until they are broken down. This increases the potential for toxicity since it's easier for the body to build up stores of the fat-soluble vitamins.

Vitamin A

Vitamin A, or retinol, is needed for the maintenance of a wide variety of body cells. As a result, a deficiency of this vitamin results in abnormalities in the skin and in bone development, and problems in the respiratory, urogenital, and gastrointestinal tracts. Since many of the tissues (membranes) that form a barrier against invasion by microorganisms rely on vitamin A, its deficiency leaves people more susceptible to infection. Vitamin A also plays a special metabolic role in our vision, and its deficiency affects how well we see, particularly in the dark. Severe deficiency can even lead to blindness.

Studies conducted during the past few years suggest that the vitamin A precursor, beta-carotene, may play a role in diminishing the risk of some cancers, in particular lung cancer (see chapter 20). Although the studies are promising, the connection has yet to be firmly established.

A number of animal foods are rich in vitamin A; these include cheese, eggs, butter, chicken, and liver. Plants don't contain vitamin A, but yellow, orange, and some dark-green leafy vegetables and fruits—such as carrots, cantaloupe, spinach, and broccoli—contain beta-carotene, which is converted to vitamin A in the body. Margarines and some other foods are fortified with vitamin A.

If you eat excessive amounts of carotene-rich foods, your skin can turn yellow, a condition that is relatively harmless. However, taking doses of vitamin A in retinol supplements that greatly exceed the RDA can be dangerous, since your body stores excessive amounts of the vitamin in your liver. In fact, the federal government has restricted the dosage allowed for vitamin A capsules. Symptoms of toxicity include fatigue, severe headaches, blurred vision, insomnia, loss of body hair, menstrual irregularities, skin rashes, and joint pain. In severe cases, excess consumption can lead to brain and nervous system damage, abnormal bone growth, and liver damage.

Vitamin D

Vitamin D is crucial in the formation of bones and teeth. The nutrient aids in the absorption and utilization of calcium. Vitamin D deficiency is manifested in children who have stunted bone growth, bone malformations (rickets), and malformed teeth. In adults, vitamin D deficiency, called osteomalacia, may lead to a tendency for bone fractures and muscle spasms.

For the majority of us, vitamin D-fortified milk is the most practical way to meet our dietary needs. The few other foods that provide vitamin D are not usually consumed in great enough quantities. Sun exposure results in the formation of the vitamin in the skin; for many people it is the primary source of vitamin D.

People who might be concerned that too much sun is not good for them can take heart from the results of a study conducted by Dr. Michael Holick, who is on the faculties of the Boston University School of Medicine and the Tufts University School of Nutrition. Dr. Holick conducted research with older white people in Boston to determine how much sun exposure was needed to meet their vitamin D requirements. He found that mild exposure of the hands, arms, and face for ten to fifteen minutes, two to three times a week, was sufficient, although the amount of pollution in the air seems to affect how much light, and therefore vitamin D, is available. Be advised that too much sun is known to have many damaging effects; you should not bake in the sun with the intention of loading up on vitamin D.

Since vitamin D enhances the body's absorption and utilization of calcium, excessive amounts of vitamin D supplements may result in irreversible calcification of soft tissues. The pathological changes can be particularly serious if they occur in the heart, kidneys, or lungs.

Vitamin E

The exact nature of the function vitamin E plays in the body is still unclear. However, it is known to act as an antioxidant—that is, it protects other substances from destructive oxidative reactions. For example, oils or fats, particularly those that are polyunsaturated, are subject to oxidative changes that lead to rancidity. The same kind of chemical changes take place in body tissues, so vitamin E requirements are increased by the consumption of diets high in polyunsaturated fats. Fortunately, many of these fats are rich sources of the vitamin.

Vitamin E also protects the walls of the red blood cells from becoming fragile. Thus, the vitamin appears to make the cell membranes more stable, and it prevents tissues from becoming damaged.

Most American diets meet the RDA for vitamin E because it is so widely distributed in foods. Some people who have deficiencies in their ability to absorb and digest fats (such as those with liver disease) may require supplements of vitamin E or other fat-soluble vitamins, even though their diets appear adequate. But most people do not need vitamin E supplements since the vitamin is abundant in vegetable oils, whole-grain products, wheat germ, liver, nuts, and leafy green vegetables.

In recent years, a number of bogus health claims have been made concerning the value of vitamin E supplements as protectors against heart disease and other conditions. This promotion has resulted in wide use of vitamin E supplements, in spite of the fact that the biomedical community has been outspoken in denigrating their use. However, recently there have been new studies indicating that vitamin E might serve as a protection against some cancers or may enhance the immune response to certain diseases. It is possible that the requirements for vitamin E will be reconsidered if the evidence proves compelling enough.

Vitamin K

Vitamin K is essential for the synthesis of at least four of the thirteen proteins needed to make blood clot. Without it, blood would fail to coagulate at the site of an injury and the victim could bleed to death.

The RDA for vitamin K was first established in 1989. Setting a dietary requirement for the vitamin was complicated by the fact that the vitamin is synthesized in large amounts by intestinal bacteria. Vitamin K-rich foods include dark-green leafy vegetables, liver, and egg yolks.

People taking antibiotics may be at risk for vitamin K deficiency because antibiotics can destroy the intestinal bacteria that produce it. The case for this likelihood was made in a recent report in the *Journal of the American Medical Association*. Researchers at a hospital in Galveston, Texas, dis-covered 42 patients on antibiotics who developed bleeding disorders, all of which were linked with a deficiency in vitamin K.

There are a variety of conditions that may result in a malabsorption of vitamin K. As a result, surgeons and dentists usually do a medical history before operating or extracting teeth to determine if a patient is vitamin K-deficient. In some cases, blood clotting tests may be conducted.

Infants are particularly susceptible to vitamin K deficiency because their immature digestive tracts do not contain any of the vitamin K-producing bacteria, and breast milk is a poor source of the nutrient. For this reason, infants frequently receive an injection of vitamin K at birth.

Macrominerals

Minerals are inorganic dietary elements that are necessary for health. Some are required in large amounts (called macrominerals) and some in small quantities (called trace minerals), but the amount required does not imply the degree of importance to the diet. They are *all* essential.

Three macrominerals have been found to be essential in established amounts and are included in the RDAs. These are calcium, magnesium, and phosphorus. Three others, potassium, sodium, and chloride are also essential, functioning as agents that help maintain the body's fluid balance. But since requirements for these three minerals vary markedly under conditions that effect body-water loss (such as sweating), RDAs have not been established for them.

Calcium, magnesium, and phosphorus are complementary minerals that work together metabolically. In addition, each one performs particular functions in the body.

Calcium

Calcium is known to be essential for building bones and teeth and for maintaining bone strength. Much research has been done on the role of calcium in preventing bone loss, or osteoporosis, especially in women. Although the adult RDA is set at 800 milligrams, the requirement for youths is listed at 1,200 milligrams to support their growth.

Large numbers of Americans do not consume the RDA for calcium—particularly adults, and especially women over 50, who frequently consume less than half the RDA. Many people avoid calcium-rich dairy foods because of their high fat content, even though low-fat dairy products contain equally high levels of calcium. Strict vegetarians who have eliminated dairy products from their diets have few food sources for calcium, and supplements are often recommended to help them meet their daily requirements. Like other mineral nutrients, calcium in supplements always comes in combination with other chemicals, since pure minerals are often not chemically stable or available in foods. The most common forms are calcium carbonate, calcium lactate, calcium gluconate, dicalcium phosphate, and oyster shell (basically calcium carbonate). Current evidence suggests that the body absorbs each of these equally well. They can be purchased in tablet, capsule, powder, or liquid form. However, not all are equal from a practical standpoint. For example, while calcium carbonate contains 40 percent calcium, calcium gluconate contains only 9 percent. And some natural sources like bone meal and dolomite may be contaminated with heavy metals like lead or mercury.

Recently, D. Mark Hegsted, M.D., visiting professor of nutritional biochemistry at Tufts and professor emeritus at Harvard University, expressed the need for caution when fortifying foods with calcium, pointing out that there is still no final proof that a high-calcium diet can definitely prevent osteoporosis. Indeed, epidemiologic studies show that in countries where consumption of high-protein dairy products (and therefore calcium) is high, such as the United States and New Zealand, the incidence of hip fratures is greater than anywhere else in the world.

Further, recent studies indicate that, after menopause, even supplementation with high doses of the mineral (2,000 milligrams or more per day) may not be particularly effective in slowing bone loss. In fact, scientists report in the *New England Journal of Medicine* that, in the early years after menopause when the rate of bone loss is greatest, administration of the hormone estrogen may be much better at "saving" bone than large doses of calcium.

There are several factors that must be considered in discussing the calcium requirements of the elderly. One is that protein foods, which Americans consume in much higher quantities than they need, cause an increase in the amount of calcium excreted in the urine, probably affecting calcium requirements. Research has also shown that osteoporosis may be affected by heredity or related to a lack of exercise and is not a condition that can be avoided simply by consuming more calcium.

It is important to be educated about the various effects of available calcium supplements, since not all are equally advantageous. Calcium carbonate is the substance that contains the highest concentration of calcium. Sources of calcium carbonate include some antacids and ground oyster shells. It is also available in synthetic forms. The calcium in "natural" and synthetic forms are practically the same as dietary supplements containing calcium carbonate, although they are labeled as drugs. While it's true that the body needs small amounts of acid to absorb calcium, antacids taken in the recommended dosages will not upset the acid balance needed for absorption.

A majority of over-the-counter antacids, such as Rolaids, DiGel, Maalox, Mylanta, and Gelusil, do not contain calcium carbonate. They contain aluminum instead. Dosages larger than the recommended limit can bind phosphorus and increase calcium excretion, increasing the risk for bone disease, especially for the elderly.

A number of calcium supplements come with other nutrients, in particular vitamin D, which is needed for the body to properly absorb and metabolize calcium. With these supplements, it is important to be sure that you don't exceed the RDA for vitamin D in order to satisfy the RDA for calcium, since an overdose of vitamin D has toxic side effects.

There may be negative effects for some people who consume large amounts of calcium. The use of large amounts of calcium supplements may increase the incidence of kidney stone disease. In one major study conducted at the Massachusetts General Hospital, it was found that about 5 percent of patients with kidney stone disease stopped making kidney stones when their calcium intakes were decreased.

Phosphorus

Phosphorus is needed to build and strengthen bones and teeth and is also involved in the formation of genetic material, cell membranes, and many enzymes. It is very important in energy metabolism. It is not common for Americans to suffer phosphorus deficiencies since it is abundant in meats, and also because they consume large amounts of soft drinks that contain phosphoric acid. But the ratio of calcium to phosphorus in the diet is important to proper bone formation, and nutritionists are growing increasingly concerned about the declining ratio of calcium to phosphorus, particularly in the diets of American children, who consume large quantities of soft drinks, sometimes as a replacement for milk.

Phosphorus deficiency, which leads to bone pain, weakness, and appetite loss, can be caused by an overuse of antacids over a long period of time.

Magnesium

Magnesium, a component of many enzyme systems, is particularly important to the normal functioning of nerves and muscles. When inadequate amounts of magnesium are present in the diet, symptoms include weakness, muscle spasms, irregular heart beat, and leg cramps. Ordinarily, magnesium deficiency is rare in healthy people, since magnesium is found in so many vegetables, grains, and legumes. However, alcoholics frequently appear deficient in this mineral. Because magnesium salts are often poorly absorbed, they act as cathartics, attracting water to the gastrointestinal tract.

Many years of animal and human studies on the effects of magnesium have led scientists to conclude that relatively small amounts of the mineral will prevent most people with a history of recurrent calcium oxalate kidney stone disease from making new stones.

Sodium, Potassium, and Chloride

Many people think of sodium as a nonnutritious dietary element, but it's actually an essential mineral that acts, in combination with potassium and chloride, to maintain the balance of our body fluids. Sodium mainly operates in the fluid outside cells and potassium mainly operates in the fluid inside cells.

Sodium cannot be stored or manufactured in the body and must be consumed in food. It is available in abundant supply in vegetables, animal foods, and in some drinking water, and our bodily requirement of 200 milligrams a day is easily satisfied from these sources. However, the average American consumes less than one-half of his or her sodium this way. The remainder comes from heavy use of salt (a combination of 40 percent sodium and 60 percent chloride), and from the sodium compounds that are used as a flavoring agent in processed foods.

Excessive sodium intake upsets the fluid balance in the body and can cause a number of serious problems. One danger of too much sodium is that it draws water and potassium out of the cells, where it is needed to maintain the electrolyte balance.

A related effect of excessive sodium is a condition called edema, which is the collection of water in and around body tissues. Women have a tendency to retain sodium and suffer mild cases of edema prior to the start of their menstrual periods, and many pregnant women suffer the condition.

A high sodium diet may also be dangerous for people with high blood pressure (hypertension), but only some people are "salt sensitive," in that their blood pressures are seriously affected by the amount of sodium they take in. Even people who are not salt sensitive will show at least some blood pressure response to increased amounts of dietary salt. For those who are salt sensitive, the benefits of decreasing sodium in the diet can be tremendous. As a case in point, one-third of a group of hypertensives at Indiana University's Hypertension Research Center lowered the levels of sodium in their diets and were able to cut down on the amount of blood pressure medication they required in only seven months.

Nutritionists agree that, salt sensitive or not, most Americans could benefit from cutting down on the amount of salt they sprinkle on food and avoiding high-sodium processed foods.

Trace Minerals

Trace minerals are crucial to health, serving as catalysts for many life-sustaining cellular processes. Yet only in the past thirty years have scientists begun to understand the metabolic function they play in humans.

There are four essential trace minerals for which RDAs have been established. They are iron, zinc, iodine, and selenium. The RDA for selenium was just established in 1989. There are five others for which RDAs have not yet been determined, but which are known to be important and for which "safe and adequate" daily ranges of intake have been estimated. These are copper, manganese, fluoride, chromium, and molybdenum. At least five to seven others are known to be needed in amounts that have not yet been quantified. No doubt these numbers will change as further research is done. Zinc was added to the RDAs as

recently as 1974, and the six for which ranges have been given were included only in 1980. Scientists are still in the process of identifying and quantifying important trace minerals, and it is likely that new discoveries will be made in the coming years. For example, there is evidence that selenium and arsenic, clearly poisonous at high levels, are essential at small levels. And there even appears to be a need for minerals such as nickel and silicon, the latter being one of the most ubiquitous elements on the planet.

Because trace minerals find their way into so many different types of food, it might seem that Americans, who have such an abundant food supply, need not be concerned about getting sufficient amounts. What's more, each of us has built-in homeostatic biochemical mechanisms that, up to a point, make it possible to more efficiently absorb the minerals and other nutrients we consume when we are deficient in them. We are also somewhat protected from toxicity by our ability to store or excrete those we consume in greater quantities than we need.

Still, as researchers dig deeper into the questions of trace element nutrition, it is clear that our food sources and eating patterns are such that many of us are not eating adequate amounts of the trace minerals. There is much still to learn about how trace minerals interact with each other and with other nutrients to help maintain health and prevent disease.

However, it is important to remember that minerals, vitamins, and other nutrients do not operate independently of one another. It is not enough to concentrate on the intake of any one, since their proper functioning depends on maintaining the delicate balance among them.

Iron

Iron is absorbed through the intestines and picked up by the bloodstream. About 70 percent of the iron we absorb ends up in hemoglobin, a protein that releases oxygen to body cells for energy production and other metabolic functions

Checklist: Are You Iron-Rich?

1. Do you regularly consume meats _____ Yes _____ No
Red meats are the best sources of heme iron, and animal protein facilitates the absorption of nonheme iron. Poultry and fish contain heme iron, but the amount is lower. Liver is one of the richest sources, but it is very high in cholesterol. You can diminish the calorie-fat-cholesterol toll on most iron-rich proteins by selecting lean cuts, removing visible fat and broiling them.

2. Are fruits and vegetables among your food favorites? _____ Yes _____ No
Consuming foods rich in vitamin C—citrus fruits and juices, dark-green vegetables, cauliflower, cabbage, tomatoes, cantaloupe, and strawberries—can substantially increase absorption of nonheme iron. But you must consume them at the same time you eat the iron-containing foods.

3. Do you look for enriched products when you buy processed foods?
_____ Yes _____ No
Many refined products are enriched to include iron. For example, almost all processed flours, baking mixes, and cereals have added iron. When purchasing these products, check the labels to find those that have the most.

4. Do you ever cook in iron pans? _____ Yes _____ No
When you cook acidic foods, such as tomato sauce, in iron pans, some of the iron leaches into the food, providing an additional iron source for your diet.

5. Are you a coffee or tea drinker? _____ Yes _____ No
When consumed with a meal, coffee can decrease iron absorption by as much as 39 percent; tea can decrease absorption by 87 percent. The culprit is not caffeine but other substances in the beverages. Poor iron absorption occurs only when coffee or tea are consumed along with the iron source. And one study showed that including vitamin C in the same meal helps improve iron absorption.

6. Are you a high-fiber eater? _____ Yes _____ No
If you normally consume very little iron but consume very large quantities of high-fiber foods, the bran and substances in the fiber can interfere with the absorption of iron. If your diet is well-rounded, with adequate amounts of both iron and fiber, this factor isn't important.

and gives color to the red blood cells. About 4 percent of absorbed iron goes into myoglobin, another protein that transfers oxygen to muscle cells. Some of the remaining iron is involved in important cellular chemical reactions responsible for energy metabolism. The amount of iron that the body absorbs depends primarily on the type and source of iron consumed. The intestines increase or decrease absorption according to the body's need. People who are iron-deficient may absorb two to three times as much iron as those who have adequate levels.

Long-term iron deficiency results in iron-deficiency anemia, a condition in which the blood hemoglobin levels drop and red blood cells become small and pale. The symptoms of iron deficiency usually appear slowly and can include fatigue, irritability, headaches, lack of energy, and tingling in the hands and feet. In some cases, a bizarre craving called pica leads people to consume dirt, clay, ice, laundry starch, and other nonfood substances.

Anemia impairs the ability to do physical and possibly mental work. In one study, when anemic tea pickers were given iron supplements, they were able to pick far more leaves per day. And another study showed that anemic workers, who were originally seen as lazy and unintelligent by their supervisors, came to be viewed as more motivated, bright, and productive after they were given iron supplements. It is now thought that iron deficiency leading to anemia may negatively affect learning ability and the ability to fight infection.

There are many food sources for iron, but it is absorbed more efficiently from some foods than from others. Iron is best absorbed from animal foods, such as beef, beef liver, chicken, tuna, and shrimp. This iron is known as heme iron. Iron found in plant foods, such as dried beans, nuts, whole grains, and dried fruits, is called nonheme iron and is absorbed less efficiently. Iron that is added to processed foods is much like nonheme iron.

It should be noted that tea and coffee contain substances that inhibit iron absorption, and that eating a vitamin C-rich food at the same meal with iron will enhance the absorption of nonheme iron. Moreover, the presence of heme iron in the meal will enhance the absorption of nonheme iron. For example, the nonheme iron content of beans in a bowl of chili will be better assimilated if the chili also contains even a little ground beef.

Blood loss caused by a heavy menstrual flow, gastrointestinal disease, surgery, and too-frequent blood donations can result in iron deficiency. The iron problems of young women are not simply due to loss of menstrual blood. Iron deficiency in a young woman may stem from a combination of low iron intake, heavy menstrual periods, repeated dieting, and too little vitamin C. Recent studies have shown that the average American woman consumes only about 60 percent of the RDA for iron.

While deficiency, not toxicity, is usually the problem with iron, toxicity can be seen in some people who have a hereditary defect that causes their bodies to store too much and also in people who ingest too much iron in supplement form. Overabundance of iron can manifest itself in liver damage and damage to other tissues. In addition, excessive amounts of iron can reduce the body's ability to use other trace minerals.

Zinc

Zinc is the second most abundant trace mineral in the body next to iron, and it serves a number of functions vital to life. It is involved in the breakdown and utilization of carbohydrates and the synthesis of proteins. It is also required for the replication of DNA, the genetic material that determines the function of every living cell. Zinc is necessary for normal growth and development in children. It is also important for the health of such diverse cells as those of the taste buds, the lining of the gastrointestinal tract, the immune system, and the retina of the eye, as well as for the production of sperm and the male sex hormone testosterone. The exact way in which zinc functions has not been determined, but, in part, it exhibits its effects by being an essential component of a variety of enzymes involved in cellular reactions.

The absorption of zinc from foods is affected by its interaction with other trace minerals and by the existence of absorption-impairing substances in some foods—most specifically, whole-grain foods and soy protein. Taking this into account, zinc is found in rich supply in meats and poultry (especially the dark meat), oysters, eggs, and legumes.

Since available zinc stores are limited and it is continually being excreted from the body in feces, sweat, and urine, inadequate dietary intake over an extended period of time can result in a state of chronic deficiency. This deficiency was first delineated in rural areas of the Middle East, where it produced a syndrome of stunted growth and impaired sexual development in boys.

Other manifestations of severe zinc deficiency include loss of appetite, impaired mental ability, emotional disorders, tremors, a slowdown in the healing of wounds and burns, poor night vision, loss of a sense of taste, and pustular skin rashes on the arms, legs, mouth, and genital region. The effects of a mild deficiency are more subtle. In children, there might be a less extreme form of physical retardation. In adults, there might be a decline in male sperm count, combined with a reduction in the amount of testosterone produced; a higher level of blood ammonia, which is a toxic by-product of the breakdown of protein; and the inability to maintain a constant body weight.

Zinc deficiency can be particularly serious during pregnancy, resulting in prolonged gestation and labor, and creating risks to the fetus toward the end of pregnancy. Laboratory studies have shown that pregnant animals fed a zinc-deficient diet have a much higher incidence of deformed and stillborn offspring. Similar results have been reported among women with inadequate zinc in their diets.

There are several groups of people who run a risk of zinc deficiency. Heavy drinkers often suffer zinc deficiency because alcohol speeds the rate at which zinc is lost from the body in the urine. Drinking alcohol is particularly hazardous during pregnancy because it not only enhances zinc excretion but impairs the transport of zinc across the placenta to the developing fetus. Indeed, fetal alcohol syndrome—a cluster of birth defects that include mental retardation in the children of women who drink excessively during pregnancy —is in part linked to the depletion of zinc in fetal tissues.

Some athletes run the risk of zinc deficiency because of the large amounts of zinc that are excreted in sweat. Studies of male long-distance runners disclosed that their average blood level of zinc was 20 percent below the normal value. The problem may be heightened by the fact that endurance athletes often eat large quantities of high-energy carbohydrate foods, such as fruit, yogurt, bread, and pasta, none of which contains much zinc.

Vegetarians have a difficult time satisfying the RDA for zinc when their diets lack animal protein or dairy products. Fruits and vegetables do not contain much zinc, and, although whole-grain foods are good sources, they contain substances called phytates that bind the mineral and impede its absorption into the body. Soy protein also contains large amounts of phytates, as well as phosphorous-containing substances that impair zinc absorption. For this reason, even if a vegetarian consumes the RDA for zinc, it may not be sufficient.

Women who are breast feeding may need zinc supplements to assure that their milk contains adequate amounts of the mineral.

Zinc is not very toxic unless it is taken in extremely high doses. In one study, eleven healthy men who consumed 300 milligrams of zinc daily (twenty times the RDA) were studied for six weeks. The results, published in the *Journal of the American Medical Association,* indicated that zinc at that dosage level impaired the function of white blood cells—the cells that fight infection. Moreover, the volunteers' blood levels of HDL cholesterol, the type believed to protect against heart disease, were lowered. LDL cholesterol, the kind that predisposes people to heart problems, was raised.

Lower levels of zinc were not seen to be as harmful. In another study, 44 men were given about 30 milligrams of zinc or a placebo every day for eight weeks. Eating these levels of zinc did not change the HDL or LDL cholesterol.

Selenium

Selenium was identified as an essential nutrient in the 1950s. Before that, selenium was believed to be toxic at any level. Now it is known that selenium is crucial for the proper functioning of the heart muscle and protects against toxic doses of the heavy metals cadmium, mercury, and silver. In addition, the data presented in some very preliminary studies suggest that selenium may help ward off certain forms of cancer. However, it is easy to reach a toxic level of selenium. High levels of selenium may increase dental cavities and cause skin lesions.

In 1989, selenium was added to the Recommended Dietary Allowance for Americans. It is found naturally in fish, meat, breads, and cereal.

Iodine

Iodine is part of the hormone thyroxine, produced by the thyroid gland. This hormone is important in the regulation of the body's energy metabolism. The RDA for iodine is only 0.15 mg, a smaller quantity than the recommendation for every vitamin except B-12. It is amazing how biologically important such tiny amounts of some nutrients can be.

A deficiency in iodine results in goiter, an enlargement of the thyroid as it tries to accommodate for the deficiency. A chronic deficiency will result in the destruction of the gland. Infants born to mothers who have iodine deficiency sometimes suffer from cretinism, characterized by retarded growth and mental development, as well as a low metabolic rate. Cretins have protruding abdomens, swollen features, thick lips, and enlarged tongues.

For a variety of reasons, some people may produce excess thyroxine. The condition is serious and may be treated by drugs that lower thyroxine levels. In some cases, the treatment may be to destroy the thyroid by radioactive iodine, as was the case with First Lady Barbara Bush, or to remove the thyroid surgically. Fortunately, thyroxine is synthesized inexpensively and people lacking the hormone can restore normal function when they're given thyroxine orally.

The primary natural source of iodine is seafood, especially saltwater fish. There was a time when goiter was epidemic in the midwestern United States because the soil was deficient in iodine. Today, most table salt in the United States is iodized, and the deficiency is much less common.

Copper

Although RDAs for copper have not yet been determined, a "safe and adequate" intake of the mineral has been set at 2 to 3 mg per day for adults. Copper is needed for the synthesis of hemoglobin, a central component of red blood cells; the manufacture of collagen, a protein that helps make up connective tissue; and the maintenance of the protective sheath that surrounds nerve fibers. Copper is also essential for the proper functioning of the heart.

Some recent evidence indicates that just a slight copper deficiency may cause an elevation in blood cholesterol levels. One researcher who placed a man on a low-copper diet found that his cholesterol level rose from 206 to 235 after only a few months. The man's cholesterol dropped back down to 200 once he resumed eating a diet with an adequate amount of copper.

Copper is available in whole-grain foods, liver, kidney, osyters, and nuts. According to Leslie Klevay, M.D., research medical officer at the USDA Human Nutrition Research Center in Grand Forks, North Dakota, as many as 75 percent of American diets include less than 2 mg of copper. But insufficient levels of copper in the diet may be caused by factors other than not eating enough copper-rich foods. Taking huge amounts of vitamin C or zinc, for example, interferes with the body's ability to use the mineral.

Other Important Trace Minerals

The functions of several other trace minerals have been studied.

Fluoride was the subject of heated debate in recent decades, when scientists announced that it might play a role in preventing dental cavities. Fluoride deficiency leads to dental decay and bone loss, and it might even be related to osteoporosis. Today, most water in the United States has been fluoridated, with the result that many American children are growing up free of dental cavities.

It appears that a form of chromium, called trivalent chromium, in a complex containing niacin and some amino acids, assists the activity of the hormone insulin in regulating glucose and lipid metabolism. Chromium may also play a role in helping to solve medical problems related to diabetes and heart disease, and it may be involved in DNA and RNA metabolism. Sources of chromium include meat, cheese, brewer's yeast, dried beans, and whole-grain products.

Manganese is involved in protein and energy metabolism and is essential for normal bone structure and the functioning of the nervous system. To date, manganese deficiency has never been observed in humans. Its sources include legumes and whole grains.

Molybdenum has been found to be a component of several of the body's enzymes, and it too has never been found to be deficient in humans. Molybdenum occurs in meats, grains, and legumes.

Water: The Most Important Nutrient

You won't find water listed on nutrient charts, but everyone knows that we can't live without it. In fact, while we can survive for extended periods of time without many vitamins and minerals, it takes only a few days without water to lead to death.

Water is a colorless compound of hydrogen and oxygen that virtually every cell in the body needs to survive; it contains no calories. Even tissues that are not thought of as "watery" contain large amounts of this substance. For instance, water makes up about three-fourths of the brain and muscles, and bone is more than one-fifth water. In all, water accounts for about one-half to two-thirds of the body's makeup. Men have more water than women per pound, since they have proportionately less fat, and fat tissue holds less water than lean tissue.

One of water's many essential tasks as a solvent and carrier is to carry nutrients and oxygen to all parts of the body through the blood and lymphatic systems. In addition, it plays an important role in maintaining body temperature; the heat released when we lose water through perspiration helps keep us cool. Water also removes metabolic waste by way of urine and sweat, lubricates the joints, gives form to the cells, surrounds and protects a fetus, and serves as the medium for thousands of life-supporting chemical reactions that are constantly taking place inside our bodies.

The average adult consumes and excretes about two and a half to three quarts of water each day. People who live in hot climates or whose jobs or hobbies involve strenuous physical exercise need to consume more. Thirst is generally a good indicator of when the body needs water. It is regulated by the sodium concentration in the blood; when the sodium level of blood rises, receptors in the brain's hypothalamus gland trigger a thirst sensation. In addition, "thirsty" blood draws water from the salivary glands, which accounts for the dry mouth. When there is a need for water, the kidneys excrete less urine.

Thirst cannot be relied on as the perfect indicator of water requirements. It is possible to quench your thirst without putting back into your body the amount of water you need. That's the reason you're advised to drink 6 to 8 glasses of fluid every day, whether you're thirsty or not. This recommendation has special implications for the elderly, as there is evidence that they are less

► NUTRITION QUIZ ◄

Check Your Vitamin-Mineral IQ

How much do you know about which foods are the best sources for the vitamins and minerals you need? Rate the following foods in order of their quality in providing nutrients: 1 = best source, 2 = medium source, 3 = least effective source.

For vitamin C
_____ apple
_____ grapefruit
_____ banana

For iron
_____ cheddar cheese
_____ round steak
_____ cod

For vitamin A
_____ corn
_____ asparagus
_____ broccoli

For calcium
_____ skim milk
_____ whole milk
_____ plain yogurt

For vitamin B-12
_____ kidney beans
_____ lentils
_____ peas

For thiamin
_____ enriched white rice
_____ mashed potatoes
_____ cooked tomatoes

For vitamin E
_____ butter
_____ shortening
_____ corn oil

For potassium
_____ grapefruit juice
_____ tomato juice
_____ grape juice

For zinc
_____ beef liver
_____ chicken breast
_____ ground beef

For riboflavin
_____ orange juice
_____ whole milk
_____ beer

ANSWERS

Vitamin C (2,3,1). Grapefruit is rich in vitamin C, as are all citrus fruits. Apple-a-day adherents might be surprised to learn that apples are not rich sources of the vitamin.

Iron (2,3,1). Red meats are high in the form of iron that is readily used by the body. Dairy products tend to be low in the mineral.

Vitamin A (3,2,1). Deep green and orange color should be your guide in selecting plant foods for vitamin A.

Calcium (all three foods are equally good sources of calcium). Low-fat dairy foods maintain as much calcium as whole-milk foods.

Vitamin B-12 (none of these foods offers vitamin B-12). It's available only from animal sources.

Thiamin (1,2,3). Enriched grain products and whole-grains are good sources of thiamin.

Vitamin E (3, 2,1). Vegetable oils are the best sources. Although shortening and margarine contain E, some of it is lost in the processing.

Potassium (2, 1, 3). Tomato juice is the richest in potassium, but each of these foods contains significant amounts of the mineral.

Zinc (1, 3, 2). Beef liver has far more zinc than the other two. All red meats are considered good sources of the mineral.

Riboflavin (2, 1, 3). Milk is the only good source listed.

likely to get thirst signals when their bodies need water. People who eat high-salt or high-protein diets have an increased need for water to maintain electrolyte balance and to help their kidneys flush out the excess salt and the waste products of protein metabolism. Drinking water past the point of thirst also reduces the risk of dehydration for people who live in extremely hot climates, as well as for athletes and laborers who sweat excessively. It's almost impossible to take in too much water, since the body is very efficient at getting rid of what it doesn't need.

Most of the water we consume comes from beverages, including juice, milk, and soft drinks. Coffee, tea, and alcoholic beverages also supply water, but these substances are diuretics and they increase loss of water through the kidneys. Solid foods also contribute substantially to our daily water intake. Most fruits are more than 80 percent water, and even foods that don't seem juicy or moist supply us with large amounts. For example, cooked lean beef is 60 percent water, bread is about one-third water, and butter is roughly 15 percent water. In addition, when foods are metabolized to provide energy, significant amounts of water are produced.

Is all water the same? Water is always composed of two parts hydrogen to one part oxygen, but the composition of the water we drink is affected by where it comes from and how it is processed. It can be hard or soft, carbonated or still, "natural" or "modified." The source of water might be buried deep within the earth's surface, or it might be a reservoir or pond. Since water is an excellent solvent, it often contains minerals, in some cases toxic.

Many people believe that bottled water is safer than tap water, and the subject is open to debate. Following are differences between the two.

Tap Water

Public water systems provide 90 percent of the American population with drinking water. Close to half of our municipal tap water comes from surface water, such as rivers and streams. The rest comes from groundwater, including wells, springs, and aquifers, which are areas of porous rock, sand, or gravel that are fed by rain and snow. In some regions the water is naturally hard; it contains comparatively high concentrations of minerals, notably calcium and magnesium. Soft water has higher levels of sodium. You can find out how hard or soft your water is from your water utility.

Many people prefer soft water for a number of

reasons. It makes soap lather better and leaves less of a ring around the tub. It also gets clothes cleaner. Some municipalities (and individuals) soften their water by removing calcium and magnesium and adding sodium, in what is known as an ion exchange process. From a nutritional standpoint, this practice has drawbacks. For one thing, our diets are already quite high in sodium and, while the levels in most water supplies don't add up to much, we don't need more, especially at the expense of minerals, like calcium and magnesium.

Water may pick up undesirable metals like lead from the pipes. Lead is more soluble in hot water than it is in cold water, so if you have a lead pipe problem, you might want to consider only using cold water for drinking and cooking, and running it first before use.

Along with the differences in mineral concentration, water has varying levels of heavy metals, microorganisms, and organic compounds. These must be filtered out (or, in the case of microorganisms, killed by disinfection) to the point where they do not endanger human health. The filtering process is nothing new; humans have been cleaning their drinking water for thousands of years. Pictures of water-clarifying apparatus have been found on Egyptian walls that date back to 1500 BC, and a Sanskrit quotation from as early as 200 BC talks about appropriate methods for filtering water.

Concern for the purity of drinking water remains high today. The composition that comes out of the tap is regulated by state and local law and the Environmental Protection Agency (EPA) under the provisions of the Safe Drinking Water Act of 1974, a law that sets minimum quality standards for drinking water. One of the agency's requirements is that tap water must be treated, if necessary, to prevent contamination from bacteria, insuring against outbreaks of waterborne diseases. Several amendments to the Safe Drinking Water Act have strengthened the provisions for water filtering and have added provisions for better protection of our groundwater resources.

Much of the tap water in the United States is disinfected with chlorine. Although chlorine kills many bacteria, it has been found to react with organic compounds to form what are known as trihalomethanes, which are suspected of causing cancer or genetic mutations that promote cancer. For this reason, the EPA restricts the level of trihalomethanes in municipal drinking water to 0.10 milligrams per liter, or 100 parts per billion. At that level or below, scientists believe that water is perfectly safe for humans.

The EPA has also set limits for many other contaminants that are found in drinking water, including mercury, nitrate, and silver, as well as pesticides and radioactivity. It is the responsibility of the water utilities to monitor the level of contaminants in the water and periodically report to the state or, in some cases, the federal government. If the water is deemed unsafe to drink, consumers must receive notification through the media and be given instructions on necessary precautions, such as boiling their water or using bottled water.

The Fluoride Factor

It has been nearly 50 years since Grand Rapids, Michigan, became the first town to fluoridate its water supply. Since then, it has been well established that fluoride helps strengthen teeth and prevent cavities, and fluoridation has been endorsed by several health organizations, including the American Dental Association and the American Medical Association. Yet many municipal water supplies remain unfluoridated. Part of the reason is the efforts of antifluoridation activisits, who use the nonsensical arguments that fluoride promotes cancer, sickle-cell anemia, and even AIDS.

It is true that dental fluorosis, a harmless, if unsightly, mottling of the teeth, has been seen in communities where the naturally occurring fluoride in the water is more than several parts per million. But when fluoride is added to water, it is in much lower concentrations, and children who live in areas where the water is fluoridated have many fewer cavities than those who don't. Further, there is no evidence that properly fluoridated water is injurious to the public's health.

To find out if your tap water is fluoridated, you can contact your local water department or the state board of health. Based on the amount of fluoride in your water, your dentist should be able to tell you whether your child needs fluoride supplements. The American Dental Association recommends that in areas where the fluoridation concentration is less than 0.7 parts per million, children should be given fluoride supplements from birth to 13 years of age.

If your water comes from a well, you should have it analyzed by a laboratory. Also, private wells are not covered by the Safe Drinking Water Act, so well water should be tested for bacteria and contaminants.

Bottled Water

Minimum standards for the quality of bottled water are set by the Food and Drug Administration (FDA) and match the standards set for municipal water supplies. There are several different types of bottled water.

Natural water is water that has been unmodified by mineral addition or depletion.

Naturally sparkling water has enough carbon dioxide to be bubbly without the introduction of outside chemicals.

Sparkling water has been made effervescent by the injection of carbon dioxide from an outside source.

Spring water naturally flows out of the earth at a particular spot and is bottled at or near its source. Like natural water, it is not altered by the addition or deletion of minerals.

Drinking water is usually noncarbonated, or still. It is generally used as an alternative to tap water, although its sources might be the municipal water supply.

Purified water has been demineralized. When it is vaporized and recondensed it is called *distilled water*.

Mineral water is an imprecise term since, with the exception of purified and distilled, all water has minerals. According to the International Bottled Water Association, mineral water contains not less than 500 parts per million (about one-eighth teaspoon per quart) of total dissolved minerals.

Seltzer is usually tap water that has been injected with carbon dioxide.

Club soda is also artificially carbonated, but it contains added salts and minerals. The FDA regulates club soda, seltzer, and naturally sparkling water under the guidelines for soda water (like colas), not bottled water. Manufacturers may add up to 0.02 percent caffeine and 0.5 percent alcohol by weight.

Supplements: Separating Myth and Reality

Certain vitamin and mineral substances have been popularized as having near-magical abilities in preventing or curing disease, improving performance, or otherwise benefiting people, usually in higher than recommended dosages. It is easy to see why consumers might be attracted to the idea of popping a pill to eliminate stress, cure baldness, become more sexy, or prevent the effects of more severe ailments. According to the FDA, four out of ten Americans over the age of 16 take at least one supplement a day, and approximately one in ten people take five or more supplements daily. And one supplement taker in eight is a heavy user—someone who consumes an average of eight times the RDA.

What are the facts behind the many myths about

supplement taking? How can you decide whether or not you need supplements?

The first thing to consider is if you might be at risk for nutrient deficiencies that could warrant supplementation. Fortunately, most people in the United States get all the nutrients they need from the abundant food supply. But if you omit a major food group from your regular diet, you may need a supplement. For example, if you're a confirmed vegetable-hater, your diet may be lacking in vitamin A or vitamin C, although you may not necessarily need supplements since many of our foods are fortified with these vitamins.

There are several groups of people who might need supplements.

▶ If you are frequently on a low-calorie diet, as are many women and adolescent girls, you may need a multi–vitamin/mineral supplement, particularly if your usual diet includes no more than 1,200 calories. In fact, government surveys have shown that many American women have low intakes of vitamins A, C, and B-6, calcium, iron, and magnesium. Because of menstrual losses, women also have difficulty obtaining enough dietary iron.

▶ Heavy smokers and drinkers may also have special needs. Regular smoking may increase the need for vitamin C. In addition, heavy alcohol consumption can increase the need for vitamins B-6 and B-12, thiamin, riboflavin, and folic acid, as well as magnesium and zinc. The increased need of alcoholics is partly metabolic and partly because a large consumption of nonnutritive calories in the form of alcohol precludes the consumption of adequate amounts of nutritious foods.

▶ Because the physiological changes of pregnancy and lactation increase the need for a number of nutrients, pregnant or nursing mothers should ask their physicians about the possible need for a supplement. It is well accepted that pregnant women need an iron supplement. And if they don't eat well, a combination vitamin/mineral supplement may also be in order.

▶ Some elderly people don't get enough of the nutrients they need from food, either because they can't physically get the food they need, can't financially afford it, or are unable to prepare it. Moreover, accommodating the low calorie needs of the aged means cutting back on foods in general, which may result in inadequate nutrient intake. Problems with chewing or swallowing, digestive disturbances, and medications can contribute to changes in an elderly person's appetite and eating habits that might also lead to nutrient deficiencies.

▶ Drug-nutrient interactions may lead to vitamin/mineral deficiencies. The risk is greater for people who have marginal diets or who have diseases or injuries that may increase nutrient needs. Both over-the-counter and prescription drugs can alter your nutritional requirements. If you take a lot of aspirin, for example, you may need more vitamin K. And the continuous use of antacids can increase the need for some minerals. Ask your physician or pharmacist whether or not there are drug-nutrient interactions with the medication you use regularly.

Even if you fall into any of these nutritionally risky categories, it is best to try to get your missing nutrients from natural food sources before you start taking supplements. But when considering supplements, the first rule of thumb is to avoid taking doses of isolated nutrients unless they have been prescribed for a specific medical reason. One possible exception is calcium, since multi–vitamin/mineral supplements do not supply the RDA of this nutrient. But large amounts of some nutrients can upset the balance of other nutrients in the body. For example, too much vitamin C may interfere with copper metabolism, and calcium supplements may interfere with the normal absorption of phosphorus. In addition, as we have seen, large doses of some nutrients can produce toxicity.

When selecting a supplement, the sensible guide is to choose a combination multi–vitamin/mineral supplement that contains a variety of vitamins and minerals in amounts no greater than 100 percent of the RDA. Because it is unlikely that your body needs more than that, the high potency supplements are of little value.

Supplement labels express nutrient levels in two ways: One is a quantity measure—for example, milligrams (mg) or International Units (IU); the other is the percentage of the U.S. Recommended Daily Allowance (USRDA). Whereas Recommended Dietary Allowance (RDA) values vary according to sex, age, and certain circumstances, the USRDA generally represents the highest value for any group (see chapter 7). However, the RDA, not the USRDA, is a more appropriate standard for children and pregnant and lactating women. Avoid supplements that use the term "minimum daily requirement" because this comparison system is no longer used and the products may be out of date.

Don't be fooled into thinking that expensive supplements are best. Given two choices with the same nutrients, the less expensive one will meet your needs just as well. Added ingredients such as choline, inositol, and PABA only increase the cost. Except for people with special medical needs, there is no dietary need for them.

There are a number of prevailing myths regarding supplement use. Let's look at what they are and at the facts behind them.

Myth: Supplements are necessary because people's nutrient needs vary and the RDAs can't always account for individual needs.

The Facts: The RDAs *do* take individual variations into account. The Food and Nutrition Board of the National Academy of Sciences sets the RDAs well above actual requirements so that the needs of all healthy people are satisfied, even those with larger than average requirements. For example, about 1,670 to 2,000 IU daily of vitamin A have been found necessary to sustain an adequate concentration of the vitamin in the blood and to prevent all symptoms of vitamin A deficiency. Yet the RDA for vitamin A is set far above this level, at 4,000 IU for women and 5,000 IU for men, in order to allow for individual needs and for a reserve store of vitamin A in the liver and other tissues. The same is true for other nutrients. Because the RDAs cover the needs of the entire healthy population, they are in excess of nearly every individual's needs.

Myth: Water-soluble vitamins must be replaced every day since they are not stored in the body.

The Facts: Although water-soluble vitamins are not retained in the body as long as fat-soluble vitamins, they are preserved in organs and tissues for weeks, months, and sometimes years, depending on the vitamin. If they weren't, there would be a high incidence of vitamin deficiency disease in the United States, since many people go for short periods without consuming adequate amounts. Specifically, several weeks must go by without vitamin B-1 before symptoms of thiamin deficiency occur, and about five years of vitamin B-12 deprivation must pass before signs of a vitamin B-12 deficiency develop. Even symptoms of scurvy won't occur for about 16 weeks if a healthy person consumes no vitamin C.

Myth: Vitamin C may prevent cancer and cardiovascular disease.

The Facts: Most studies that reveal a possible link between vitamin C and the prevention of cancer have shown that it is difficult to isolate the vitamin as the sole protective ingredient. However, there are some studies that suggest that vitamin C and some other, as yet undefined, dietary antioxidants may play an unquantified role in protecting against cancer. And some people already stricken with cancer have been reported to have low blood levels of vitamin C. But this might be because they are eating less food, particularly less vitamin C-rich foods. There is no evidence that large doses of the vitamin can prolong a cancer patient's life. False hopes may have been raised when a report in the mid-1970s indicated that people with terminal cancer lived an average of about 300 days longer when they took 10,000 milligrams daily of vitamin C. But this claim lacked credibility, as it was based on inadequate data. More recent studies conducted at the Mayo clinic showed that people with advanced cancer, given either vitamin C or a placebo, lived the same amount of time.

Research on the connection between cardiovascular disease and ascorbic acid has failed to show beneficial links. It is true that cholesterol metabolism appears to be impaired in people with vitamin C deficiency and that some heart attack victims have been found to have low blood levels of the vitamin. But that does not mean that overdosing with vitamin C will prevent heart disease. In fact, studies demonstrating that large intakes of ascorbic acid lower cholesterol in some patients are countered by others that reveal an increase of blood cholesterol or no effect at all. Limited research shows that there may be a connection between vitamin C and HDL-containing cholesterol, the kind of cholesterol that protects against heart disease. But, to date, not nearly enough evidence is available to warrant taking vitamin C supplements in an effort to prevent cardiovascular disease.

Myth: Megadoses of vitamin C will prevent and cure colds.

The Facts: The notion that large doses of vitamin C can prevent or cure colds has been popular since Linus Pauling first published *Vitamin C and the Common Cold* in 1970. But scientific studies have not confirmed Dr. Pauling's assertions. For example, after pooling the data from eight well-designed scientific studies on ascorbic acid and colds, Dr. Thomas C. Chalmers of New York's Mount Sinai Medical Center concluded in the *American Journal of Medicine* that people who took vitamin C rather than a placebo had only about one-tenth fewer colds per year. And their colds lasted an average of one-tenth less time than those of people who took a placebo in place of a supplement.

Myth: If you're tired or run down, vitamin B-12 supplements will boost your energy.

The Facts: Some practitioners of vitamin therapy give vitamin B-12 shots to their patients, and many people report feeling more energetic as a result. However, there is no proof that B-12 can cure fatigue, except in cases of pernicious anemia. Most Americans have many years worth of vitamin B-12 stored in their livers, so a vitamin B-12 shot or pill is like a drop in the river.

Myth: Zinc supplements will cure impotence or otherwise improve sexual prowess.

The Facts: That zinc has been touted as a sexual aid probably stems from the finding that some adolescent boys in the Middle East suffered from stunted growth and arrested sexual development as a result of deficiency in the mineral. When the young men were given zinc supplements, they began to grow again and to mature sexually. But zinc deficiency and subsequent supplementation with that mineral have nothing to do with an otherwise healthy man's sexual potency.

Myth: Vegetarians need a variety of supplements to compensate for the absence of meat in their diets.

The Facts: According to Albert Sanchea, Ph.D., of Loma Linda University, an institution in southern California where much of the nation's research on vegetarianism is conducted, the supplement needs of vegetarians vary according to the regimen. People who avoid only red meat do not need supplements because poultry and fish provide all the nutrients that red meat does. Lacto-ovo vegetarians—those who eschew all meat, poultry, and fish, but do eat dairy products and eggs—do not need supplements either. However, strict vegetarians who do not eat any kind of dairy food, eggs, meat, poultry, or fish, should gauge the amount of vitamin B-12 they are consuming from foods fortified with B-12, and consult qualified health professionals about their need for supplements of this nutrient, as well as calcium, iron, and zinc.

Myth: High doses of beta-carotene supplements will protect against cancer.

The Facts: It's true that some epidemiological research has suggested that groups of people who eat a relatively high amount of certain fruits and vegetables, specifically the cruciferous vegetables such as brussels sprouts and cabbage, along with dark-green- and orange-pigmented plants, appear to run a lower risk of developing cancer. But these studies examined the consumption of whole foods, not supplements. And the substance or combination of substances in these foods, including beta-carotene, vitamin C, the different fibers, and any one or more of a number of other chemicals present in fruits and vegetables, may be responsible for the apparent protection. Until the connection is firmly established, all the major health organizations involved in cancer research, including the National Cancer Institute, the American Health Foundation, and the American Cancer Society, strongly recommend eating foods containing beta-carotene rather than taking supplements in order to decrease cancer risks.

Myth: People with drinking problems should take vitamin supplements to balance the negative effects of alcohol.

The Facts: Excessive amounts of alcohol are toxic to the liver, and the damage cannot be reversed by vitamin or mineral supplements. Although a supplement might supply some of the nutrients missing from their diets as well as some of the nutrients they are not absorbing properly, supplementation will ultimately prove meaningless if heavy alcohol consumption is continued.

Myth: Vitamin E is an all-purpose miracle cure.

The Facts: Popular myth often hails vitamin E as a miracle cure for a wide variety of ailments, in-

cluding sterility, old age, menstrual disorders, heart disease, diabetes, ulcers, and muscular dystrophy, to name a few. With virtually all of these conditions, however, vitamin E has not lived up to expectations when actually put to scientific tests. One of the reasons for the distortion is that many of the claims are based on animal studies that cannot be applied to humans. For example, two of the most prevalent misconceptions are that vitamin E can cure sterility and muscular dystrophy. In fact, animal studies have shown that vitamin E-deficient rats become infertile, and that rabbits, chickens, and monkeys develop a type of muscular dystrophy when deprived of vitamin E. But in humans, other factors than vitamin E deficiency contribute to these conditions. And attempts to treat sterility and muscular dystrophy with vitamin E supplements have been unsuccessful.

One of the most exciting claims for vitamin E is that it offers a fountain of youth—that it can reverse or slow down the aging process. This claim probably derives from the fact that in both animals and humans, the normal aging process is associated with the buildup of a brown pigment called lipofuscin. The pigment accumulates rapidly in vitamin E-deficient animals. But there is no evidence that vitamin E supplements will prevent the buildup of lipofuscin in aging humans.

Curbing Supplement Abuse

Annual sales of vitamin and mineral supplements have grown substantially during the last decade. Consumers spend upwards of $3 billion each year on nutrients in the form of pills and foods that are over-fortified with nutrients, a matter that has caused concern among physicians and scientists, since megadoses of some of these substances can cause adverse side effects. Many people don't realize that taking high doses of nutrient supplements is a risky practice that can amount to a form of over-the-counter drug abuse.

The FDA is currently prohibited from setting

upper limits on allowable levels of vitamins and minerals unless adverse effects can be clearly demonstrated. In the past, the agency has had no means of keeping track of adverse reactions. In fact, during the 1970s, in response to pressure from the supplement industry, health food stores, and private citizens, Congress prohibited the FDA from interfering with the sale or dosage regulation of supplements unless such negative reactions were proven. But as the nation's doctors begin to record their patients' use of supplements, more information is becoming available. Now doctors are encouraged to report adverse reactions to vitamin and mineral pills to the FDA, just as they do for drugs.

The practice of taking nutrients in pill form is becoming so widespread that four major health organizations—the American Dietetic Association, the American Institute of Nutrition, the American Society for Clinical Nutrition, and the National Council against Health Fraud—have issued a joint statement warning Americans about the unnecessary and sometimes unsafe use of vitamin and mineral supplements.

In 1986, a panel formed by the American Dietetic Association established initial guidelines about when supplement use turns to abuse. Panel members agreed that they saw no harm in taking daily multi–vitamin/mineral preparations that contained 100 percent of the RDA. However, they documented serious side effects from higher doses of certain nutrients. For example, vitamin A, if taken at a daily level of 25,000 IU, a level believed to be safe by many vitamin enthusiasts, may cause permanent liver damage after seven to ten years of use.

If you are in the habit of taking a multi–vitamin/mineral supplement containing RDA levels of nutrients every day, we wouldn't presume to tell you to stop taking it, or suggest that it doesn't really make you feel better. We would only encourage you to consider it a supplement, not a substitute, for the rich variety of vitamin-and-mineral-packed foods available in the American diet.

7

The Recommended
Dietary Allowances

The Recommended Dietary Allowances (RDAs) are standards set for the daily intake of various nutrients, and they're considered to be adequate quantities for practically all healthy people.

The RDAs are based on the recommendation of the nutritional scientists who comprise the Food and Nutrition Board of the National Academy of Sciences-National Research Council. They are defined as "the levels of intake of essential nutrients considered, in the judgment of the Food and Nutrition Board on the basis of available scientific knowledge, to be adequate to meet the known nutritional needs of practically all healthy persons." The RDAs are reestablished approximately every five years. The latest RDAs were published in 1989.

To arrive at these recommendations, the Food and Nutrition Board appoints committees of scientists to review scientific literature from around the world on the nutrient requirements of people, paying particular attention to new findings since the last RDAs were published. The research they look at includes studies of individuals who are deficient in particular nutrients and those who are not. They also consider studies in which scientists have determined nutrient requirements in groups of people of different ages and sex.

From these and other studies, the committee can estimate the average daily requirement for each nutrient. Of course, people vary in their needs, so before the scientists come up with a final number, they increase the figures to account for the needs of people with high requirements. The figures allow for the body's inefficient use of certain nutrients as they appear in particular foods; for example, the RDA for iron allows for the fact that only about 10 percent of the iron we eat is absorbed.

The RDA values for nutrients vary according to age and sex, and are also altered for pregnant and breast-feeding women. In total, there are 15 different recommendations by age (two for infants, three for children, five for males 11 years and older, and five for females 11 years and older), in addition to the three special categories of pregnant and breast-feeding women.

The nutrients for which RDAs exist are protein, most fat- and water-soluble vitamins, and seven minerals. For most groupings, there is considered to be a "reference," or typical, person for whom recommendations are made. For example, the "reference" woman is 5'4" tall and weighs 120 pounds. Obviously, not all women are this size. And some nutrient requirements, such as those for the B vitamins, depend on both size and activity level.

The RDAs are not intended to be requirements; they are merely offered as guidelines for meeting the needs of most people. Common sense should be your guide as you review the RDAs. If you were to consume less than a particular nutrient's RDA for a day, a week, or even a month, it probably would do no harm. However, the risk increases with time, depending on how much below the RDA you go, and the state of your stores of the nutrient. Also, many people safely consume more than the RDA, although the RDA committee states that they've seen no evidence of benefits gained from overconsumption. In some cases, toxicity can result when consumption greatly exceeds the RDA, particularly for fat-soluble vitamins such as A and D.

The 1989 recommendations include the suggestion that cigarette smokers consume 100 milligrams per day of vitamin C.

When we look for nutrient information on a food label, we don't find the RDAs listed. Practically, there isn't enough space on food labels to list the RDA for all 18 categories, so the Food and Drug Administration has developed the U.S. Recommended Daily Allowances (USRDAs). Usually, the USRDA figures are the highest RDA for each nutrient. For example, the USRDA for iron is 15 milligrams (the amount suggested for women), not 10 milligrams (the amount suggested for men). Normally, what you see on labels is the USRDA for people age four and up. There are three other less commonly used USRDAs: one for infants up to one year old, found on baby food and certain supplements; one for children from one to four years old; and one for pregnant and lactating women.

What the RDAs Don't Cover

RDAs exist for nutrients when there are reliable, quantifiable data. But there are essential nutrients for which these data do not exist. For a number of vitamins and minerals, "safe and adequate" ranges have been devised by the RDA committee.

These figures give the minimum amounts believed to prevent deficiencies and the maximum amounts believed to be needed and, in the case of potential toxicity, safe.

Another essential nutrient for which there is no RDA is water. It's difficult to specify an ideal amount because needs vary greatly according to climate, activity level, and the amount of salt consumed. In addition, certain illnesses and medications, as well as high protein diets, can markedly increase the amount of water one should drink. Fortunately, except for elderly people and athletes, thirst is usually a reliable indicator that the body's water level has fallen too low. (See chapter 24 for further information on the nutritional needs of athletes and chapter 17 for dietary guidelines for the elderly.)

Beside lacking numbers for various substances classified as "required" nutrients, the RDAs also do not list such food components as fiber or water. Nor do they address many pertinent issues, such as how much salt intake is suggested, the number of calories, or the amount of complex carbohydrates, fat, and dietary fiber that is needed for a healthy diet. As far as these other components are concerned, Tufts agrees with the recommendations presented in the 1989 report by the National Research Council, *Diet and Health: Implications for Reducing Chronic Disease Risk.* According to the report, which was based on a

SAFE AND ADEQUATE NUTRIENT RANGES

Biotin	100–200 ug
Pantotheenic acid	4–7 mg
Copper	2–3 mg
Manganese	2.5–5 mg
Fluoride	1.5–4 mg
Chromium	0.05–0.2 mg
Molybdenum	0.15–0.5 mg
Sodium	1,100–3,300 mg
Potassium	1,875–5,625 mg
Chloride	1,700–5,100 mg

review of more than 5,000 studies, by following their guidelines Americans could reduce the risk of heart disease by at least 20 percent, and also reduce the risk of cancer, strokes, high blood pressure, osteoporosis, liver disease, and obesity. The recommendations include:

▶ Limit fats to 30 percent of daily calories, with saturated fats making up no more than 10 percent of total daily calories.

▶ Maintain dietary cholesterol intake below 300 milligrams daily.

▶ Consume at least 55 percent of daily calories in the form of complex carbohydrates.

▶ Consume the RDA for protein, but no more than twice that amount.

▶ Avoid the use of vitamin and mineral supplements, instead consuming the daily requirements in the form of a varied diet.

▶ Limit daily alcohol intake to less than one ounce, the equivalent of two beers or two small glasses of wine.

```
┌─────────────────────────────────────────────┐
│                     Key                      │
│                                              │
│  µg = microgram (one millionth of a gram)    │
│  mg = milligram (equal to 1,0000             │
│         micrograms)                          │
│  g  = gram (equal to 1,000 milligrams)       │
│  kg = kilogram (equal to 1,000 grams)        │
│                                              │
│  Heights and weights are averages based on   │
│  the "reference" person in the particular    │
│  category.                                   │
└─────────────────────────────────────────────┘
```

The 18 RDA Breakdowns

Following are the 1989 Recommended Dietary Allowances for 18 categories. We have presented them in a manner that should be easier for you to follow than the standard chart format.

1. Infants—Birth to 6 Months
Height: 24 inches   Weight: 13 pounds

Fat-Soluble Vitamins

Vitamin A	Vitamin D	Vitamin E	Vitamin K
375 µg	7.5 µg	3 mg	5 µg

Water-Soluble Vitamins

Vitamin C	B Vitamins					
30 mg	Thiamin	Riboflavin	Niacin	B-6	Folacin	B-12*
	0.3 µg	0.4 mg	5 mg	0.3 mg	25 µg	0.3 µg

Minerals

Calcium	Phosphorus	Magnesium	Iron	Zinc	Iodine	Selenium
400 mg	300 mg	40 mg	6 mg	5 mg	40 µg	10 µg

Protein
13 g

2. Infants—6 Months to 1 Year
Height: 28 inches
Weight: 20 pounds

Fat-Soluble Vitamins

Vitamin A	Vitamin D	Vitamin E	Vitamin K
375 µg	10 µg	4 mg	10 µg

Water-Soluble Vitamins

Vitamin C	B Vitamins					
35 mg	Thiamin	Riboflavin	Niacin	B-6	Folacin	B-12
	0.4 µg	0.5 mg	9 mg	0.6 mg	35 µg	0.5 µg

* The recommended dietary allowance for vitamin B-12 in infants is based on average concentrations of the vitamin in human milk. The allowances after weaning are based on energy intake (as recommended by the American Academy of Pediatrics) and consideration of other factors, such as intestinal absorption.

Minerals

Calcium	Phosphorus	Magnesium	Iron	Zinc	Iodine	Selenium
600 mg	500 mg	60 mg	10 mg	5 mg	50 mg	15 μg

Protein

14 g

3. Children—1 to 3 Years
Height: 2'11"
Weight: 29 pounds

Fat-Soluble Vitamins

Vitamin A	Vitamin D	Vitamin E	Vitamin K
400 μg	10 μg	6 mg	15 μg

Water-Soluble Vitamins

Vitamin C	B Vitamins					
	Thiamin	Riboflavin	Niacin	B-6	Folacin	B-12
40 mg	0.7 μg	0.8 mg	9 mg	1.0 mg	50 μg	0.7 μg

Minerals

Calcium	Phosphorus	Magnesium	Iron	Zinc	Iodine	Selenium
800 mg	800 mg	80 mg	10 mg	10 mg	70 μg	20 μg

Protein

16 g

4. Children—4 to 6 Years
Height: 3'8"
Weight: 44 pounds

Fat-Soluble Vitamins

Vitamin A	Vitamin D	Vitamin E	Vitamin K
500 μg	10 μg	7 mg	20 μg

Water-Soluble Vitamins

Vitamin C	B Vitamins					
	Thiamin	Riboflavin	Niacin	B-6	Folacin	B-12
45 mg	0.9 μg	1.1 mg	12 mg	1.1 mg	75 μg	1.0 μg

Minerals

Calcium	Phosphorus	Magnesium	Iron	Zinc	Iodine	Selenium
800 mg	800 mg	120 mg	10 mg	10 mg	90 μg	20 μg

Protein

24 g

5. Children—7 to 10 Years
Height: 4'4"
Weight: 62 pounds

Fat-Soluble Vitamins

Vitamin A	Vitamin D	Vitamin E	Vitamin K
700 μg	10 μg	7 mg	30 μg

Water-Soluble Vitamins

Vitamin C
45 mg

	B Vitamins				
Thiamin	Riboflavin	Niacin	B-6	Folacin	B-12
1.0 μg	1.2 mg	13 mg	1.4 mg	100 μg	1.4 μg

Minerals

Calcium	Phosphorus	Magnesium	Iron	Zinc	Iodine	Selenium
800 mg	800 mg	170 mg	10 mg	10 mg	120 mg	30 μg

Protein
26 g

6. Adolescent Males—11 to 14 Years
Height: 5'2"
Weight: 99 pounds

Fat-Soluble Vitamins

Vitamin A	Vitamin D	Vitamin E	Vitamin K
1 mg	10 μg	10 mg	45 μg

Water-Soluble Vitamins

Vitamin C
50 mg

	B Vitamins				
Thiamin	Riboflavin	Niacin	B-6	Folacin	B-12
1.3 μg	1.5 mg	17 mg	1.7 mg	150 μg	2.0 μg

Minerals

Calcium	Phosphorus	Magnesium	Iron	Zinc	Iodine	Selenium
1,200 mg	1,200 mg	270 mg	12 mg	15 mg	150 μg	40 μg

Protein
45 g

7. Adolescent Females—11 to 14 Years
Height: 5'2"
Weight: 101 pounds

Fat-Soluble Vitamins

Vitamin A	Vitamin D	Vitamin E	Vitamin K
800 μg	10 μg	8 mg	45 mg

Water-Soluble Vitamins

Vitamin C
50 mg

	B Vitamins				
Thiamin	Riboflavin	Niacin	B-6	Folacin	B-12
1.1 μg	1.3 mg	15 mg	1.4 mg	150 μg	2.0 μg

Minerals

Calcium	Phosphorus	Magnesium	Iron	Zinc	Iodine	Selenium
1,200 mg	1,200 mg	280 mg	15 mg	12 mg	150 μg	45 μg

Protein
46 g

8. Adolescent Males—15 to 18 Years
Height: 5'9"
Weight: 145 pounds

Fat-Soluble Vitamins

Vitamin A	Vitamin D	Vitamin E	Vitamin K
1 mg	10 μg	10 mg	65 μg

Water-Soluble Vitamins

Vitamin C	B Vitamins					
	Thiamin	Riboflavin	Niacin	B-6	Folacin	B-12
60 mg	1.5 μg	1.8 mg	20 mg	2 mg	200 μg	2 μg

Minerals

Calcium	Phosphorus	Magnesium	Iron	Zinc	Iodine	Selenium
1,200 mg	1,200 mg	400 mg	12 mg	15 mg	150 μg	50 μg

Protein
59 g

9. Adolescent Females—15 to 18 Years
Height: 5'4"
Weight: 120 pounds

Fat-Soluble Vitamins

Vitamin A	Vitamin D	Vitamin E	Vitamin K
800 mg	10 μg	8 mg	55 μg

Water-Soluble Vitamins

Vitamin C	B Vitamins					
	Thiamin	Riboflavin	Niacin	B-6	Folacin	B-12
60 mg	1.1 mg	1.3 mg	15 mg	1.5 mg	180 μg	2 μg

Minerals

Calcium	Phosphorus	Magnesium	Iron	Zinc	Iodine	Selenium
1,200 mg	1,200 mg	300 mg	15 mg	12 mg	150 μg	50 μg

Protein
44 g

10. Adult Males—19 to 24 Years
Height: 5'10"
Weight: 160 pounds

Fat-Soluble Vitamins

Vitamin A	Vitamin D	Vitamin E	Vitamin K
1 mg	10 μg	10 mg	70 μg

Water-Soluble Vitamins

Vitamin C	B Vitamins					
	Thiamin	Riboflavin	Niacin	B-6	Folacin	B-12
60 mg	1.5 μg	1.7 mg	19 mg	2.0 mg	200 μg	2.0 μg

Minerals

Calcium	Phosphorus	Magnesium	Iron	Zinc	Iodine	Selenium
1,200 mg	1,200 mg	350 mg	10 mg	15 mg	150 μg	70 μg

Protein

53 g

11. Adult Females—19 to 24 Years
Height: 5′4″
Weight: 128 pounds

Fat-Soluble Vitamins

Vitamin A	Vitamin D	Vitamin E	Vitamin K
800 μg	10 μg	8 mg	60 mg

Water-Soluble Vitamins

Vitamin C	B Vitamins					
	Thiamin	Riboflavin	Niacin	B-6	Folacin	B-12
60 mg	1.1 mg	1.3 mg	15 mg	1.6 mg	180 μg	2.0 μg

Minerals

Calcium	Phosphorus	Magnesium	Iron	Zinc	Iodine	Selenium
1,200 mg	1,200 mg	280 mg	15 mg	12 mg	150 μg	55 μg

Protein

46 g

12. Adult Males—25 to 50 Years
Height: 5′10″
Weight: 174 pounds

Fat-Soluble Vitamins

Vitamin A	Vitamin D	Vitamin E	Vitamin K
1 mg	5 μg	10 mg	80 μg

Water-Soluble Vitamins

Vitamin C	B Vitamins					
	Thiamin	Riboflavin	Niacin	B-6	Folacin	B-12
60 mg	1.5 μg	1.7 mg	19 mg	2.0 mg	200 μg	2.0 μg

Minerals

Calcium	Phosphorus	Magnesium	Iron	Zinc	Iodine	Selenium
800 mg	800 mg	350 mg	10 mg	15 mg	150 μg	70 μg

Protein

63 g

13. Adult Females—25 to 50 Years
Height: 5′4″
Weight: 136 pounds

Fat-Soluble Vitamins

Vitamin A	Vitamin D	Vitamin E	Vitamin K
800 μg	5 μg	8 mg	65 μg

Water-Soluble Vitamins

Vitamin C	B Vitamins					
60 mg	Thiamin	Riboflavin	Niacin	B-6	Folacin	B-12
	1.1 μg	1.3 mg	15 mg	1.6 mg	180 μg	2.0 μg

Minerals

Calcium	Phosphorus	Magnesium	Iron	Zinc	Iodine	Selenium
800 mg	800 mg	280 mg	15 mg	12 mg	150 μg	55 μg

Protein
50 g

14. Adult Males—51-Plus Years
Height: 5'10"
Weight: 170 pounds

Fat-Soluble Vitamins

Vitamin A	Vitamin D	Vitamin E	Vitamin K
1 mg	5 μg	10 mg	80 μg

Water-Soluble Vitamins

Vitamin C	B Vitamins					
60 mg	Thiamin	Riboflavin	Niacin	B-6	Folacin	B-12
	1.2 μg	1.4 mg	15 mg	2.0 mg	200 μg	2 μg

Minerals

Calcium	Phosphorus	Magnesium	Iron	Zinc	Iodine	Selenium
800 mg	800 mg	350 mg	10 mg	15 mg	150 μg	70 μg

Protein
63 g

15. Adult Females—51-Plus Years
Height: 5'4"
Weight: 143 pounds

Fat-Soluble Vitamins

Vitamin A	Vitamin D	Vitamin E	Vitamin K
800 μg	5 mg	8 mg	65 μg

Water-Soluble Vitamins

Vitamin C	B Vitamins					
60 mg	Thiamin	Riboflavin	Niacin	B-6	Folacin	B-12
	1 mg	1.2 mg	13 mg	1.6 mg	180 μg	2.0 μg

Minerals

Calcium	Phosphorus	Magnesium	Iron	Zinc	Iodine	Selenium
800 mg	800 mg	280 mg	10 mg	12 mg	150 μg	55 μg

Protein
50 g

16. Pregnant Women

Fat-Soluble Vitamins

Vitamin A	Vitamin D	Vitamin E	Vitamin K
800 µg	10 µg	10 mg	65 µg

Water-Soluble Vitamins

Vitamin C	B Vitamins					
	Thiamin	Riboflavin	Niacin	B-6	Folacin	B-12
70 mg	1.5 µg	1.6 mg	17 mg	2.2 µg	400 µg	2.2 µg

Minerals

Calcium	Phosphorus	Magnesium	Iron	Zinc	Iodine	Selenium
1,200 mg	1,200 mg	320 mg	30 mg	15 mg	175 µg	65 µg

Protein
60 g

17. Lactating Mothers, First Six Months

Fat-Soluble Vitamins

Vitamin A	Vitamin D	Vitamin E	Vitamin K
1.3 mg	10 µg	12 mg	65 µg

Water-Soluble Vitamins

Vitamin C	B Vitamins					
	Thiamin	Riboflavin	Niacin	B-6	Folacin	B-12
95 mg	1.6 µg	1.8 mg	20 mg	2.1 mg	280 µg	2.6 µg

Minerals

Calcium	Phosphorus	Magnesium	Iron	Zinc	Iodine	Selenium
1,200 mg	1,200 mg	355 mg	15 mg	19 mg	200 µg	75 µg

Protein
63 g

18. Lactating Mothers, Second Six Months

Fat-Soluble Vitamins

Vitamin A	Vitamin D	Vitamin E	Vitamin K
1.2 mg	10 µg	11 mg	65 µg

Water-Soluble Vitamins

Vitamin C	B Vitamins					
	Thiamin	Riboflavin	Niacin	B-6	Folacin	B-12
90 mg	1.6 µg	1.7 µg	20 mg	2.1 mg	260 µg	2.6 µg

Minerals

Calcium	Phosphorus	Magnesium	Iron	Zinc	Iodine	Selenium
1,200 mg	1,200 mg	340 mg	15 mg	16 mg	200 µg	75 µg

Protein
62 g

8

Red Flags in the Food Supply

Some people approach nutrition as though they were entering a mine field where danger lurks at every turn. Others find themselves caught up in a constant swirl of confusion as they try to sort through the bombardment of conflicting information. Nutritional experts seem to be constantly flip-flopping on whether or not certain substances are good, bad, or indifferent. In particular, there are three areas of dietary concern that are the subject of ongoing study and speculation. They have to do with caffeine, alcohol, and other nonnutritive substances, such as additives and food substitutes. (A fourth and sometimes related concern regarding safety and the use of pesticides is addressed in chapter 13.)

All three of these so-called "red flags" are part of the everyday lives of a majority of Americans. For millions of people, caffeine, in the forms of coffee, tea, and soda, is a necessary part of the day, as is an evening cocktail or a glass of wine at dinner. And nearly all of us consume additives to some extent.

Like many areas in the complex world of nutrition, we find some ambiguity in the evidence about the relative dangers or benefits of these substances. Our basic recommendations are threefold: First, that you take to heart the advice of health professionals; second, that you keep the information, especially about additives, in perspective and avoid placing "good or evil" labels

on them; and third, that you consider this material in light of the other information contained in this section on the constituents of a well-balanced, healthy diet.

Sorting Out the Caffeine Controversy

After more than thirty years of research, the reviews are still mixed on the relative hazards and benefits of caffeine, the substance millions of Americans depend on for a quick energy boost. During the past decade, many people have cut back on caffeine because of the speculation that it might be a contributor to a variety of health problems, including heart disease, cancer, fibrocystic breast disease, and birth defects. The most well-publicized studies have linked caffeine consumption with heart disease. But the studies are far from conclusive since it is nearly impossible to do controlled research on the effects of solitary substances.

One widely reported study tracked the coffee drinking habits of more than a thousand male graduates of Johns Hopkins Medical School for up to 25 years. Thomas A. Pearson, M.D., Andrea LaCroix, Ph.D., and their colleagues found that the more coffee the men drank, the higher the incidence of heart disease. At greatest risk were those who drank at least five cups a day; their rate of heart disease was two and a half times the rate for men who did not drink coffee.

The researchers' findings took into account the effects of smoking, high blood pressure, and variations in blood cholesterol when the men were young—all factors that might enhance the susceptibility to heart disease. But the analysis did not take into account exercise, stress, or diet, three further aspects that play a role in heart health, but which are difficult to measure over the course of many years. So it is possible that the heavy coffee drinkers were under more pressure, exercised less, or ate more fatty foods than the other men. Further, the study lumped together those who drank five cups of coffee a day with those who consumed very large quantities—ten to twenty cups a day. It was also difficult to isolate caffeine as the culprit since coffee contains many other chemical substances.

Other attempts to study the effects of caffeine have had similar drawbacks. Many have not defined the size of a cup when evaluating coffee drinking, or compared findings about caffeinated-coffee drinkers with decaffeinated-coffee drinkers. Results are also clouded when the method of brewing is considered. For example, a group of Norwegian coffee drinkers was found to have increased levels of blood cholesterol. But in Norway, people tend to add coffee grounds directly to boiling water and steep them for some time, so the results of that study are not necessarily applicable to Americans who use automatic drip coffee makers, instant coffee, and electric percolators.

For the time being, there is no definitive evidence that moderate amounts of caffeine are a problem for most people, but it is easier to evaluate the facts when you understand what happens to caffeine after you've consumed it.

The Nature and Role of Caffeine

Caffeine is one of a group of compounds called methylxanthines, which occur naturally in more than sixty species of plants. The most familiar sources of caffeine are coffee beans, cola nuts, cocoa beans, and tea leaves. Coffee is the nation's greatest source of caffeine, with soft drinks ranked second, followed by tea and chocolate.

Many people are unaware of all the places caffeine shows up. It is also found in some cold medications, allergy pills, diet pills, and headache remedies. Sometimes coffee is used as a flavoring agent in baked goods, frozen desserts, and puddings.

Foods and beverages containing caffeine are often consumed as "pick-me-ups" to get that extra lift that helps you have a sharper focus in performing mental and physical tasks. These "upper" effects stem from caffeine's ability to act as a stimulant to the central nervous system. In this respect, the caffeine levels in one or two cups of coffee can increase alertness. Caffeine can also cause a number of other reactions, depending on how much you consume, how high your caffeine tolerance is, and other individual factors. It can increase heartbeat and urine production, and it can open up some blood vessels while constricting others. Caffeine promotes the stomach's output of acid. However, since decaffeinated coffee also produces acid secretion, there are other substances in coffee apart from caffeine that are responsible for this.

What Are Caffeine's Risks?

People who consume large amounts of caffeine may experience insomnia, heartbeat irregularities, and diarrhea. Even moderate consumption of caffeine can lead to irritability, headaches, trembling, and nervousness. In fact, a symptom likened to an anxiety neurosis, termed "caffeinism," has been shown to disappear in people who eliminate caffeine-containing foods and beverages. But since caffeine's effects are highly individual, it may cause problems for some people and not for others. People who are used to consuming a fair amount tend to develop a tolerance and be less susceptible to caffeine's effects.

Children may be more vulnerable to caffeine-related problems, particularly through some sodas which contain only about one-third the caffeine of coffee but still enough to create problems. Laurence Finberg, M.D., former chairman of the committee on nutrition at the American Academy of Pediatrics, recommends that children who drink soda consume no more than two twelve-ounce cans of caffeine-containing soda a day.

Caffeine can pose problems for certain people on medications. This was discovered when Dr. Michael Simmons and his colleagues at UCLA found that caffeine from as little as three cups of coffee increased the potency of asthma medications containing theophylline, since this substance is structurally similar to caffeine.

Controversy about the effects of caffeine have focused on certain types of medical problems:

Caffeine and birth defects: The Food and Drug Administration (FDA) has advised that pregnant women avoid or use sparingly foods that contain caffeine, since caffeine passes through the placenta and enters the unborn infant's body. This warning is based on research conducted by the agency that showed that caffeine, when fed to rats, caused birth defects and delayed bone development in fetuses. It is not known how these findings might apply to humans, but the FDA issued the warning because of the widespread use of caffeine-containing beverages in the United States.

Many researchers criticized one of the FDA's studies, since the rats were force-fed exceedingly high amounts of caffeine. In a later study, the rats were given varying levels of caffeine in their water throughout the day. Ultimately, no birth defects were seen unless the pregnant rats consumed caffeine levels equivalent to 18 or more cups of coffee a day.

In early 1982, a team of Harvard scientists published in the *New England Journal of Medicine* their study on the effects of caffeine on the outcome of pregnancy in more than 12,000 women. The researchers found no link between the amount of coffee consumed and birth defects. Additional studies in the United States and Finland reached the same conclusion. However, even if conflicts remain, since caffeine contains no inherent value as a nutritional substance, it would be advisable for pregnant women to proceed with caution in its use.

There is early evidence that caffeine may also contribute to infertility in some women. Researchers at the National Institute of Environmental Health Sciences of the National Institutes of Health studied a group of women who were trying to get pregnant. Those who consumed more than 100 milligrams of caffeine a day (comparable to one cup of coffee or two cans of caffeinated soda) were only half as likely to become pregnant in a given month as women who consumed less caffeine. Age, frequency of sexual intercourse, alcohol use, and smoking were all factored into the study. While the study is far from conclusive, women who want to get pregnant might consider cutting down on caffeine consumption.

Caffeine and nursing babies: Again, there is no firm evidence relating caffeine consumption to problems for the babies of breast-feeding mothers. In fact, one study showed that there was little pass-along to babies of coffee-drinking mothers. Ceston Berlin, Jr., M.D., and colleagues from the Hershey Medical Center in Pennsylvania, studied the metabolism and transfer of caffeine in fifteen nursing mothers who had been instructed to drink their preferred caffeine-containing beverage in the usual amounts. Thirteen women were accustomed to drinking one to three cups of coffee a day, and two were used to drinking six cups of coffee a day. On the day of the study, the amount of caffeine the women consumed at one time ranged from 36 to 335 milligrams. The caffeine in their breast milk was measured over the course of twelve hours and their infants were fed according to their usual schedules. To determine how much caffeine was reaching the babies, the researchers tested their urine.

Four of the mothers who drank less than 100 milligrams of caffeine had none in their breast milk. Caffeine rapidly appeared in the milk of the other mothers and peaked within an hour, yet none was detected in the urine of the babies. The researchers estimated that only 0.06 to 1.5 percent of the caffeine the mothers drank was available to the infants. Their conclusion was that "the modest use of caffeinated beverages does not appear to present a hazard to the nursing infant."

However, researchers acknowledged that the mothers in the study consumed a single dose of caffeine, and they raised the possibility that frequent intakes, particularly in amounts greater than 150 milligrams, might cause a cumulative effect.

Caffeine and fibrocystic breast disease: Fibrocystic breast disease is a painful, noncancerous breast condition that occurs in approximately 10 to 20 percent of women. Some evidence suggests that removing all methylxanthines, including caffeine, from the diet helps control or cure the painful breast lumps.

Dr. John Minton, a specialist in breast disorders at the Ohio State University College of Medicine, studied 47 female patients and reported that an increased risk of benign fibrocystic breast disease was proportional to the amount of caffeine consumed. As a result, he advised women with the condition to eliminate caffeine from their diet.

Some researchers believe this caution may be premature. Critics of Minton's work identified factors other than diet, such as age, number of children, and previous history of benign breast disease, that may influence the course of fibrocystic breast disease. A later study of 323 women with the condition and nearly 1,500 without it showed no association between the consumption of caffeine and benign fibrocystic disease.

Caffeine and heart disease: The debate over the possible association between heavy consumption of coffee and cardiovascular disease has been going on for more than three decades. The difficulty in reaching a firm conclusion stems from differences in the results of clinical and epidemiologic studies that observe the health habits of large populations.

During 1972 and 1973, researchers at the Boston University Medical Center published their findings on the relationship between drinking coffee and the incidences of heart attacks. They reported a 60 percent greater risk of heart attack for those consuming more than six cups of coffee per day. But since the research team, headed by Dr. Hershel Jick, found no link between tea consumption and heart disease, it is unlikely that caffeine alone is the culprit. Further, the study did not evaluate the effects of such factors as diet, exercise, and personality type.

Other studies contradict the findings of Jick and his colleagues. The well-respected and highly publicized Framingham Heart Study has found no association between coffee consumption and the increased risk of heart problems. But caffeine has not escaped all blame when it comes to heart conditions. Researchers at Ohio State University Hospital investigated the role caffeine might have in producing arrhythmias, which are irregular heartbeats. After receiving the amount of caffeine in two cups of brewed coffee, three heart patients experienced an increased heart rate, and six patients had arrhythmias. Three of the healthy volunteers also had arrhythmias after receiving coffee. The researchers concluded that caffeine has the potential to induce heartbeat irregularities, especially in patients with existing heart problems.

Another study examined coffee consumption and its effects on blood cholesterol in more than 14,500 Norwegian men and women. The study concluded that as coffee consumption increased, so did blood cholesterol levels. For those who drank one to four cups of coffee a day, blood cholesterol was more than 5 percent higher than that of noncoffee drinkers. And those who drank nine or more cups a day showed blood cholesterol levels that were about 14 percent higher than those of people who drank less than one daily cup of coffee.

The Norwegian study created such a stir that a public health warning was issued in the Federal Republic of Germany. It also caused a storm of criticism from research and medical groups. Criticisms included charges that the study failed to account fully for such factors as stress and certain other dietary components that can affect blood cholesterol. Further, while two groups found an association between coffee or caffeine consumption and blood cholesterol, three other research groups did not. Some experts believe that the different results obtained from laboratory to laboratory might in part be related to the way coffee is grown and prepared.

Caffeine and cancer. In 1981, a team of scientists at the Harvard School of Public Health reported an increased risk of pancreatic cancer among coffee drinkers. However, the study had a number of serious limitations and was strongly criticized. The Harvard researchers later retracted their findings until further study could be completed.

What To Do

Evidence seems to suggest that, like most things, caffeine consumption in moderation is unlikely to pose health risks for otherwise healthy people. However, it would be wise for pregnant women and heart patients to discuss caffeine use with their physicians. Further, those on medications should find out what potential effects caffeine might have when consumed along with the drugs.

What About Decaffeination?

Traditionally, products have been decaffeinated using an agent called methylene chloride. Although this substance is still allowed by the FDA, many companies have turned to safer methods. Methylene chloride is used to extract the caffeine from coffee beans, but it has been found to cause cancer when inhaled in large amounts by laboratory animals.

Since the chemical has been banned in hair spray, why is the FDA allowing its use in coffee? According to FDA officials, the amount of methylene chloride in decaffeinated coffee is negligible. Even if someone drinks as many as five five-ounce cups of coffee a day, there is only a one in a million chance that the risk of cancer will increase. However, public interest groups disagree with this line of thinking, arguing that even minimum amounts of a substance associated with cancer risk should not be used, especially if safe alternatives are available.

Some coffee producers are doing just that. They are using ethyl acetate, a substance that occurs naturally in fruits and vegetables, to extract the caffeine from coffee beans. Ethyl acetate is also used to decaffeinate tea. Others use a combination of water and carbon dioxide or water and coffee oils that have been pressed from other coffee beans.

Of the major brands, Folgers decaffeinates with ethyl acetate. Sanka, Taster's Choice, Hills Brothers (if the container is marked "natural"), and Nestle Decaf apply either the carbon dioxide or coffee oil method. Brim, Yuban, and Maxwell House continue to use the methylene chloride method. (Since these brands might have changed since press time, be sure to check the package labels before making a purchase.)

The Pros and Cons of Drinking Alcohol

Recent reports that drinking in moderation may actually be good for you have created quite a stir. According to some studies, having one or two drinks a day may protect people from developing heart disease. But there are many flaws to the research picture. For one thing, behavioral studies are difficult to measure. For example, in one study, the categories used were "teetotaler," "moderate drinker," and "heavy drinker." There was no effort to distinguish a person who had

MEASURE YOUR CAFFEINE INTAKE

Beverages	Caffeine (milligrams)	Beverages	Caffeine (milligrams)
Coffee		Squirt	0
(5-oz. cup)		Sunkist Orange, regular	0
regular, drip	110–150	diet	0
percolated	64–124		
instant	40–108		
decaffeinated, ground	2–5	**Nonprescription Drugs**	
instant	2		
		Cold Remedies	
Tea		(standard dose)	
(loose or bags, 5-oz. cup)		Dristan	32
1 minute brew	9–33	Coryban-D	30
3 minute brew	20–46	Triaminicin	30
5 minute brew	20–50		
		Diuretics	
Tea Products		(standard dose)	
instant (5-oz. cup)	12–28	Aqua-ban	200
iced (12-oz. can)	22–36	Permathene H-20ff	200
		Pre-Mens Forte	100
Cocoa			
(made from mix)		**Pain Relievers**	
milk chocolate (1 oz.)	6	(standard dose)	
baking chocolate (1 oz.)	35	Excedrin	130
		Midol	65
Soft Drinks		Anacin	64
(12-oz. cans)		Aspirin, plain (any brand)	0
Dr. Pepper	61		
Colas, regular	30–46	**Stimulants**	
diet	2–58	(standard dose)	
caffeine-free	0	Caffedrin Capsules	200
Mountain Dew	52	NoDoz Tablets	200
Mellow Yellow	51	Vivarin Tablets	200
Tab	44		
Fresca	0	**Weight Control Aids**	
Hires Root Beer	0	(daily dose)	
7-Up, regular	0	Prolamine	280
diet	0	Dexatrim	200
Sprite	0	Dietac	200

never consumed alcoholic beverages from, say, a recovering alcoholic who did not currently drink. Nor do the studies take into account other factors, such as cigarette smoking, which, in combination with alcohol, appears to substantially increase risk factors.

Another study, analyzing data on approximately 5,000 adults from Framingham, Massachusetts, over a 22-year period, revealed that men who had one or two drinks a week had a lower mortality rate than heavy drinkers or those who did not drink at all. However, these studies are not considered conclusive, since other factors might be at play. For example, it is possible that men who drink in small amounts tend to have life-styles or personalities that increase longevity.

Even if moderate drinking was shown conclusively to reduce the risk of heart disease, most health professionals would be hesitant to make an across-the-board recommendation since there are plenty of reasons not to drink. For example, research indicates that people who have one to three drinks a day have a 60 percent higher risk of developing oral cancer than nondrinkers. For people who drink that amount and smoke one to two packs of cigarettes a day, the risk is three times greater than for smokers who do not drink. Furthermore, given the fact that there are an estimated 18 million Americans with alcohol problems, health professionals are not anxious to promote drinking.

Nevertheless, among people who do drink, some research indicates that beer may benefit certain individuals. Johns Hopkins Medical Institutions sponsored a widely publicized study on the drinking habits and illness of 17,000 people. Alex Richman, M.D., and his colleagues found that people who preferred beer over other alcoholic beverages said they were ill much less often than the researchers expected. They had fewer doctor's visits, spent fewer days sick in bed, and lost fewer days from work or school. Those who drank one or two beers a day reported the lowest incidences of illness. Once the level reached 35 beers a week, the apparent health benefits were canceled out.

People in the study who drank different alcoholic beverages—namely, wine and distilled spirits—reported being ill only 1 to 2 percent less than expected, so it may be that some ingredient in beer other than alcohol helps keep beer drinkers healthy. However, these studies shouldn't lead to the conclusion that it's a good idea to drink beer.

There's simply not enough data available to warrant the statement that a couple of drinks a day can be considered beneficial to health. In order to fully understand the role of alcohol in the diet, it is important to know what happens in your body once it is consumed.

What Does Alcohol Do?

Unlike protein, fat, and carbohydrate, all of which must pass from the stomach to the small intestine before being absorbed into the bloodstream, about 20 percent of the alcohol we consume goes directly from the stomach to the blood. That's because alcohol molecules are so small that the intestine does not need to break all of them down into smaller components before they enter the circulatory system. Most of the remaining alcohol that does not pass straight from the stomach to the blood goes through the wall of the small intestine.

In the bloodstream, the body handles alcohol (or, more precisely, ethyl alcohol or ethanol) much as it would a drug, quickly setting about its elimination. About 3 percent leaves the body unmetabolized via urine, perspiration, and expired air. The rest, formerly thought to be almost exclusively metabolized by the liver, is now believed to be processed in significant amounts in the stomach and small intestines of men after it is consumed. Much less is metabolized this way in women, so if the same amount of alcohol is consumed by men and women of the same size, more gets into the bloodstream of women. Since usually men are larger than women, these two factors make women less able to "hold their liquor" than men.

Since the intestine can metabolize only about seven grams (or a quarter of an ounce) of alcohol an hour, it starts to accumulate in the bloodstream and affect the brain and other organs if it's consumed at a faster rate. In the brain, alcohol acts as a narcotic, actually putting nerve cells "to sleep." This anesthetic effect begins in areas of the brain that control behavior, which is why people who are drinking tend to be less inhibited.

As blood alcohol levels rise, other brain centers become depressed. The result is that speech becomes slurred, vision blurred, and walking diffi-cult. If one drinks to the point of passing out, it means the entire conscious brain has effectively dozed off. It's even possible to shut down the brain's unconscious centers, such as those that control breathing and heart rate, if enough alco-hol is consumed.

Alcohol: The Nutritional Issues

According to the 1988 Surgeon General's Report on Nutrition and Health, "social" drinkers do not seem to suffer any notable nutritional deficien-cies. The report cited two important studies. In one, three groups of nonalcoholics kept diaries of what they ate over a period of six to twelve months, and 79 percent of them reported con-suming alcohol on half or more of the days. For 22 percent of the drinkers, alcohol contributed approximately 10 percent of average daily calo-ries; for another 23 percent, it contributed from 5 to 10 percent of daily calories. Alcohol accounted for less than five percent of daily calories for the remaining fifty-five percent. It was found that, as the proportion of calories from alcohol in-creased, the protein intake underwent little change, and the overall quality of the diet could not be related to the consumption of alcohol.

In a second study, conducted with upper-mid-dle-class people in southern California, it was found that alcohol did not replace calories de-rived from other nutrients.

The surgeon general concludes that nutritional issues are not pressing for the average healthy person who consumes moderate amounts of al-cohol.

But what constitutes a "moderate" amount of drinking? For one thing, alcohol's effect is highly individual; its influence depends on your body size, your metabolism, what or whether you've eaten recently, and the medication you're taking. If consumed with food, one or two drinks usually won't cause major problems (unless you're driv-ing a car). But what constitutes a drink? Many peo-

HOW MUCH ALCOHOL IS IN A DRINK?

Beverage	Amount Equal to One Ounce of Absolute Alcohol
80-proof liquor	two 1.5-oz. shots
beer	two 12-oz. cans or bottles
sherry	two 3-oz. glasses
table wine	two 4-oz. glasses

ple don't measure, and might be consuming far more than one or two. See the guideline above.

Alcohol is also loaded with calories, and they're "empty" calories in that they provide no nutrients. Take note of the approximate calorie count of your favorite drinks, listed below.

Who Should Avoid Alcohol?

While a drink or two a day probably won't cause problems for most normal people, there are sev-

WILL DRINKING MAKE YOU FAT?

Drink	Amount	Approximate Calories
beer or ale	12 oz.	150
light beer	12 oz.	100
liquor (gin, rum, brandy, bourbon, scotch, vodka)		
80 proof	1.5 oz.	100
100 proof	1.5 oz.	125
champagne, dry	3 oz.	80
cold duck wine	3 oz.	90
cordials, liqueurs	1 oz.	80–120
wine (dry red, white, rosé)	6 oz.	130–150
light wine	6 oz.	90
eggnog, with 1 oz. rum	½ cup	235
hot toddy or grog, with 1 shot of liquor	1 cup	115
hot buttered rum	½ cup	260

eral categories of people who should proceed with caution or avoid alcohol consumption altogether. These include:

Pregnant women: Many authorities, including the U.S. surgeon general and the American Medical Association, feel it is best for mothers-to-be to avoid alcohol, since it reaches the baby's blood at the same concentration as the mother's within 15 minutes of her taking a drink. At very high levels of chronic intake, alcohol causes a number of defects, known as fetal alcohol syndrome. But even moderate drinking may be linked to miscarriages, stillbirths, and low birth weight.

Breast-feeding mothers: There are some theories that new mothers who are having difficulty breast-feeding should have a glass or two of wine to help them relax. However, alcohol can be counterproductive to this end since it can inhibit the "letdown" reflex that leads to milk secretion. The alcohol also passes into the mother's milk. And although the level of alcohol in the milk is lower than in the mother's blood, the infant can become intoxicated even if the mother has only had a couple of drinks. For these reasons, nursing mothers should avoid alcohol or be sure to consume it well before nursing time.

People on medication: Since alcohol can have the same effect as a drug when it is consumed, it is wise for people taking any form of medication to check with their physicians before drinking. Even a single drink may increase or decrease the potency of some medications.

Diabetics: Diabetics should consult with their doctors before drinking even in moderate amounts, since alcohol can interfere with blood sugar metabolism. In addition, it can raise blood triglycerides. These fats, which may increase the risk of heart disease if they're excessively high, are already elevated in people with diabetes, especially if their blood sugar is poorly controlled. Small amounts of alcohol may also interact with oral medication, such as Diabenese, used to lower blood sugar, and result in flushing, nausea, rapid heart beat, or impaired speech.

People with high blood pressure: Drinking appears to be associated with the development of hypertension. Researchers at Stanford University found that as alcohol intake increased, so did blood pressure in a group of men, ages 20 and older. The alcohol-blood pressure connection was strongest after the age of 50. For women, alcohol intake was linked to high blood pressure only after age 50. Other studies have shown that, in some hypertensive people, an increase in alcohol intake definitely causes an increase in blood pressure. Thus, alcohol not only may be involved in the development of hypertension, but may also aggravate an existing condition.

In November 1989, a federally mandated warning label appeared on all containers of liquor, wine, and beer. The warning reads:

▶ Consumption of alcoholic beverages impairs your ability to drive a car or operate machinery and may cause health problems.

▶ According to the surgeon general, women should not drink alcoholic beverages during pregnancy because of the risk of birth defects.

Alcoholic Malnutrition

The nutritional balance in chronic alcoholics is upset both because they consume fewer nutrients and because excessive amounts of alcohol impede the proper absorption and utilization of the nutrients they do consume. Studies have shown that hospitalized alcoholics who derived 30 percent or more of their daily calories from alcohol showed signs of protein malnutrition, as well as deficiencies in calcium, iron, vitamins A and C, the B vitamins, in particular B-12, thiamin, and riboflavin.

In addition to symptoms associated with a poor diet, the alcoholic suffers a variety of symptoms related to the effects alcohol has on the absorption, metabolism, storage, and excretion of many nutrients.

It was once believed that the organ and tissue damage often seen in chronic alcoholics, such as cirrhosis of the liver, was primarily caused by the long-term effects of nutritional deficiencies. By the 1960s, however, medical experts had reached the conclusion that many of the clinical consequences of alcoholism were the direct result of the toxic effects of alcohol itself.

There is much that remains unknown about the specific relationship between alcoholism and the activity of nutrients in the body. Most of the studies have focused on indigent alcoholics, who make up only 5 percent of the alcoholic population, and whose life-style and general eating patterns differ greatly from the average, more healthy population. Furthermore, the indigent alcoholics studied have been almost exclusively male.

Avoiding the Post-Party Blues

Many of America's favorite holiday and celebrative occasions take place around food and abundant drinking, and it is a common plight for even the most moderate of drinkers to succumb to the festivities and imbibe "one too many." It's easy to see how this can happen when you consider that it takes an average size man about two hours to burn off the fourteen grams of alcohol contained in one drink. Three or four drinks over an evening's time can present problems, especially if you're not accustomed to drinking. Ironically, the body builds a tolerance for alcohol consumption, so the light drinker becomes drunk on less alcohol than the heavy drinker.

If you drink, it is best not to do so on an empty stomach. Food acts as a kind of barrier between the alcohol and the stomach wall, decreasing the absorption there. Food also postpones the emptying of the stomach's contents into the small intestine, where most of the alcohol is absorbed into the bloodstream. And food appears to stimulate enzymes in the stomach and small intestine

that help break down some of the alcohol before it reaches the bloodstream and travels to the brain.

Diluting drinks can also help. Although sparkling water and other carbonated mixers—as opposed to plain water and juices—can hasten alcohol absorption, this is more likely to happen on an empty stomach. "Nursing" a drink is another good way to avoid getting drunk. Or alternate alcoholic drinks with club soda, juices, or water.

Once alcohol enters the bloodstream, there is no way to speed up its metabolism. Drinking coffee, taking cold showers, or walking around the block may wake you up, but they will not make you less inebriated. For full sobriety, nature must take its course.

Of course, if you do have too much to drink, you're likely to be saddled with the infamous "morning after" hangover. The metabolic reasons for the headache, nausea, irritability, and fatigue that drinkers suffer when they've had too much are not understood, although the accompanying thirst is the result of alcohol's diuretic effect.

It is possible that some types of liquor bring on more serious hangovers than others. One study showed that, in descending order, brandy, red wine, rum, whiskey, white wine and gin caused the worst hangovers. This difference in the aftereffects of alcohol might be caused by congeners, a large number of diverse chemicals that are the by-products of distillation and fermentation. It appears that the more congeners a liquor has, the worse the hangover.

Can Nonfoods Be Beneficial?

In addition to coffee, tea, and alcohol, we consume many other substances that contain no naturally occurring nutrients. Many of them are added to foods to preserve, color, flavor, stabilize, or replace substances lost in processing. Others are designed as substitutes for foods that, for a variety of reasons, some people are unable or unwilling to eat in their natural form. The most common examples of food substitutes are artificial sweeteners and, more recently, artificial fats.

Many people assume that our food supply would be healthier without these nonnutrients. It is in response to this assumption that many food manufacturers label their products with terms such as "no preservatives" or "no artificial ingredients." But do artificial food substances necessarily compromise the nutritional quality of our diets? Scientists who have devoted many years to the study of this question have found that, for the most part, FDA-approved additives do not. The choice is left up to you. However, before you jump on the "no additive-no substitute" bandwagon, it is important that you understand all sides of the issue, including some surprising nutritional benefits of additives and substitutes.

The Additive Debate

It is estimated that nearly 3,000 chemical and natural substances are added to foods during processing, and the federal government keeps close tabs on their use. The Food, Drug, and Cosmetic Act was passed by Congress in 1938, prohibiting the marketing of foods containing toxic substances. Since that time, amendments have been passed to clarify specific issues, such as the 1958 Food Additive Amendment, which stated that no additive could be used in any amount that had been shown to cause cancer in animal or other studies. However, the Food Additive Amendment exempted 670 substances that were classified as "Generally Recognized as Safe" (GRAS), based on scientific studies and other data. GRAS substances were not always trouble-free, however. Saccharin had to be taken off the list in the early 1970s when it was found to cause cancer in laboratory animals.

Many consumers are alarmed by the intimidating words that appear on food labels and are loathe to consume products that contain such scary-sounding ingredients as "L-lysine mono-

hydrochloride" or "apocarotenal." What they might not know is that many of these are naturally occurring substances. L-lysine monohydrochloride, for example, is simply a form of the amino acid lysine, one of the building blocks of protein that is in short supply in most grains. Quaker Oats adds it to *Life* cereal to give it higher protein quality. Apocarotenal is a member of the carotene family of plant pigments found throughout nature, some of which are converted by the body into vitamin A. Kraft uses it to add color to its Velveeta cheese food product.

Over the years, there have been a number of hotly staged controversies over particular additives, and a number of them have been removed from the food supply. However, in spite of the questions that still remain, we do know that, as a category, additives are not "bad." In fact, overall, they have a number of benefits:

▶ Additives prevent spoilage and the accompanying bacterial ailments associated with eating spoiled foods.

▶ Additives allow a year-round supply of nutritious fruits and vegetables that would otherwise be available only during a given season.

▶ Foods containing certain additives may be tastier and of a consistent quality.

▶ Foods fortified with vitamin and mineral additives help some people, who might otherwise suffer deficiencies, meet their daily requirement for essential nutrients.

▶ Overall, they make more foods available in greater varieties to more people.

Much as the natural-food enthusiasts might hope for a return to the "good old days" of unprocessed, additive-free foods, such a state would leave many people with inadequate diets. In the long run, it appears that most additives do more good than harm. According to a major report prepared in 1989 by the Committee on Diet and Health of the National Research Council, there is no data to support the opinion that Americans suffer nutritionally from the presence of nonnutritive substances in their diets. In fact, the committee noted, "Exposure to individual nonnutritive chemicals, in the minute quantities normally present in the average diet, is unlikely to contribute to the overall cancer risk to humans in the United States.... The life span of humans in Western countries is steadily increasing, and age-specific mortalities from most common cancers such as breast and colon cancer show no increases (or decreases) over the past generation. These facts suggest that our society as a whole is not facing a health crisis posed by environmental agents."

Nevertheless, the debate goes on regarding certain additives common to the American food supply.

After many years of debate, the FDA banned the use of sulfite preservatives in fresh fruits and vegetables (except potatoes), but it appears likely that they'll continue to be allowed elsewhere. Almost half the adverse reactions to sulfites, including hives, shortness of breath, and even death, have been linked to their use in fruits and vegetables —and these are most commonly experienced by asthmatics. The FDA estimates that about 80,000 to 100,000 people in the United States are sensitive to sulfites.

However, products that contain at least 10 parts per million of sulfites are required to state their presence on the label. Look for the names sulfur dioxide, potassium metabisulfite, sodium metabisulfite, potassium bisulfite, sodium bisulfite, or sodium sulfite on the ingredients list.

Concern over sulfites in wine and beer (put there to prevent the growth of molds and bacteria) have led the Federal Bureau of Alcohol, Tobacco, and Firearms, which monitors these products, to require labels that say "contains sulfites" on cans and bottles. However, because this ruling went into effect in January 1988, products bottled before that do not contain the warning.

Nitrates, additive substances that inhibit the growth of bacteria that cause botulism in foods and are used for curing bacon and other processed meats, have also been the subject of debate because, during frying and digestion, nitrates are converted to nitrosamines, which have been shown to cause cancer in laboratory animals. At present, there has been no action taken to discontinue their use.

Some people may choose to avoid foods containing certain additives because they add to the sodium content of foods or because they have food sensitivities to these substances. Monosodium glutamate (MSG) is one such substance. MSG, which is the sodium salt of glutamic acid, naturally occurs in many foods, such as tomato sauce and cheese. It is also frequently used as a flavor enhancer.

Substituting Nonfoods for Foods

Perhaps the most concerted effort related to nonfood substances has been focused on artificial sweeteners.

In the early 1950s, the Food and Drug Administration approved an artificial sweetener called cyclamate. Cyclamate-sweetened foods and beverages became popular, as did a cyclamate-based artificial sweetener called Sweet 'n Low.

Cyclamate, sometimes combined with saccharin, became the country's most popular sugar substitute, sweetening canned goods, baked goods, bacon, toothpaste, mouthwash, lipstick, and cereal, as well as diet and nondiet beverages. It wasn't until 1969 that the FDA banned cyclamate, after research showed that it caused bladder tumors in laboratory rats who were fed large amounts. Saccharin then became the substitute of choice and also the subject of continued controversy after laboratory rats, also fed large amounts of the substance, developed bladder cancer.

In 1981, the FDA approved a new sugar substitute, aspartame, marketed as NutraSweet. Aspartame is comprised of the amino acids aspartic acid and phenylalanine, which are found in large quantities in most proteins. Today, more than 100 products contain aspartame, but it too has been the subject of some controversy. Various claims have been made concerning possible damaging effects from aspartame, but they have failed to stand up under careful scientific investigation. To date, most of the antiaspartame evidence has been anecdotal, not scientific. That is, people said they developed headaches or other symptoms, but there was no independent verification of the claims. In fact, when researchers at Johns Hopkins Medical Center conducted a double-blind study, using aspartame and placebos, the subjects taking aspartame reported no more headaches than those taking placebos.

The FDA has set guidelines regarding an acceptable daily intake (ADI) for aspartame, and research has shown that most people consume well below the ADI. For example, a 150-pound adult would have to drink about 17 cans of soda sweetened with aspartame to meet the ADI: a 40-pound child would have to drink four to five cans.

Some people are concerned about the effects of the amino acid phenylalanine on a particular group of people who lack the enzyme to metabolize it normally. The condition, called phenylketonuria, or PKU, is rare, but the danger exists that children with PKU could suffer neurologic damage from aspartame. (They suffer similar damage from eating protein foods.) Because of this, aspartame products contain the warning, "Phenylketonurics: Contains Phenylalanine."

For people who do not have this condition, there is no evidence that moderate amounts of aspartame in the diet are harmful.

In 1988, the FDA approved a new artificial sweetener for use in dry-food products and for sale in powder and tablet form. The new sweetener, marketed under the name Sunette, is known as acesulfame K. According to the FDA, four long-term animal studies showed no toxic effects from the substance. But the Center for Science in the Public Interest disputed this with two studies. In one, rats fed acesulfame K developed more tumors than those who were not given the substance. In another study, a group of diabetic rats experienced a rise in blood cholesterol after

being fed the sweetener. The results of these tests are being examined to determine their validity.

If you're concerned about the potential dangers of artificial sweeteners, you might ask yourself why you're using them. Chances are, you're interested in their "calorie-saving" properties. But as you swig your artificially sweetened soda, consider this: Several studies have demonstrated that people who "save" calories by drinking artificially sweetened sodas, usually add them elsewhere. So far, no one has shown that people who substitute sugar (only 16 calories a teaspoon) for these substances lose more weight than other people.

Manufacturers are also currently testing several different kinds of fat substitutes, which include both synthetic varieties and substitutes made from naturally occurring food substances. Olestra, being tested by Procter & Gamble, is composed mainly of sucrose and vegetable oil, bonded together into molecules that are too large to be digested. Because it cannot be digested, it adds no calories. It has been suggested that it might inhibit the absorption of cholesterol from other foods, but this is yet to be fully determined, and it may reduce the absorption of fat soluble vitamins.

Simplesse, produced by NutraSweet, has been approved for distribution. It is composed of whey protein from milk or egg whites. Unlike Olestra, it's utilized by the body, but reduces calorie consumption since it can replace 27 calories of fat with 4 calories of high-quality protein.

While these "fake fats" are still open to scrutiny they certainly have the potential to provide real benefits in helping people cut down on fat and cholesterol. One caution might be that, if people can eat as much as they want of ice cream, candy, rich sauces, and the like, might this not lead to their cutting down on high-carbohydrate, high-fiber foods? Human nature being what it is, if the artificial fats are approved and catch on, medical experts and nutritionists will probably need to firmly reestablish the necessity of eating a variety of wholesome foods.

There are many gray areas concerning food additives and substitutes, and the FDA's reviewing process of currently available products moves very slowly. However, we agree with the FDA that the majority of additives are safe and play an important role in our diets. In fact, the FDA ranks additives last on a list of things to be concerned about in food, with such issues as bacterial contamination and nutrient deficiencies ranking higher. As a consumer, your best defense is to be as aware as possible about common nonfood substances and the role they play in foods.

COMMON FOOD ADDITIVES AT A GLANCE

Category	Examples	Dietary Contribution
		(+) = positive role (−) = other considerations
Preservatives	BHA, BHT, calcium propionate, sodium propionate, sodium benzoate, sorbic acid, sodium nitrate, sulfites	+ Increase food shelf-life + Prevent spoilage + Increase availability of perishable foods + Sometimes add nutrients (calcium propionate is a good source of calcium) − nitrates can be converted into nitrosamines in the body; being studied as a factor in cancer − sulfites cause reactions in some people, especially asthmatics; banned in fresh fruits and vegetables (except potatoes)
Flavoring agents	Spices, essential oils, MSG, vanillin, limonene, GMP	+ replace natural flavors lost in processing + enhance flavors + create new flavors − some people sensitive to MSG − GMP, found in many prepared soups, converts to uric acid in the body and should be avoided by people with gout or other excess-uric acid diseases
Coloring agents	Annatto, caramel, beta-carotene, dyes	+ provide rich colors that consumers associate with foods (e.g., yellow butter, green mint) − Five dyes have been approved as safe; others have been banned—red dyes no. 2 and no. 4
Sweeteners	Saccharin, aspartame	+ noncaloric sweetening − possible cancer link to saccharin products must contain warning − aspartame may cause symptoms in people with genetic disorder known phenylketonuria

Category	Examples	Dietary Contribution
		(+) = positive role (−) = other considerations
Emulsifiers	lecithin, monoglycerides, diglycerides, polysorbates	+ prevent separation of oil and water + enhance flavor + retard spoilage − polysorbates are limited by FDA, contain very small amounts of carcinogens
Texturizers and stabilizers	gelatin, pectin, carrrageenan, cellulose gum, modified starches, sodium alginate	+ add "body" and thicken foods + improve flavor/texture + prevent canned foods from separating − safe in small quantities; in larger amounts might replace needed nutrients

PART TWO

Eating Better in America

Food is basic to life, but there are many factors that dictate what we eat, how our food is prepared, and the ways we incorporate eating into our social rituals. We do not eat simply to fuel our bodily operations; if that were the case, we might already have developed nutrition capsules to circumvent the complex business of procuring, preparing, and eating food. Instead, eating is a central and valued human activity whose contexts include custom, religion, family tradition, health, pleasure, and life-style.

In recent times, the availability of nutritional information has heightened consumer awareness of the ways food relates to health and fitness. This is a positive trend, but sound nutrition does not exist in a vacuum. There can exist no fixed list of good foods or bad foods. Nor is there a simple set of rules that can guarantee a perfect nutritional balance that applies to everyone. Nutrition goals must encompass the full range of social, psychological, historical, and economic considerations with which people live.

If there is flexibility in the idea of what good nutrition is, there are firm statements we can make about what good nutrition is not:

Good nutrition is not torture: It does not mean deprivation or being forced to eat foods one dislikes. The "no pain, no gain" philosophy of health is not only unnecessary, but often leads to a reverse effect. The fact is that good nutrition can coexist with the pleasure of eating.

Good nutrition is not a magic formula: We cannot guarantee a certain level of health or longevity by virtue of what we eat. It's true that there are scientific judgments about certain foods. These dietary guidelines help us make choices, but they are not rigid standards that apply to every individual in every situation.

Good nutrition need not be costly: It does not require the purchase of special foods, expensive supplements, or unusual appliances. A healthy diet can easily be maintained on even a modest food budget.

Good nutrition is not dull: Some people see nutrition as a clinical eating experience, at odds with the notion that food gives pleasure. But sound nutritional advice can be expressed in ways that allow people to fully enjoy food without constantly analyzing it.

In our daily lives, nutrition is a dynamic force, not a static one. It is an exercise in problem solving, a way of taking into account all our needs and evolving an eating style that fits them.

Making Better Choices

Our life-styles dictate many things about the way we eat, and these life-styles are determined by a variety of factors—family, ethnic background, the influence of media, daily schedules, and peers. There is no reason most people can't develop a diet that both suits their life-styles and meets all of their nutritional needs.

For example, as we examine what people eat, we see that almost everyone consumes food from grains, primarily wheat, rice, and corn. These foods may differ in the way they are prepared, but they supply basically the same kind of nutrients. A corn tortilla and a bowl of spaghetti aren't that different in their nutritional effects; neither are a serving of rice and a slice of bread. Their consumption reflects our diet preferences, but none of the choices are superior to the others.

Within the context of the diet you have chosen, nutrition boils down to making the best possible choices rather than imposing restrictions. We know, for example, that Americans spend nearly $15 billion every year on frozen foods. The best nutritional approach is to determine which frozen foods make the best choices. We also know that at least one-third of all Americans patronize a restaurant (half of them "fast" food restaurants) at least once a day. The best nutritional approach describes how to make choices from restaurant menus.

To be sure, there are concerns about the American diet. The Surgeon General's Report on Nutrition and Health, released in the summer of 1988, warned that while most Americans can now avoid the deficiency diseases that were once common, an overconsumption of certain dietary components—notably fat and especially saturated fat—have increased their risk for chronic diseases such as coronary heart disease, some types of cancer, diabetes, high blood pressure, and obesity. According to the Department of Health and Human Services, dietary influences play a role in five of the nation's ten leading causes of death: heart disease, cancer, stroke, diabetes, and atherosclerosis (clogged arteries).

It is easy to feel a sense of panic when reports such as these are published. This panic is fueled by the absence of practical guidelines that educate people in how to make the eating decisions in their everyday lives that will eliminate health risks and promote vitality.

Nutrition in the Real World

Consumer confusion is the natural fallout of a health industry that stresses information over practical application. Consumers are assaulted with facts, theories, warnings, and impressions about diet, but are usually left with very little in the way of simple, realistic guidelines for eating that can be followed in the normal course of life.

Practical nutrition relates to people and the ways they live. In this section, we focus on the life-styles of Americans. We provide hundreds of practical guidelines for purchasing and preparing healthy foods. Since more than half the foods Americans eat come in packages, we describe how to read package labels for nutrition. We address the very real concerns people have about the safety of the food supply. And we offer practical advice for the millions of people who eat out in restaurants. More than anything, this section will debunk the myth that painful sacrifices must accompany healthy eating.

9

A Healthy Cook's Kitchen

Americans may be dining out in greater numbers than ever, but the home kitchen is still the focus of most family meals. In its 1988 survey on eating trends, the National Restaurant Association found that 7 out of 10 meals are still prepared at home. Indeed, there has been something of a revival of home cooking in recent years, a fact born out by burgeoning cookbook sales.

Many people find great pleasure in creating imaginative and delicious meals. And the pleasure can be enhanced when you know you're promoting health at the same time.

Make Home Cooking a Nutritional Delight

If you are a lover of gourmet cooking and eating, or even simply a lover of food, you may wonder if your enjoyment of culinary delights is at odds with your desire for nutritious cuisine. The good news is that adopting healthy cooking techniques need not doom you to tiny portions of bland foods. On the contrary, foods prepared with nutrition in mind can satisfy the most exotic palate. Once you discover the simple techniques and have the right tools on hand, it can be fun to discover the many ways you can imaginatively prepare foods that provide a good nutritional balance and that are low in calories, fat, cholesterol, and sodium—without sacrificing the pleasure of eating.

Variety Improves Your Meals in Two Ways

The first step is to make sure that your meal plans include plenty of variety to guarantee that you're getting the appropriate range of nutrients. In doing so, you will add enjoyment to your diet, because food is best enjoyed in its full range of tastes, textures, colors, and styles.

The U.S. Department of Agriculture has established recommendations on food intake for the average American. These guidelines are in no way intended as "rules" for a perfect diet. Rather, they're designed to help people get the right balance of nutrients. The recommendations are based on four basic food groups, summarized in the accompanying table.

Small Changes Go a Long Way

Changes in your cooking style can provide you and your family with a diet that may protect against heart disease, hypertension, and possibly cancer. It can also help you to restrict calories

▶ NUTRITION QUIZ ◀

Test Your Food Savvy

With all the new findings about fish oil and fiber, the controversies about calcium, the recommendations about fat, and the myriad other nutrition notes that cross your path every day, it's hard to keep track of some of the basic facts and figures about nutrition. Take this quiz to assess your nutrition knowledge.

1. Which of these foods is highest in fat?
   (a) 1 tablespoon of peanut butter   (b) ¼ cup of sunflower seeds   (c) 5 shortbread cookies

2. For adults, the recommended dietary allowance for calcium is:
   (a) 800 milligrams   (b) 1,000 milligrams   (c) 1,500 milligrams

3. Which fish is highest in omega-3 fatty acids?
   (a) salmon   (b) rainbow trout   (c) haddock

4. Spinach is a particularly good source of:
   (a) calcium   (b) vitamin A   (c) iron

5. Which is the best source of water-soluble fiber?
   (a) wheat bran   (b) oat bran   (c) oatmeal

6. Which of the following foods is richest in the iron the body absorbs most efficiently (heme iron):
   (a) iron-fortified cereal   (b) red snapper   (c) tofu

7. A baked potato best meets our need for:
   (a) vitamin C   (b) vitamin B-6   (c) protein

8. Which of these nuts contains the least fat?
   (a) peanuts   (b) macadamia nuts   (c) chestnuts

ANSWERS:

1. (b) Although all foods listed are high in fat, sunflower seeds top the list with more than 15 grams (equal to 135 calories) in a ¼ cup serving. One tablespoon of peanut butter contains approximately 8 grams of fat. Five shortbread cookies have 11.5 grams.

2. (a)—with a caveat. The current RDA for calcium is 800 milligrams for adults, with the exception of pregnant women and breastfeeding mothers, whose allowance is recommended at 1,200 milligrams per day.

3. (a) Salmon, one of the richest sources of omega-3 fatty acids, contains 1 to 1½ grams in a 3½ ounce serving. Fresh rainbow or brook trout is also a rich source of

omega-3 fatty acids, with nearly ¾ gram in a 3½ ounce portion. All three fish mentioned are good, low-calorie sources of protein.

4. **(b)** Spinach, like other darker salad greens, packs more nutrients than the light-colored varieties such as iceberg lettuce. It is richest in vitamin A because it is high in beta-carotene, which is converted to vitamin A in the body. A ½ cup serving provides more than 100 percent of the RDA. Contrary to popular belief, spinach is not a very good source of iron or calcium.

5. **(b)** Oat bran (the outer husk or shell of the oat grain) is the richest source of water-soluble fiber. Oatmeal, which is huskless, has only about half as much soluble fiber as the bran portion. Wheat bran contains mainly insoluble fiber, which increases the bulk of the stool and helps prevent constipation.

6. **(b)** Animal foods (fish, meat, and poultry) contain heme iron, of which the body absorbs roughly 25 percent. Cereals, grains, and vegetables contain nonheme iron, of which the body absorbs only 3 to 8 percent. But when foods with nonheme iron are eaten in combination with foods that contain heme iron, the amount of iron that is absorbed from them increases.

7. **(a)** One medium-sized potato (with many of its nutrients concentrated just under the skin) contains more than a third of the body's daily requirements for vitamin C. Potatoes are also a good source of vitamin B-6, providing more than 20 percent of the RDA for this nutrient. In addition, they supply 6 percent of the RDA for protein, along with smaller amounts of other nutrients.

8. **(c)** Three small chestnuts contain only 29 calories and less than ½ gram of fat. Sixteen shelled, roasted peanuts, which weigh the same amount, have 85 calories, 65 of which come from fat. Macadamia nuts top the list. Six of them contain 109 calories, nearly all of which come from fat.

while you eat hearty portions of foods that are tasty and good for you.

The way you set up your kitchen for healthy cooking depends on your personal living style, your family makeup, and your particular health and fitness concerns. Even if you're a minimalist cook, you can add quality to your meals (both nutritionally and in terms of taste) by doing some basic planning and preparation. It's not necessary to completely overhaul your diet and totally re-stock your kitchen overnight. Begin by making small changes. If you find it difficult, for example, to juggle many nutritional recommendations at once, choose one or two that are particularly im-portant and focus on them, adding other changes over time. Don't forget that food can be fun. If you approach dietary changes with a heavy heart and feelings of deprivation, your good intentions aren't likely to last. When you're making food sub-stitutions, be sure to choose the foods you enjoy.

You'll be pleasantly surprised to learn how easy it is to incorporate nutrition into your day without making any drastic changes. In fact, the simplest substitutions can dramatically improve your food intake. To demonstrate, if you were to make the following minor changes in your cooking, your calorie savings would be quite substantial, and nearly all the calories saved are from fat.

BALANCE YOUR DIET

Milk Group

Recommended Intake
3 servings/day for children
4 servings/day for adolescents
2 servings/day for adults

Sample Servings
1 cup milk or yogurt
1 cup cottage cheese
1 oz. cheddar cheese
1½ cups ice cream
(Note: If you are watching your fat and calorie intake, substitute low-fat milk and cheeses, and use ice milk or frozen yogurt instead of ice cream.)

Meat Group

Recommended Intake
2 servings per day

Sample Servings
2 oz. lean meat, fish, or poultry
2 eggs
2 oz. cheese
1 cup cooked dried beans or peas
4 tbsp. peanut butter
2 oz. nuts
(Note: If you are watching your cholesterol, consume eggs in moderation. Fat watchers should use low-fat cheese and lean cuts of meat, and monitor their intake of nuts and nut foods, which are very high in fat.)

Vegetable and Fruit Group

Recommended Intake
4 servings daily, including a citrus fruit or other fruit or vegetable high in vitamin C, and a deep-green or yellow-orange vegetable for vitamin A

Sample Servings
1 cup raw fruits or vegetables
½ cup cooked fruits or vegetables
½ cup juice

Bread and Cereal Group

Recommended Intake
4 or more servings daily

Sample Servings
1 slice bread or roll
1 tortilla
1 cup dry cereal
½ cup cooked cereal or grits
½ cup cooked rice or pasta

Other Foods
Includes high-calorie foods with limited or no nutritional value, like fats, oils, alcohol, salad dressings, sweets, and high-fat snacks. These foods should be eaten in moderation.

Stock Your Kitchen for Health

You can have a nutrition-at-your-fingertips kitchen once you stock your larder with supportive cooking ingredients and diet-conscious cooking aids. Chances are, you will already have on hand some of the items we'll talk about here, but maybe you've never understood their benefits. The following information and checklists will establish some ground rules for your healthy kitchen. Start slowly and gradually to set up your kitchen, experimenting with cooking ingredients and equipment to find those that suit you best. We're not going to tell you that all of them are essential for every kitchen. It really depends on how much you cook and the kinds of foods you like to eat. And even if you don't do a lot of home cooking, you're sure to find some quick and easy ways to improve both the nutrition and the enjoyment you get from your diet.

FAT-SAVING SUBSTITUTIONS

Substitute	For	Calories Saved
1 cup low-fat milk (1%)	1 cup whole milk	50
1 cup skim evaporated milk	1 cup heavy cream	640
1 cup plain low-fat yogurt	1 cup sour cream	375
1 cup blended low-fat cottage cheese	1 cup sour cream	305
1 cup plain low-fat yogurt	1 cup regular mayonnaise	1,455
1 cup part-skim ricotta cheese	1 cup whole-milk ricotta cheese	90
1 cup white sauce, made with low-fat milk, 2 tablespoons flour, no fat	1 cup whole-milk white sauce made with 2 tablespoons flour and 2 tablespoons butter	250
¼ cup diet margarine	¼ cup regular margarine	205
½ cup reduced-calorie mayonnaise	½ cup regular mayonnaise	480

Fill Your Pantry with Nature's Best

Most people who cook stock their kitchens with a certain number of "cooking basics," such as flour, sugar, and rice. Start with an examination of your kitchen's staples to find the items for which you can substitute better choices. Here are some suggestions:

▶ Long- or short-grain brown rice without the bran removed is a better choice than white rice, primarily because of its high fiber content.

▶ Whole-grain flours (such as whole wheat, buckwheat, rye, and oat flour) are better choices than refined grains, primarily because they're high in fiber. These flours are also a very good source of B vitamins. Some, like soy flour, are excellent sources of protein. Be aware that these drier, heavier flours may change the way you prepare recipes that call for refined flours. Some cooks find that a satisfying compromise is to mix a whole grain flour half and half with a refined flour.

▶ Legumes (beans, peas, and lentils) are good sources of protein for those who want to reduce their fat intake by sometimes substituting a non-meat main course. Legumes can also be superior sources of B vitamins, iron, and calcium. Use them to make hearty soups and stews, casseroles, and salads. The most commonly used legumes include black beans, black-eyed peas, kidney beans, lentil beans, lima beans, navy beans, pinto beans, soybeans, split peas, and whole peas. (Be sure to store legumes in tightly covered containers in a cool, dry place to preserve nutrients and prevent rancidity.)

▶ Most vegetable oils—such as safflower, sunflower, and corn—are high in polyunsaturated fats, which may help lower cholesterol. The exceptions (notably palm and coconut oils) are rarely used in home cooking. Vegetable oils will last up to one year, and olive oil six months, if stored at room temperature. With refrigeration, they will last a month or two longer.

▶ Use sparingly those condiments that are high in sodium and/or fat. Worcestershire sauce, soy sauce, and bouillon are examples of condiments with a particularly high sodium content. Mayonnaise and cream-based sauces have a high fat content. Better choices include vinegar, tomato paste, lemon juice, lime juice, and mustard. Ketchup is moderately high in sodium (unless you choose a no-salt brand) and it usually contains sugar, but it's okay for occasional use in small amounts.

Cut the Salt and Add Flavor

We have become so accustomed to the flavor of salty foods that many people assume they wouldn't enjoy food without having the salt shaker handy. In reality, by using salt as your primary flavoring agent, you are not only increasing your daily sodium intake, you are also potentially masking the flavors of many foods, not to mention missing out on the wonderful taste enhancement that herbs and spices can provide.

If the world of herbs and spices is a new one for you, you're in for a treat. The range of flavors is as varied as you want it to be. The table below lists common spices, along with the foods they most perfectly compliment.

Liquid flavorings (extracts) can also add zest to foods, reducing the necessity of adding sugars or sauces that are high in fat and calories. Just a drop or two of these intense flavors can punch up a salt- or sugar-free dish. You can purchase common extracts in the supermarket (usually in the baked-goods section), but for the more exotic varieties, you may have to try specialty bakeries or gourmet shops.

Extracts are usually sold in tiny bottles that con-

SPICE UP A LOW-SALT DIET

Allspice	fish, eggs, soups, stews, carrots, tomatoes, winter squash	Ginger	poultry, pork, fish, fruit
Anise	poultry, coleslaw, desserts, baked goods	Horseradish	beef, fish, green salad
		Marjoram	beef, poultry, fish, eggs, eggplant, summer squash, tomatoes
Basil	beef, poultry, lamb, fish, eggs, soups, green beans, green salad, peas, spinach, summer squash, tomatoes, zucchini	Mint	beef, lamb, fish, carrots, peas, spinach, fruit
		Mustard Seed	beef, pork, green salad, beans
Bay Leaves	poultry, fish, soups, spaghetti, tomatoes	Nutmeg	poultry, fruit, desserts, baked goods, cottage cheese
Caraway Seed	asparagus, cabbage, carrots, green beans, fruit, baked goods	Onion	beef, poultry, fish, soups, eggs, salads, tomatoes
Cardamom	poultry, cabbage, fruit	Oregano	eggs, soups, green salad, tomatoes, pasta dishes
Celery Seed	beef, pork, fish, eggs		
Chervil	poultry, fish, eggs, soups, carrots, green salad	Paprika	poultry, fish, coleslaw
		Parsley	beef, poultry, pork, lamb, fish, soups, salads, peas
Chives	beef, poulty, fish, soups, cottage cheese	Poppy Seed	green salad, fruit, baked goods
Cinnamon	poultry, pork, lamb, fruit, desserts, baked goods	Rosemary	poultry, lamb, fish, pasta, spinach, potatoes, fruit
Clove	poultry, pork, fish, tomatoes	Sage	beef, poultry, fish, eggplant, peas, tomatoes, rice, pasta
Coriander	pork, zucchini	Savory	fish, eggs, green beans
Cumin	beef, eggs, beans	Sesame Seed	poultry, bread, salads, casseroles
Dill	lamb, fish, soups, carrots, coleslaw, green salad, peas, summer squash, tomatoes	Tarragon	poultry, pasta, fish, green salad
		Thyme	poultry, fish, soups, carrots, peas, tomatoes
Fennel	fish		
Garlic	beef, pork, lamb, poultry, fish, beans, rice, salads		

Try Flavors You Like in These Ways:	
Almond	
Anise (licorice flavor)	
Apricot	added to dessert recipes
Blackberry	added to plain seltzer
Blueberry	added to coffee
Cherry	mixed with yogurt
Chocolate	rubbed into meats before
Cinnamon	cooking
Clove	mixed into salads
Lemon	added to milk
Lime	added to vegetable dishes
Maple	mixed into fruit compotes
Mint	added to vanilla ice cream or
Orange	ice milk
Peppermint	dashed into plain tea
Raspberry	added to cold fruit and
Root beer	vegetable soups
Spearmint	mixed with yogurt dips
Strawberry	
Vanilla	
Walnut	

tain from two to four ounces, but a little bit goes a long way. The flavors listed above may be used in a wide variety of creative ways.

If you enjoy ethnic cooking or like to make your own sauces and dressings, these ingredients are often used to create favorite seasonings:

Barbecue seasoning: celery seeds, cayenne, clove, coriander, garlic, nutmeg, onion, chili powder, hickory flavor

Cajun spice: paprika, garlic, onion, cumin, chilis, oregano, parsley, pepper, basil, thyme, marjoram, rosemary, cayenne pepper

Curry: cumin, coriander, cayenne, tumeric, fenugreek, garlic, ginger, cloves, pepper

Italian seasoning: savory, oregano, marjoram, sage, thyme, sweet basil, rosemary

Mexican seasoning: chilis, garlic, onion, paprika, cumin, bay, parsley, oregano, celery seed, cayenne

Pizza seasoning: onion, fennel, oregano, garlic, basil, parsley, marjoram, celery flakes, thyme

Poultry seasoning: marjoram, parsley, savory, sage, thyme

Salad seasoning: basil, tarragon, dill, chervil, parsley

Salsa: onion, celery, parsley, cumin, garlic, oregano, cayenne pepper

While you're spicing up your diet, be careful that you don't inadvertently choose seasonings that contain large amounts of sodium. These include:

Garlic salt: 1,850 mg in 1 teaspoon. (Use garlic powder, which contains only 1 mg of sodium per teaspoon.)

Meat tenderizer: 1,750 mg in 1 teaspoon.

Onion salt: 1,620 mg in 1 teaspoon. (Use onion powder, which contains only 1 mg of sodium per teaspoon.)

(Note: Salt substitutes don't contain sodium, but they don't taste just like salt either. You might enjoy experimenting with the wide variety of spices and seasonings that are available.)

Nutrition-Wise Kitchen Tools

The tools you use for cooking can be nutritional helpmates. The equipment you buy depends to a large extent on how much time you spend in the kitchen and the kinds of foods you tend to prepare. There are literally hundreds of cooking materials from which to choose, from basic essentials to luxury appliances to colorful but not particularly useful gadgets. Stocking your kitchen with health-enhancing cooking tools will not guarantee good nutrition, but some tools will enable you to make small changes in your everyday meal preparation that, over time, can add up to a more nutritious diet. Every healthy kitchen should have the following basics:

NONSTICK PANS

Use. All-purpose pans for sautéing meats and vegetables, "frying" eggs, and making omelettes.

Nutrition Benefit. Allows foods to be fried with the use of very small amounts of butter or oil. You may also use a nonstick spray, such as Pam.

VEGETABLE STEAMER

Use. An inexpensive, usually metal, insert that, when placed inside of cooking pots, holds vegetables above the water. Vegetables are cooked with a moist steam heat.

Nutrition Benefit. Limits the nutrient loss that occurs when vegetables are submerged in water while cooking.

KITCHEN SCALE

Use. Weighing food portions—usually meat, poultry, fish, and cheese. A small, inexpensive postage-style scale (for weights of 1 to 10 ounces) is sufficient.

Nutrition Benefit. Many people have trouble calculating portion sizes, often overestimating the amount of food that constitutes a 4- or 5-ounce serving. A scale can be particularly helpful if you're watching your calories and/or want to better control your intake of fatty foods.

The following items can also be used to enhance the nutritional quality of your food, or to provide you with easy options for preparing more healthful meals.

BLENDER OR FOOD PROCESSOR

Use. Mixes, purees, chops, slices, and grates foods. Food processors are equipped for more purposes than blenders and are better at tasks such as very fine grating and chopping.

Nutrition Benefit. Can simplify home cooking and make nutritional drinks, soups, and vegetable-pureed gravy stock.

JUICER

Use. Squeezes and liquifies fresh fruits and vegetables, creating fresh juice.

Nutrition Benefit. Makes it easy to keep fresh fruit and vegetable juices available, cutting down on commercial brands that may contain extra sugar or salt.

EGG CODDLER

Use. Cooks eggs in a style similar to poaching.

Nutrition Benefit. There's no need to use butter or oil. Coddling is easier than poaching and allows spices and other chopped ingredients to be added to the egg.

WOK

Use. Stir-frying meats and vegetables.

Nutrition Benefit. A little oil is used, but not as much as required for pan frying, and the intense heat cooks foods fast. This is a very healthy way to cook vegetables, since the longer they cook, the more nutrients are depleted.

SKIMMER/STRAINER

Use. Removes congealed-fat from the tops of stews and soups that have been stored in the refrigerator or freezer. Also allows skimming of fat from the top of broths while cooking. (You can do this with a spoon, too, but a skimmer makes it easier.)

Nutrition Benefit. Substantially reduces fat content and reduces the number of calories in soups and stews.

MICROWAVE OVEN

Use. Fast cooking for most foods.

Nutrition Benefit. Since moist heat is used, there is no need to use butter or oil. Also, the fast cooking helps preserve vitamins and minerals in foods.

HOT-AIR POPCORN POPPER

Use. Pops corn.

Nutrition Benefit. Keeps popcorn snack low in calories and free for fat, since no oil or butter is required.

One Key to Nourishment Lies in the Cooking

Even if you've carried home grocery bags full of "healthy" foods, it's possible to at least partially sabotage your good intentions by using the wrong method of cooking. Begin to train yourself to think of the process of preparation as an integral part of what makes a food "good." For example, rather than thinking "A potato is nutritious," think "A potato baked in its skin is nutritious." The methods you use to prepare your foods can make a big difference in their nutritional value. And the preferred methods do not necessarily take more time; in some cases, they take less. Here is some cooking wisdom for your favorite foods.

Keep Vegetables Packed with Nutrients

Before cooking begins, fresh vegetables must be washed thoroughly, even when you buy them "washed" in the supermarket. As you remove all dirt, you will also remove surface pesticides. Run vegetables in a heavy stream of water, whether they're to be cooked or eaten raw. Scrub hard-surfaced items with a vegetable brush. Separate the leaves of leafy vegetables and immerse them in a sinkful of water. Lift them out while the dirty water drains, repeating the process more than once, if necessary. Avoid soaking vegetables as this promotes a loss of nutrients.

As you prepare your vegetables for cooking, minimize chopping and peeling, since vitamins are lost when the surface is exposed. Using a sharp knife, cut vegetables into uniform pieces that will all cook at the same rate. Try to cook vegetables with jackets and skins intact, peeling afterward. Be sure to cover and refrigerate anything you don't use right away.

When vegetables are being cooked, their enemies are light, heat, air, and water. Light destroys the B-vitamin riboflavin, as well as vitamin A; heat wreaks havoc with vitamin C, thiamin, and folic acid; air breaks down vitamins C, E, and K; and

water leaches out water-soluble vitamins and some minerals. The end result to shoot for with any cooking method is vegetables that are tender-crisp, not soggy or mushy. You can accomplish this goal using any of the following procedures:

▶ Cook in a pan with a tight-fitting lid, using only a small amount of water in the bottom. For best results, bring water to a boil, add vegetables, cover, and quickly return to the boil. Then lower heat and gently cook for a few minutes.

▶ Steam using a vegetable steamer, in a pot with a lid that fits. Don't allow the vegetables to touch the water or pack them so tightly that steam can't circulate.

▶ Stir-fry a dish for a family of four with only a tablespoon or two of oil. Make sure the oil is hot (but not smoking) before you add the vegetables.

▶ Pressure cook, following the directions on the appliance. Be careful not to overcook, or you'll lose both nutrients and crisp texture. You may find that young, tender vegetables need less time than is recommended.

▶ Microwave with one or two tablespoons of water in a covered, microwave-safe container. The microwave creates a moist, hot atmosphere that conducts heat from one area to another. You'll need to experiment for different types of vegetables and quantities.

The least effective cooking method for retaining nutrients in vegetables is to boil them in large quantities of water. However, if you do this, save the water for use in soups, stews, and gravies to recover some of the vitamin and mineral loss.

Once your vegetables are cooked, serve them right away; nutrient loss occurs when they sit on a warming tray or at room temperature. In fact, two-to-three-day-old leftovers can lose as much as half their vitamin C.

Acids, such as vinegar and lemon juice, will not destroy nutrients, but it is better to add them after cooking to avoid a hard-textured surface on the vegetables.

Use Methods that Cook Meat Lean

Good ways to cook meat and poultry include roasting, baking, broiling, and stir-frying. These methods require the addition of little or no fat and even help drain off some of the fat contained in the meat. With the development of crisping trays and other specialty microwaving dishes, it will soon become more common to microwave meats. This is also a low-fat method.

▶ Roasting is a dry-heat cooking method. Beef, pork, and lamb usually won't require basting because of their fat content, which renders them self-basting. If very lean items require basting, use nonfat substances like wine, vinegar, and lemon juice. Be sure to place the meat on a rack in the roasting pan so excess fat can drip away during cooking. Baking is also a dry-heat cooking method for meat, poultry, fish, and casseroles. Some baking dishes (such as glass bakeware) require greasing to prevent food from sticking.

▶ Broiling is done under very high, direct heat. Be sure to place meat on a rack that allows the fat to drip away during cooking. If you choose to marinate the meat before cooking, try fruit juices like lemon, lime, or grape, or dry wine.

▶ Stir-frying is a very fast, very hot method. Although a little oil is required, it is not enough to cause concern, and because foods are constantly moving around in the pan, they absorb very little fat.

Trim the obvious fat from meat and remove the whitish fat pads from under the skin, especially in poultry. One fatless method for browning meat and poultry is to pan-broil them in nonstick pans. The least healthful methods of preparing meat and poultry are frying and batter frying. Also, if you stew meat or slow-cook it in a Crockpot, reduce the fat content by skimming the top of the broth occasionally while it's cooking.

Enhance the Value of Fish

It appears that eating one or two fish meals a week may cut the risk of cardiovascular disease for some people. Both lean and oily fish varieties are good; some of the oils in fish like salmon, trout, and mackerel, known as omega-3 fatty acids, may be associated with a lowered risk of heart disease.

Prepare fish with an eye to protecting its health benefits. The amount of fat that a fish naturally contains should determine the way it is cooked. Fattier fish, such as salmon and trout, can be grilled or broiled. Leaner fish, such as flounder and haddock, do better with moist cooking methods, such as poaching or microwaving. Incorporate these tips into your fish preparation:

▶ The mistake cooks make most often is to overcook fish, rendering it dry and tough. You can tell when fish is ready simply by looking at it: Once it loses its translucence and becomes opaque, it is probably ready. Test it with a fork; if it is flakey to the touch, remove it from the oven.

▶ Fish responds best to slow-cooking methods, using low temperatures. For baking, set the oven at 350°F, baste the fish with a dab of oil and a little lemon juice, and bake for about 20 to 25 minutes. If you choose to broil your fish, be sure to watch it carefully. Broiling is a fast-cooking method, and an extra minute can spell disaster.

▶ Use low-fat ingredients to make a delicious liquid for poaching. The best include tomato juice, lemon or lime juice, and wine. Vegetable bouillon is also a good low-fat option, although it is higher in sodium than the others. When poaching, keep the heat at a temperature that just barely simmers the liquid, and cover the pan with a lid.

Pasta Made Perfect

With its impressive range of shapes, sizes, and colors, pasta can really jazz up your table. And since pasta is free of cholesterol and saturated fat, it makes for a nutritious, satisfying meal.

The most healthy way to eat pasta is *al dente,* tender but firm. Many cooks make the mistake of overcooking the noodles, thus letting vitamins leach out into the water. Rinsing after cooking also tends to wash away nutrients, particularly the B vitamins, so pasta should never be rinsed unless a recipe specifically calls for it.

Since pasta is eaten with either a sauce or dressing, you'll want to be attentive to the ingredients in the sauce you choose. A creamy, high-fat sauce can severely undercut pasta's natural low-fat properties. Use simple tomato, vegetable, or fish sauces, and take advantage of the many seasonings that enhance the flavor of pasta.

We suggest using low-fat cottage cheese, skim milk, or yogurt instead of sour cream for flour and whole-milk sauces. Whenever possible, use polyunsaturated margarine instead of butter.

Remember: To keep down the calories, flavor pasta with the sauce, don't drown it.

Delicious Diets Full of Beans

High in protein, vitamins, and fiber, and low in salt and fat, beans taste great in soups, salads, and casseroles. Because of their high protein content, beans are often used as a main-course meat substitute for people who are interested in reducing fat and cholesterol.

Before cooking beans, rinse them well and remove misshapen or discolored beans. Most beans need to be presoaked before cooking. If you place them in a large pot of cold water and let it stand overnight, beans will soften yet retain their shape. A quicker method can be used if you don't care about the beans breaking apart in water. Place them in a saucepan and cover with water by about 2 inches. Bring to a boil over medium heat, then simmer for 2 to 3 minutes. Turn off the heat, cover, and let stand for 1 to 2 hours before cooking.

Be prepared to cook the beans for a while before you add other ingredients. As they cook, remove the residue that floats to the top of the water

with a strainer, and add water as needed so that the beans are always covered.

How do you know when your beans are ready? A slight cracking in the skin usually indicates that they're done. Of course, the fool-proof method is to taste the bean. When beans are cooked whole, they should be tender, but not mushy.

Bean eaters often complain of problems with gas after a meal. To eliminate some of the gas-forming ingredients, drain the water after beans have finished soaking, refill the saucepan with fresh water, and simmer until tender.

If you are not accustomed to eating beans, incorporating them gradually into your diet will give your intestines a chance to adapt to this new carbohydrate source and help cut down on gas problems.

Make Your Own Hearty Soups

Many people shy away from making soups from scratch because they think it's too time consuming or complicated. But homemade soups can be relatively easy to prepare, and are worth the effort from the standpoints of both taste and nutrition. These ten basic techniques are all you need to know to prepare mouth-watering and super-healthy soups.

▶ Make your stock by simmering vegetables, bones, and spices together in water over a gentle heat, barely boiling. Stock is easy to make, since ingredients don't have to be measured, and almost any vegetable is suitable: onions, carrots, and garlic, as well as flavorful but otherwise discarded parts like celery tops, tomato, and potato peels, and parsley stems.

▶ Leave vegetables and trimmings in large pieces. Add bones (shank and knuckle bones have the most flavor, but others, including poultry carcasses, make delicious stock), bay leaves, and a few crushed peppercorns. Cover with water in a large pot and simmer for an hour or two.

▶ "Degrease" the stock before use by chilling it and then lifting off the hardened top (fat) layer. Alternately, fat-free broth can be made by omitting bones and meat, and fat-reduced broth can be made by trimming the fat as closely as possible before cooking.

▶ If making broth from scratch takes more time than you want to spend, commercial broths —also called consommé, bouillon, or broth—can be used. They come bottled, canned, or in concentrated dry cubes or granules. Be aware, though, that many commercial stocks are quite salty. As a rule of thumb, check to see that "chicken broth" or "beef broth" is listed as one of the first ingredients on the label, not salt or animal fat.

▶ After you have prepared the stock, sauté chopped onions, garlic, and celery in a large kettle, using a little olive oil. You can minimize the amount of oil you need to use by covering the vegetables during part of the sauté to retain moisture and prevent sticking. Then add your stock.

▶ Next, plan on an assortment of goods for substance. By including beans, peas, or other legumes in the same soup with grains and vegetables you increase the fiber and protein value of your soup. A little meat, poultry, or seafood will then go a long way.

▶ Time your additions to the soup pot according to how long items take to cook. Raw meats (which should be quickly browned beforehand) and long-cooking grains and vegetables should go in first. To preserve texture and nutrients, add fresh or frozen fast-cooking vegetables shortly before serving.

▶ Always simmer the soup gently, since a vigorous boil will break up the ingredients and cloud the mixture, in addition to diminishing the flavor. You can tell that you've got a good simmer when the bubbles that form in the bottom of the pot rise slowly, barely breaking the surface. Once simmering, the pot can be left on its own.

Yellow Pea and Spinach Soup

Yield: 8 servings, just under 1 cup each
Per serving: Calories: 130
          Fat: 18%
          Sodium: 211 mg
          Fiber: 3.6 g

½ cup chopped onion
2 tsp. minced garlic
2 tsp. olive oil
1 cup yellow split peas, washed
4 cups chicken broth (no added salt)
2 cups water
10 oz. package frozen, chopped spinach
½ tsp. salt (optional)
⅛ tsp. pepper

Sauté onion and garlic in olive oil in a large pot, covered. Add yellow split peas, chicken broth, and water. Bring them to a boil, then lower heat and simmer for 30 minutes. Add spinach, salt, and pepper and continue simmering for 30 more minutes.

▶ Add seasonings during the second half of cooking because they intensify as liquid evaporates. Fresh herbs, such as parsley, dill, thyme, oregano, and marjoram, may be left whole and tied together in what is known as a bouquet garni, for easy removal, or they may be chopped and sprinkled into the soup.

▶ To thicken the soup, add a little grated raw potato, barley, peas, rice, oatmeal, or oat bran, then simmer a bit longer. Pureed vegetables can also be used to thicken a soup.

Dress Your Salad Well

Many a salad has been marred by an overdose of dressing, tipping the calorie balance from modest to excess by its richness. As many calorie watchers know, even the simplest vinaigrette has 90 to 100 calories per tablespoon, and a single tablespoon doesn't go far on the average salad. The problem is that most salad dressings are laden with fat, and fat calories mount quickly. To be sure, a number of reduced-fat versions are available commercially. While a few are delicious, some are high in salt, and other rely on tasteless gums ands fillers as replacements for oil.

Why not try making your own salad dressing? It's easy to prepare one that is both tasty and high in quality ingredients. Good oil, fine vinegar, and fresh seasonings are all readily available in supermarkets. The rich flavor of these select ingredients allows *less* to taste like *more,* and that helps you keep the fat and calorie content of your salads under control.

PICKING YOUR INGREDIENTS

For oil, choose one that is labeled "unrefined," "virgin," or "cold-pressed." It will have more color and taste of the grain, nut, or seed from which it originated, making a more savory dressing. (The more often the oil is "pressed," the more it loses its original composition.) In addition to unrefined olive oil, sesame seed oil and nut oils like hazelnut and walnut are especially rich. Granted, these oils tend to be more costly. But you can make them stretch farther by blending them with a neutral-tasting but more economical oil like soybean, corn, safflower, or sunflower.

Today's markets feature a wide variety of flavorful vinegars that will spark up a dressing. Delicious varieties include balsamic and rice- or fruit-flavored versions, such as raspberry, blueberry, or black currant. Fine red and white wine vinegars also make rich dressing flavors.

You might also make a habit of using fresh seasonings to enrich the flavor of your dressing. For example, try minced garlic clove instead of garlic powder or salt. Whenever possible, use fresh herbs instead of dried. Good salad choices include basil, chervil, chives, coriander, dill, fennel, marjoram, mint, oregano, parsley, rosemary, summer savory, tarragon, and thyme.

MAKING YOUR DRESSING

If you want to significantly reduce the fat and calorie content of your dressing, replace one-half or more of the oil or fat in traditional recipes with low-fat ingredients or "expanders." In noncreamy dressings, use fruit juices (like tomato or lemon), water, ketchup, or broth for part of the oil. For creamy dressings, use low-fat yogurt, buttermilk, tofu, or cottage cheese instead of mayonnaise, sweet cream, or sour cream. For a smooth texture, swirl the dressing briefly in a blender or food processor. These techniques add body without sacrificing flavor.

If you want to cut calories even further, increase the ratios of substitute ingredients. A good rule of thumb is to start with a 1:2 ratio of vinegar or lemon juice to oil, then add varying amounts of "expanders," anywhere from about one-half to two times the volume of the vinegar and oil components.

Tips to Increase Your Cooking Savvy

A little savvy goes a long way toward more nutrition-conscious cooking. Here are simple ways that you can maintain a high level of nutrition while enjoying the foods you love.

Nutrient-Rich Vegetables and Fruits

► Keep vegetables whole until you're ready to cook them, in order to preserve water-soluble vitamins (Bs and C).

► Nutrients are lost when you peel the skins from vegetables. Try to cook them with the skins on.

► If you're concerned about the sodium content of canned vegetables, you can rinse some of the salt away with water.

► Cook vegetables covered in a small amount of water. Or use steaming, microwaving or stir-

Try These Three Lean Dressings

Each one is rich in taste and texture, but lighter in calories and sodium than regular commercial brands. To further cut fat, change the ratio of vinegar or lemon juice to oil, as described above.

Raspberry Vinaigrette

Calories: 50/tbsp.
Sodium: 60 mg/tbsp.

1 tbsp. raspberry vinegar
1 tbsp. cider vinegar
4 tbsp. vegetable oil (½ olive oil)
3 tbsp. water
1 minced garlic clove
¼ tsp. Dijon mustard
¼ tsp. salt
freshly ground black pepper to taste

Creamy Italian

Calories: 40/tbsp.
Sodium: 40 mg/tbsp.

1 tbsp. lemon juice
2 tbsp. vegetable oil (½ olive oil)
4 tbsp. low-fat yogurt
¼ tsp. oregano
⅛ tsp. salt
freshly ground black pepper to taste
⅛ tsp. sugar (optional)

Light Russian

Calories: 40/tbsp.
Sodium: 40 mg/tbsp.

1 tbsp. rice vinegar
2 tbsp. vegetable oil
1½ tbsp. ketchup
1½ tbsp. water

frying methods. When you boil vegetables in a large amount of water, vitamins and minerals are lost into the water.

▶ More than one-half the minerals in some canned vegetables can be left behind in the liquid. Save the vegetable liquid to use in soups or as a base for sauces.

▶ Use chicken broth or tomato juice, rather than butter, to cook vegetables.

▶ Broccoli and leafy green vegetables like collard greens, kale, and mustard greens are good sources of calcium. Use them to supplement other calcium sources, such as dairy foods, to meet your daily requirements.

▶ To improve your iron absorption from plant foods, serve iron-rich foods with foods rich in vitamin C, such as oranges, tomatoes, and broccoli. Vitamin C aids the absorption of iron.

▶ Eat baked potatoes with the skin. One medium-sized baked potato has 2 grams of fiber, almost twice as much as a peeled potato.

▶ Boost the fiber content of breakfast cereal by slicing a banana on top; one medium-sized banana contains 2 grams of fiber.

▶ Use fruit as a sweet, nutritious staple. Mix fresh fruit as a topping for unsweetened cereals, waffles, and baked goods (like angel food cake).

Cut the Fat in Main Courses

▶ Trim visible fat from meat before cooking.

▶ Use a light basting sauce for cooking meat, such as lemon juice or wine.

▶ Use oven bags to keep lean meat and poultry from drying out during cooking. Available in supermarkets, they can be used in both conventional ovens and microwaves.

▶ Skim the fat off the top when stewing or cooking meat in a Crockpot.

▶ If you broil regular (that is, not lean) hamburger meat well-done on a grill that allows fat to drip off, you'll end up with as little fat as you'd get from using lean ground beef, which is more expensive.

▶ To cut the grease in fried chicken, minimize the cooking time. Fat absorption is related to the time food spends in oil. After cooking, set the chicken on a paper towel to absorb surface fat. Better yet, use this low-fat cooking method: Pull the skin off before baking or broiling.

▶ Crispy baked chicken can be made by dipping chicken into water, lemon, or skim milk, then rolling it in unsalted cracker crumbs before baking. This method works well even if you pull off the skin before dipping.

▶ Create delicious, nutritious, and less fattening poultry stuffings by using larger amounts of fresh vegetables, such as celery, carrots, mushrooms, and onions, to supplement the bread.

▶ Light meat on chicken and turkey contains less fat than dark meat. (A 3½ ounce serving of light turkey meat has 25 fewer calories than a similar serving of dark meat.)

▶ Rather than purchase processed luncheon meats, which are high in fat and sodium, make your own sandwich fillings by baking turkey breast with the skin removed.

▶ For Mexican tacos and burritos, substitute home-cooked pinto beans for chopped beef. (Beware of commercial brands of pinto beans, since they're usually cooked in lard.)

▶ For homemade pizzas, replace high-fat cheese with a combination of part-skim mozzarella and freshly grated Parmesan.

▶ Create a lower-cholesterol omelette by using more egg whites than egg yolks. For example, a three-egg omelette can be made with the whites of three eggs and the yolk of one.

Better Ways to Dress Your Meals

▶ Create a pasta sauce from the saved juices of fish, scallops, clams, chicken, or vegetables. Add spices and tomato paste.

▶ Reduce the calories in coleslaw or salad dressing by "cutting" mayonnaise with low-fat yogurt.

▶ Hummus makes a satisfying and nutritious dip for vegetables and pita-bread sandwiches. It's made of cooked chick peas and sesame seeds ground with lemon juice, garlic, and a little olive oil.

▶ Four ounces of cottage cheese (with 1 percent milk fat) has only 83 calories and can be used with seasonings for vegetable dips or fruit toppings.

▶ Thicken soups with pureed vegetables, such as carrots and onions, instead of oil and flour.

▶ Choose low-sodium seasonings such as fresh garlic and onion, herbs and spices, lemon or lime juice, and vinegar.

▶ Instead of sour cream, use plain yogurt as a topping for a baked potato or fresh fruit.

▶ Reduced-calorie mayonnaise has 50 percent fewer calories than regular and is acceptable in salads and dressings. (Just be aware that it still contains the same percentage of fat, since the reduction in calories is achieved by adding water.)

General Advice

▶ Cook with a nonstick vegetable spray instead of oil.

▶ In lasagna recipes, substitute whipped cottage cheese with Italian seasonings for ricotta cheese.

▶ When possible, use only egg whites, not the whole egg, in cooking; the whites contain no cholesterol.

▶ Replace some of the flour in a muffin recipe with oat bran, which is said to help lower cholesterol.

▶ Store frozen foods at 0°F or below. A temperature of 15°F or higher can result in the loss of vitamins. For example, when stored at 15°F for six months, asparagus, peas, and lima beans lose half their vitamin C.

▶ Substitute soft frozen yogurt for ice cream. Three ounces of most brands contain 90 calories and 3 grams of fat, compared to about 160 calories and 8 grams of fat in regular ice cream (not including extra-rich premium brands).

▶ Add chopped fresh fruit to plain yogurt instead of serving ready-made fruit-filled brands.

▶ If you do purchase flavored yogurt brands, note that plain flavors such as vanilla, coffee, and lemon contain less sugar than the fruited brands.

▶ Make your own snack chips by cutting corn tortillas into quarters and baking at 350°F until crisp.

▶ Instead of serving store-bought fruit drinks, make your own by mixing equal parts sparkling water of seltzer with fresh fruit juices.

▶ Every ¼ cup of sugar (brown or white) adds nearly 200 empty calories to your recipes. You can adapt many of them by cutting the called-for sugar by 25 to 50 percent and adding cinnamon, nutmeg, vanilla, almond, or other spices and extracts to spark the flavor.

▶ Eliminate a substantial number of sugar and fat calories from cake by replacing icing with a light dusting of confectioners' sugar.

10

The Nutritional Shopping Cart

If you're like 70 percent of Americans, you make one or two major trips to the local supermarket each week. Once inside, you juggle a number of variables in making choices, including quality, convenience, nutrition, taste, presentation, and price.

Even though supermarkets are becoming bigger and expanding the number and variety of products, there is no need for you to be intimidated by the prospect of shopping for good food. It would be absurd to think that responsible shopping requires careful scrutiny of the 20,000-plus products in a given store. In fact, you probably only have 10 to 20 items on your shopping list, and many of these (particularly the nonperishable ones) don't even show up every week.

Of course, supermarkets are not designed merely to be holding tanks for food. The modern American supermarket is a cultural center, a form of entertainment, and a masterpiece in marketing.

Supermarket chains do care about nutrition—to the extent that it sells. For fundamentally, these stores are about selling food. Literally billions of dollars are spent each year in designing supermarket aisles to take advantage of every selling opportunity. The goal of the selling game is simple: to see that people leave the store with more items in their bag than they had on their list when they entered.

Every single item in the supermarket has a reason for being placed on a particular shelf, along a certain aisle, and at a certain height. Among the dozens of selling techniques that are used are:

▶ End-of-aisle displays for on-sale or featured products (which don't necessarily constitute better values than similar products)

▶ "Dumps," which are freestanding displays that feature new or special products

▶ Holiday and seasonal displays, often combining a variety of products

▶ Tasting islands, with free food samples

▶ Cross-merchandising displays that put together complementary products in an attractive way

▶ Shelf signs directing you to sale items, contests, two-for-ones, and other values

▶ Checkout aisle and counter displays for high-impulse items

Modern technology allows stores to track the sales performance of each product, by scanning for the Universal Product Code (UPC) when you make a purchase. A product that can't hold its own in the store doesn't remain on the shelf for long, since supermarketing is, in the first instance, a game of economics. The more clout a manufacturer has, the more display space their products are allotted; many supermarket suppliers pay millions of dollars per year in "retail display allowances"—a way to buy into more space and better locations.

Knowing a little about the marketing orientation of today's supermarket will help you be a smarter shopper. If you approach supermarket shopping defensively, you're more likely to make the best food choices—including the most nutritious ones. In the next chapter, we'll describe how product manufacturers have joined the marketing bandwagon by including many misleading nutritional claims on their products.

Customers Demand Nutrition and Quality

While dazzling displays, price incentives, free samples, and other marketing gimmicks are designed to get consumers to buy more, today's supermarket shopper is by no means always starstruck by gimmicks. On the contrary, consumers are more sophisticated than ever, and they're not easily swayed by marketing. In its 1988 *Trends* report on consumer attitudes and the supermarket, the Food Marketing Institute (FMI) found that consumers rank their concern about product safety and nutrition above price, storability, and ease of preparation. (The only factor that scored higher was "taste."). Almost all shoppers (93 percent) say they are "very" or "somewhat" concerned with the nutritional content of food, particularly fat content, salt/sodium content, cholesterol levels, and vitamin/mineral content.

The FMI also reports that nearly two-thirds of shoppers frequently select foods to balance their families' diets and serve nutritional snacks, such as fruits and vegetables. More than half check labels for sodium content, and nearly half check labels for calorie, fat, and protein content. (It should be noted that, along with their legitimate

nutritional concerns, consumers surveyed frequently mention "preservatives" near the top of their health concern lists. As we discuss in chapter 13, preservatives should not necessarily be considered a health concern.)

In its 1988 marketplace report, the Board on Agriculture of the National Research Council, using industry sales figures from 1985 (the most current period for which figures were available) demonstrated how supermarket buying habits have taken a turn toward nutrition. The report cited these examples:

▶ Sales of calorie- and portion-controlled frozen dinners hit an all-time high of $232 million, accounting for one-third of all frozen-food sales.

▶ Sales of dietetic and low-calorie sauces and dressings increased by nearly 10.5 percent.

▶ Sales of salt substitutes and low-sodium salt products increased by 9 percent.

▶ The food categories with the largest sales increases included fresh and frozen poultry, fresh fruits and vegetables, fresh fish and seafood, and yogurt.

▶ The food categories with the largest sales declines included fresh and frozen beef, sugar, natural cheese, fresh and cured ham and pork, and bacon.

At the other end of the spectrum, the committee observed a phenomenon that one expert referred to as "the workout/pigout paradox." That is, the phenomenal growth in popularity of what they term super-premium foods—high-cost, high-fat, and high-calorie. For example, sales of super-premium ice-cream products like Dove Bars and Haagen Dazs ice cream (both loaded with butterfat) increased by 20 percent.

Supermarkets Get Healthy

To a large degree, the nation's supermarket chains are attempting to respond to their nutrition-conscious public. One important way this response is being demonstrated is in consumer education. Chains like Xtra Super Food Centers (Florida), Giant Foods, Inc. (Washington, D.C.), A & P Stores (New Jersey) and Stop & Shop (New England), have instituted shelf-labeling programs to alert consumers to foods that are low in calories, sodium, cholesterol, and fat.

Manufacturers are getting involved, too. One effective program, jointly sponsored by the National Livestock and Meat Board and the Food Marketing Institute, provides point-of-purchase information on the nutritional makeup of various cuts of meat, along with suggestions for preparation and cooking. And the National Dairy Board sponsors a calcium education program that includes booklets keyed to different age groups, with information about specific dairy products.

These are positive signs that nutrition is gradually becoming an integral part of the food shopping experience. But the primary responsibility for filling the shopping cart with the best variety of healthy foods still rests with the customer. The following sections provide practical advice and information that will make that task easier.

Begin with a Good List

Your shopping trip will be more nutritionally effective if you use a little creativity in creating your shopping list.

First, set it up by category. For efficiency, the categories should follow the layout of your supermarket. Place your list in a handy location, so you can add items as you notice you need them.

When you create menus for the week, keep your list nearby and write down the ingredients you'll need. On your shopping list, these ingredients should appear in the form in which you'll actually be buying them. For example, if a recipe calls for two cups of milk, write "one quart" on the list.

If you have trouble keeping track of the best nutritional selections while you're shopping, include the information right on your list. You might want to create a symbol system to remind yourself about the nutritional characteristics you're looking for in certain foods. For instance, dairy foods might be checked for fat and cholesterol, breads for fiber, and sauces for sugar and sodium. If you know that certain brands meet your nutritional standards, write the brand names on your list.

Tip Sheets for Smart Shoppers

Dairy Products

NUTRITIONAL BENEFITS

Milk products are excellent sources of protein, calcium, the B vitamins, and vitamin A. Low-fat milk is usually fortified with A (since fat-soluble vitamins are lost in the defatting process), and most milk is fortified with vitamin D (which aids the absorption of calcium). According to government figures, milk and milk products account for more than 75% of the calcium available in our food supply. Calcium intake is considered to be one of the major factors in the prevention of osteoporosis (the loss of bone mass that most commonly afflicts postmenopausal women). One cup of low-fat (1%) milk contains 300 milligrams of calcium.

NUTRITIONAL CAUTIONS

Whole-milk dairy products are high in saturated fat, a problem for those concerned with cholesterol levels. The high fat content shows up in the calorie total, too. For example, 8 ounces of low-fat (1%) milk has 100 calories, compared with 150 calories for whole milk. Hard cheeses such as cheddar, made from whole milk, typically contain

How Americans Use Milk Products

According to the 1988 report of the Board on Agriculture of the National Research Council, Americans have gradually changed their consumption habits for milk products during the past twenty years.

Product	1965 (in pounds)	1985 (in pounds)
Whole milk	236.5	116.5
Low-fat milk	10.9	85.0
Skim milk	12.6	13.0
Butter	6.4	5.1
Whole-milk cheese	9.6	22.4
Cottage cheese	4.7	4.1
Yogurt	0.3	4.0

Sources: Adapted from K. Bunch & G. Simon, eds., 1985 "Food Consumption, Prices and Expenditures, 1964–1984"; Statistical Bulletin 736, Economic Research Service, USDA.

more saturated fat than meat products. Cheeses made from skim milk have less fat; the leanest are cottage cheeses made with 1% fat.

Fortunately, there are low-fat substitutes for nearly all high-fat dairy products, and these are becoming the staples of the average household. (Per capita sales of low-fat milk increased more than 680 percent in the twenty year period from 1965 to 1985.)

SHOPPING TIPS

▶ Check the labels on low-fat and skim milk to be sure they have been fortified with vitamins A and D. These fat-soluble vitamins are lost in the defatting process.

▶ If you're eliminating cream in order to cut your fat intake, don't use nondairy substitutes. They're frequently made with palm and coconut oils, both high in saturated fat. Nonfat dry milk or 1% liquid skim milk are acceptable alternatives.

▶ If milk cartons are stacked in the display case, select the ones near the bottom. Those on top may not be getting cooled properly. Always check the "sell by" date on the carton.

▶ Buy milk right before you're ready to pay. The less time it remains unrefrigerated, the better.

▶ Flavored yogurts, such as vanilla or coffee, contain some sugar, and the fruit-filled brands contain even more. They also have more calories, up to 250. You're better off buying plain yogurt and adding your own fruit and flavorings. The chart on p. 105 shows the nutritional variables in the most popular yogurt brands.

BEST CHOICES

MILK

skim milk (no fat)

low-fat (1%)

buttermilk

COMPARE YOUR FAVORITE YOGURT BRANDS

Brand	Calories	Fat Calories (%)	Brand	Calories	Fat Calories (%)
Breyers, 8 oz.			Hearty Nuts & Raisins,	260	10
Plain	190	38	Mixed Berries,		
Blueberry	260	21	Orchard Fruit		
Strawberry	270	17	Vanilla	270	17
Vanilla Bean	230	27	Original (all)	240	11
Brown Cow Farm, 8 oz.			**Dannon Nonfat, 8 oz.**		
Plain	190	52	Plain	110	0
Blueberry	230	31	**Light n' Lively Lowfat, 8 oz.**		
Raspberry, Strawberry	223	32	Red Raspberry	230	8
Vanilla	250	36	Strawberry	240	8
Brown Cow Farm, Lowfat, 6 oz.			**Weight Watchers Nonfat**		
Plain	94	19	Plain, 8 oz.	90	*
Blueberry	133	14	Flavored, 8 oz.	150	*
Strawberry	129	14	A la Francais, 6 oz.	150	*
Vanilla	125	14	**Whitney's, 6 oz.**		
Columbo, 8 oz.			Plain	150	42
Plain, farm-style	180	45	Fruit, most flavors	200	23
Plain, regular	150	42	Coffee, Lemon, Vanilla	200	27
Blueberry, Raspberry	230	23	**Yoplait, 6 oz.**		
French Vanilla	215	29			
Columbo, Nonfat Lite, 8 oz.			*Breakfast-style*		
Plain	110	*	Berries	230	16
Fruit, all flavors	190	*	Strawberry-Banana	240	15
Vanilla	160	*	*Custard-style*		
Dannon, Lowfat, 8 oz.			Fruit, most flavors	190	19
Plain	140	26	*Original*		
Fresh Fruit Flavors (all)	200	18	Fruit, all flavors	190	14
Coffee, Lemon, Vanilla	200	14	**Yoplait 150 Nonfat, 6 oz.**	150	*

* Contains less than 1 gram (fewer than 9 calories) of fat

COTTAGE CHEESE

low-fat

dry-curd

YOGURT

low-fat, plain

nonfat, plain

Eggs

NUTRITIONAL BENEFITS

Eggs are a good source of high quality protein, as well as a good source of vitamin A and several other micronutrients.

COMPARE THE CHEESE CHOICES

	Calories	Fat (g)	Sodium (mg)		Calories	Fat (g)	Sodium (mg)
American (1 oz.)				Philadelphia Light Neufchatel (Kraft)	80	7	115
Deluxe Pasteurized Process Cheese (Kraft)	110	9	460	Philadelphia Light Pasteurized Process Cream Cheese Product (Kraft)	60	5	160
Lite-Line Pasteurized Process Cheese Product (Borden)	50	2	410	**Mozzarella (1 oz.)**			
Low Sodium Pasteurized Process Cheese Product (Weight Watchers)	50	2	140	Low Moisture Part Skim Mozzarella (Deli-Light)	80	5	90
Pasteurized Process Cheese Product (Weight Watchers)	45	2	400	Whole-milk mozzarella	80	6	68
Singles Pasteurized Process Cheese Food (Kraft)	90	7	390	**Muenster (1 oz.)**			
				Light Imitation Low-Cholesterol Low-Sodium Cheese (Dorman's)	90	7	90
Velveeta Pasteurized Process Cheese Spread Slices (Kraft)	80	6	430	100% Natural Muenster (Kraft)	100	9	180
Cheddar (1 oz.)				**Ricotta (½ cup)**			
Cracker Barrel Sharp Cheddar Cheese (Kraft)	110	9	175	Part-Skim Milk Ricotta (Sorrentino)	170	12	100
Light Natural Reduced Fat Cheddar Cheese (Kraft)	80	5	200	Whole Milk Ricotta (Sorrentino)	200	14	56
Light Vitalait Cheese (Cabot)	70	5	170	**Spreads (1 oz.)**			
Natural Part-Skim Milk Cheese (Weight Watchers)	80	5	150	Cheez Whiz Pasteurized Process Cheese Spread (Kraft)	80	6	470
Cottage (½ cup)				Laughing Cow Pasteurized Process Cheese Spread (Bel)	70	6	310
Cottage Cheese, 4% fat (Hood)	120	5	410	Laughing Cow Reduced Calorie Wedges (Bel)	50	3	310
Dry Curd Cottage Cheese (Breakstone)	90	0	65	**Swiss (1 oz.)**			
Lite Lowfat Cottage Cheese (Cabot)	90	1	460	Light No-Salt-Added Swiss (Dorman's)	100	8	8
Creamy Cheeses (1 oz.)				Swiss Pasteurized Process Cheese Product (Weight Watchers)	50	2	400
Farmer cheese	40	3	70	100% Natural Swiss (Kraft)	110	8	40
Philadelphia Cream Cheese (Kraft)	100	10	105				

NUTRITIONAL CAUTIONS

Eggs are extremely high in cholesterol. One egg contains about 213 milligrams, more than half the limit suggested for one day. (Since the cholesterol is all in the egg yolk, the whites can be used for cooking without adding cholesterol.)

According to recent studies, raw eggs have been known to cause salmonella poisoning, and you can't be 100 percent certain of avoiding this risk. To protect yourself, avoid eating raw eggs. Be sure that the eggs you buy are not cracked or dirty. If the white is thin and runny and the yolk does not hold together when you crack the egg, it may not be perfectly fresh.

SHOPPING TIPS

▶ If you notice cartons of eggs sitting in the supermarket aisle, waiting to be shelved, do not buy them from that store. Eggs can easily spoil if they're left unrefrigerated.

▶ Always open the egg carton and take a look before you put it in your cart. Check for cleanliness and wholeness; if even one egg is cracked, select a new carton.

▶ If eggs aren't on your list because of their cholesterol content, you might want to try one of the cholesterol-free egg substitutes, usually located in the frozen-food section.

Beef and Poultry

NUTRITIONAL BENEFITS

Meat and poultry are the highest quality sources of protein available, and meat is also a good source of iron and the B vitamins.

Shifting to leaner cuts of beef can yield many benefits, including a higher concentration of the B vitamins, iron, phosphorus, and zinc. For example, the riboflavin and iron content in 100 grams of beef ranges from about 10 to 20 percent of the RDA, with increased concentration in the leaner cuts.

Poultry is a high-quality protein source that is leaner than beef, especially if the skin is removed before cooking. For example, a chicken breast without the skin is only 131 calories, with 6 grams of fat and 64 milligrams of dietary cholesterol. While the cholesterol total does not change when the skin is added, the fat total nearly doubles and the number of calories shoots up to 229.

NUTRITIONAL CAUTIONS

Because certain cuts are very high in fat (and calories), beef can be a nutritionally expensive way to get your protein if you don't stick with lean cuts. In a study by the USDA, beef was found to be the primary source of fat for most age and sex groups, particularly adult males. Many Americans should probably cut their beef intake, and all should be conscious of selecting leaner cuts and trimming visible fat. Like all organ meats, liver is high in cholesterol, although it is a very good source of iron and vitamins.

Beware of meat labeling on ground hamburger, since "lean" can mean different things at different stores. You might want to discuss with your butcher how meat is labeled. Most meat departments label according to weight, so a cut that says "85% lean meat" might actually contain more than 50 percent fat calories.

SHOPPING TIPS

▶ Examine meat for visible fat, including marbling, the thin white streaks of fat that run throughout the meat. Choose those that have the least.

▶ Check the "sell by" date to see how fresh the meat is. Hold the package to your nose and smell. It is easy to judge freshness by smell. If you think it smells "funny," but aren't sure, choose another package.

Know the meaning of the grades that are assigned to meat cuts at the slaughterhouse, according to USDA guidelines. Grades are assigned on the basis of fat content and texture. They are: *Prime* (usually has the most fat and is also the most tender); *Choice* (moderately fatty and

Chicken Versus Beef

Chicken, Roasted (no skin)		Ground Beef, Broiled (17% fat by weight)	
Serving:	1.5 oz.	Serving:	1.5 oz.
Calories	70	Calories	115
Protein	13.5 g	Protein:	11.5 g
Fat:	1.5 g	Fat:	7.5 g
Calories from fat:	19%	Calories from fat:	59%
Sodium:	27 mg	Sodium:	31.5 mg

tender; the grade most commonly sold in supermarkets—94 percent of the beef graded by the USDA is graded "choice"); and *Select* (lean).

Memorize the grading terms. They tend to be misleading and often cause consumer confusion. In a national study published in 1987, *Farm Journal* asked consumers to identify which grade of beef had the least amount of fat: 56 percent said Prime! Examples of the difference: A cut of chuck blade from the Select grade, braised, has 13 percent less total fat and saturated fatty acids and 7 percent fewer calories than a Choice cut of chuck. A Select grade indicates that the cut is almost 20 percent lower in calories and has only two-thirds the fat and saturated fatty acids of a Prime cut.

In addition, the Agriculture Department now permits beef with 10 percent fat or less to be called *lean* or *low-fat,* and beef with 5 percent fat to be called *extra-lean.* Watch for these cuts in the supermarket meat case.

▶ If you can afford it, choose ground round instead of ground chuck, or ask the butcher to grind the meat for you from the round cut of the beef.

▶ Look for labeling that gives the percentage of fat-to-lean. Remember, terms indicating leanness can vary from store to store, so even if the label says "lean," the cut may actually contain more fat than say, a select-graded meat. If you're not sure, discuss the differences with your butcher.

▶ Self-basting turkeys are often injected with oils high in saturated fat. You might be better off creating your own basting liquid with polyunsaturated oils or margarine.

▶ Since meat spoils easily, don't buy portions that are wrapped in damaged containers, with broken wrap or crushed plastic.

BEST CHOICES

BEEF

lean round

lean shoulder

lean rump

lean sirloin tips

ground round

veal (cuts with no visible fat)

LAMB

leg

PORK

center cut ham (high in sodium)

loin chops

pork tenderloin

POULTRY
chicken broiler
turkey (not self-basting)
cornish game hen

Processed Meats

NUTRITIONAL CAUTIONS
While processed meats have plenty of convenience benefits, they really don't have any sterling qualities nutritionally. On average, they provide only about half the protein value of nonprocessed meats and are very high in fat and sodium.

SHOPPING TIPS
If you do buy processed meats occasionally, some varieties are better than others, particularly lean brands of turkey and ham. Incidentally, government regulations require that meat products designated as "light," "lite," "leaner," or "lower fat" must have at least 25 percent less fat than a comparable product. Foods labeled "light" or "lite" may also have less sodium, calories, or filler than a comparable product. Compare the labels.

Most packaged meats wouldn't be recommended for a person watching calorie, cholesterol, sodium, or saturated fat content. However, some are definitely better than others. For example, a slice of Oscar Meyer bologna fashioned from beef and pork has about 90 calories, with 72 of them from fat, and 300 milligrams of sodium. On the other hand, a slice of Oscar Meyer smoked turkey breast has only about 20 calories, with half of them from fat, and 290 milligrams of sodium.

Turkey has found its way into the cold-cut section, providing a low-fat, low-calorie substitute for everything from bologna to salami to ham to hot dogs. If you buy any of these products, look for the turkey version. It will save you fat, calories, and sometimes sodium.

Fish and Shellfish

NUTRITIONAL BENEFITS
Fish and shellfish are excellent sources of high-quality protein, as well as several vitamins and minerals. Fish is low in fat, but even the fattier varieties may provide a benefit because they contain omega-3 fatty acids.

For a long time, shellfish were crossed off many shoppers' lists because of their relatively high cholesterol content. But recent data suggests that this should not be of great concern. First, what researchers formerly took to be cholesterol in mollusks (clams, oysters, mussels, scallops, and squid) is really a composite of several different kinds of sterols, and these noncholesterol sterols may actually inhibit cholesterol absorption. Even the cholesterol in crustaceans (crab, shrimp, lobster, crayfish) is very low. For example, a 1½ pound Maine lobster contains only about 140 milligrams, and Alaska king crab contains a scant 42 milligrams per 3½ ounce serving. Add the benefits of low calories and fat, and shellfish can be considered a very nutritious main course.

Nutrition Note: Kosher Meat

Kosher meat is determined by the method of slaughter. Rather than the usual method (which involves blood being spilled), the kosher technique involves drawing the blood from the animal through a salting process. For this reason, kosher meats have a much higher sodium content than nonkosher meats. Small amounts of sodium can be removed by soaking beef in water for an hour or so; this method is ineffective for chicken.

CHOOSING THE LEANEST MEATS AND POULTRY

Meat (3 oz. cooked)	Calories	Fat (%)	Cholesterol (mg)	Protein (% RDA)
sirloin tip roast, trimmed of fat	156	33	69	38
top loin steak, trimmed of fat	163	36	65	38
ground chuck	240	57	87	37
lamb chop, loin cut	184	41	81	40
leg of lamb, sirloin	175	41	79	38
veal chop, loin cut	192	36	135	44
veal cutlet, round cut	150	37	112	34
chicken breast, trimmed of skin	131	24	64	36
ham	191	26	*	51
pork tenderloin	142	26	78	38

* Figures not available

NUTRITIONAL CAUTIONS

Certain fish preparations are high in sodium. Salted, dried, and smoked fish such as smoked salmon and dried, salted mackerel should be avoided by those concerned with sodium levels. Pickled fish, such as pickled herring, may be high in both sodium and calories, especially if it is in a creamed sauce.

Caviar is a rich fish food prepared by mixing the black, gray, or golden eggs of sturgeon with salt. A one-ounce serving (one rounded tablespoon) contains almost 72 calories, nearly two-thirds of them fat. It also contains more than 400 milligrams of sodium and about 170 milligrams of cholesterol.

A composite crab substitute product called surimi is commonly sold in supermarkets as an inexpensive substitute for crab. Surimi has mixed reviews from a nutritional standpoint. While it has low levels of fat and cholesterol, it can contain up to eight times the sodium found in raw shellfish as a result of added salt and MSG. At present, surimi is the subject of major research and testing to guarantee levels of quality. Ultimately, surimi could become a top-of-the-line processed food.

Many people are currently concerned about the condition of our waters, particularly fresh-water outlets near major industrial areas. Yet incidents of contamination from fish have been rare; most reports have involved mollusks and shellfish eaten raw. Proper refrigeration before cooking and thorough cooking eliminates most of the potential danger. Popular wisdom suggests eating raw mollusks and shellfish only during cold weather months, when the water temperature falls and there is less chance of bacteria. There may be some truth to this, but there's no guarantee that raw mollusks and shellfish will be without infection, regardless of the season.

SHOPPING TIPS

▶ The best way for fish to be sold is inside glass cases, unwrapped on ice. If you can, buy from markets that display it this way, rather than purchase the prewrapped fish that is located at one end of the meat counter in most supermarkets.

▶ Don't buy prewrapped fresh or frozen fish if there are any breakages in the package.

▶ Smell fish before you buy it. If fish is fresh, it won't smell "fishy."

▶ When buying a whole fish, check for yellowing along the cut line, which indicates deterioration. A fresh whole fish will have bulging eyes, firm flesh, and a light, almost translucent, color.

▶ When you buy fresh lobster and crab, buy only live ones. Since bacteria forms very quickly, it's always best to eat these fish as soon as possible after they're cooked.

▶ Use caution when buying prepared fish dishes from deli or gourmet departments. They are really only safe to eat on the day they're prepared. Never buy cooked fish if it's displayed next to raw fish, since bacteria can be transferred from the raw to the cooked.

BEST CHOICES
The difference between lean and fatty fish is a matter of a few calories. All of these varieties are good choices nutritionally.

LEAN	*MOLLUSKS*
cod	abalone
flounder	clams
haddock	cuttlefish
monkfish	blue mussels
sea bass	oysters
pike	scallops
whiting	squid

MODERATELY LEAN	*CRUSTACEANS*
bluefin	crab
tuna	crayfish
halibut	lobster
mullet	shrimp
red snapper	
swordfish	

FATTIER
salmon
albacore tuna
mackerel
bluefish
herring
shad
trout

Canned Fish

NUTRITIONAL INFORMATION
Canned sardines, tuna, and salmon can nutritionally enhance your diet if you take certain precautions. Sardines and salmon canned with soft, edible bones are a good source of calcium. Three ounces of unboned sardines contain 371 milligrams of calcium, and 3 ounces of unboned salmon contain 167 milligrams of calcium.

Canned tuna is a staple of many American diets, but canning in oil increases the total fat content by 200 to 500 percent compared with canning in water.

SHOPPING TIPS

▶ Canned tuna labeled "white" is made only from the albacore species and is flakier and less fishy-tasting than "light" tuna, which can come from a variety of species. The word "light," in this case, has no nutritional significance. It simply refers to color.

▶ The difference between oil-packed and water-packed tuna is roughly the following: A 3½ ounce serving of oil-packed tuna contains about 300 calories and 20 grams of fat; the same serving of drained oil-packed tuna has about 200 calories and 8 grams of fat. A 3½ ounce serving of water-packed tuna has 131 calories and only about ½ gram of fat.

▶ Canned fish is generally high in sodium: a 3½ ounce serving of tuna can contain more than 600 milligrams. Some of the sodium can be washed away by rinsing the tuna, and many companies are now selling low-sodium canned fish.

▶ Boneless canned salmon doesn't have the calcium benefits of salmon with bones.

▶ Deeper-colored salmons are highest in fat and contain more omega-3 fatty acids and calories. Chinook, or king salmon, is the most oily; pink salmon is paler and has less oil; chum is the least oily. (Prices usually correspond to the oil content, with Chinook being the most costly, chum the least.

Fresh Fruit

NUTRITIONAL BENEFITS

Fruit is low in calories and sodium, high in carbohydrates and fiber, and a good source of some essential nutrients—particularly vitamins A and C and potassium. Since Vitamin C enhances the absorption of iron, it can also boost the benefits of iron intake from other foods.

NUTRITIONAL CAUTIONS

Dried fruits are higher in calories because they contain less water and are more concentrated. For example, 10 dates contain 200 calories, so, if you're watching calories, you may choose to get your potassium and iron elsewhere. Avocados are high in fat, even though it is unsaturated, and calories: one avocado contains about 300 calories. Since avocados supply only small amounts of vitamins A and C, the B vitamins, and potassium, you might want to limit your intake.

FRESH FRUIT SHOPPING GUIDE

Fruit	Best Season	Nutrients	Fruit	Best Season	Nutrients
apples	year-round	good fiber; some potassium	limes	year-round	excellent vitamin C
apricots	late spring to midsummer	excellent vitamin A	mangoes	late spring–summer	excellent vitamin A; some potassium, folic acid
bananas	year-round	excellent potassium; some vitamin A	nectarines	July–August	vitamin A, potassium; some vitamin C
blueberries	July–August	vitamin C, iron, fiber			
cantaloupe	summer	excellent vitamins A and C, potassium	oranges	autumn–spring	excellent vitamin C, potassium, folic acid
cherries	June–July	vitamins A and C	peaches	summer–early fall	vitamin A; some potassium
figs	summer–early autumn	excellent fiber, potassium; some iron	pears	late summer–winter	potassium, fiber
grapefruit	year-round	excellent vitamin C, potassium, good vitamin A (pink)	pineapples	year-round	good vitamin C
			plums	summer	vitamin A, some fiber
			raspberries	summer	good vitamin C, folic acid
grapes	year-round	fiber			
honeydew melon	summer–early autumn	good vitamin C, potassium	strawberries	late spring	excellent vitamin C; some potassium, folic acid
kiwifruit	spring–autumn	excellent vitamin C	tangerines	early winter	excellent vitamin C; some vitamin A
kumquats	winter	good vitamin C; some potassium			
lemons	year-round	excellent vitamin C	watermelon	late spring–summer	vitamins A and C

SHOPPING TIPS

▶ For most fresh fruit, a week is the upper limit for storage before it begins to spoil. Buy fruit only in quantities you can easily consume.

▶ Many fruits—such as bananas, pears, peaches, and plums—might not be quite ripe when you buy them. Allow them to ripen naturally by keeping them at room temperature.

▶ Vitamins A and C are easily destroyed in storage; eat your A- and C-rich fruits right away to get the most out of them.

▶ If possible, pick berries and cherries from a bin, rather than buying them in prewrapped packages that don't allow examination.

Canned/Frozen Fruit

NUTRITIONAL INFORMATION

Canned or frozen fruit can be used as a substitute for out-of-season fresh varieties. Frozen is usually preferable, since canned fruits sometimes contain added sugar or sugary liquids. Generally, those that don't will be labeled "unsweetened," "packed in its own juices," or "packed in fruit juice."

Fresh Vegetables

NUTRITIONAL BENEFITS

A satisfying variety of fresh vegetables is available year-round in the supermarket. Most vegetables

---

BUY FRUITS AT THEIR BEST

How do you know what to look for when you're examining fruit for quality? Follow these general guidelines to choose top-notch fresh fruits:

Fruit	Look For	Fruit	Look For
apples	strong color, firm texture, no bruises or soft spots	mangoes	orange-yellow to red skin, barely soft
apricots	golden yellow, plump, and firm; avoid if soft to the touch or wilted	nectarines	firm, slightly unripened; avoid if hard, dull, or shriveled
bananas	firm, not fully yellow	oranges	heavy, for their size (indicates juiciness), firm, with relatively smooth (not spongy) surface
blueberries	plump with strong color, no signs of mold		
cantaloupe	no stem, coarse skin, slightly soft, fresh odor	peaches	fairly firm—just a bit soft
cherries	fresh stems, plump, bright, rich color	pears	firm, but not hard; avoid if shriveled near the stem
grapefruit	heavy for their size (indicates juiciness)	pineapples	heavy for their size (indicates juiciness); deep green, fresh-looking leaves; fragrant aroma; flat, almost hollow "eyes"
grapes	rich color, plump, firmly attached to stem		
honeydew melon	creamy white surface with waxy texture	plums	slight shine, good color, barely soft to the touch
kiwifruit	hard texture indicates they're not ready to eat; ripe kiwifruit is just barely soft	raspberries	rich, scarlet color, plump, cool, dry, free from mold or bruises
		strawberries	bright red color, green caps in place, no signs of mold
lemons	heavy for their size (indicates juiciness), rich yellow color, relatively smooth	tangerines	strong, bright color, heavy for their size (indicates juiciness)
limes	heavy for their size (indicates juiciness), shiny skin	watermelon	smooth surface, filled-out shape, dull green color

How Well Do You Know Your Fruit?

1. What is the best-selling fruit in the United States year after year?

2. What popular "vegetable" is really fruit?

3. What is a drupe? Can you name three?

4. Name three fruits that are native to the continental United States.

5. Name six citrus fruits. Why are they such an important part of the American diet?

6. What popular fruit is actually an herb?

7. Can you tell if a watermelon is ripe by thumping it? By looking at the color of the rind?

8. Name a fruit—other than avocado—that is high in fat.

9. What noncitrus fruit contains more than 100 percent of the USRDA for vitamin C?

ANSWERS

1. Bananas—Over 5 billion pounds are sold each year, an average of 22.5 pounds per person.

2. The tomato—It is really the "blossom," or fruit, of the plant. Tomatos are a fair source of vitamin C and also provide vitamin A.

3. A drupe is a fruit that has a large pod or seed in the center with fleshy pulp surrounding it—Three examples are apricots, plums, and peaches.

4. Cranberries, blueberries, and concord grapes come from the continental United States—Other than these three (and some minor berries), the fruits that Americans consume were originally imported from Central and South America, Asia, and Europe.

5. Orange, lemon, lime, grapefruit, tangerine, and ugli fruit (a hybrid of a grapefruit and tangerine)—Citrus fruits are a major source of vitamin C.

6. The pineapple is an herb, or edible leaf—When a pineapple fruit is picked, another seed-leaf grows. The process is repeated time and again during the 50-year life span of the typical pineapple plant.

7. No and no—The only sure way to know if a watermelon is ripe is to see that the pulp is a rich red and the seeds are dark brown and black. Thus, it's better to buy a watermelon that has already been cut, even if it's a little more expensive.

8. The coconut—A cup of coconut milk has about twice as much as the amount in a quart of whole milk.

9. The kiwifruit—It is only about the size of a large egg, but it has almost twice as much vitamin C as several varieties of orange.

are low in calories and many are excellent sources of essential nutrients, including fiber, vitamins A and C, potassium, calcium, and iron.

NUTRITIONAL CAUTIONS

Vegetables easily lose their nutritional punch. To insure that the nutrients aren't lost in the cooking process, follow the preparation and cooking guidelines in chapter 9.

SHOPPING TIPS

▶ Try to purchase fresh vegetables at least twice a week to assure that you get the freshest available. The fresher the vegetables, the more nutrients are available to you.

▶ Avoid the precut vegetables many markets sell. They may be convenient, but more nutrients are preserved when you cut vegetables yourself, shortly before use.

▶ In general, the darker the vegetable, the better it is nutritionally. For example, pale, small carrots have far less vitamin A activity than mature, bright-orange carrots. Dark-green leafy vegetables, like spinach and leaf lettuce, are better nutritionally than light greens, like iceberg lettuce.

▶ Sometimes vegetables are marked for sale because they are old or damaged. After produce has been sitting around unrefrigerated for a few day, levels of vitamins A and C drop substantially.

▶ Check vegetables before you purchase them to be sure they don't have bruises or soft spots. Soft spots and bruises may harbor harmful bacteria.

Canned/Frozen Vegetables

NUTRITIONAL INFORMATION

Canned and frozen vegetables can be good substitutes for fresh vegetables, providing almost the same nutritional value. They are a good substitute for out-of-season varieties. Overall, more nu-trients are preserved in freezing, since the water in canned vegetables tend to leach out some of the nutrients. Always check the labels on packaged vegetables, particularly canned; the sodium content is usually high. Beware the frozen varieties with added cream or cheese sauces; they're high in calories and fat.

Legumes (dried beans, peas, lentils)

NUTRITIONAL BENEFITS

Legumes are excellent nutritional bargains. Their high protein content makes them a healthy substitute for meat, and they have the added advantage of being high in fiber. Legumes also supply essential minerals and vitamins, including iron, zinc, magnesium, phosphorus, thiamin, and niacin, as well as vitamin B-6. And legumes are a good source of complex carbohydrates.

NUTRITIONAL CAUTIONS

By themselves, legume proteins are considered "incomplete" in that they lack certain amino acids the body needs to get from food. If they are frequently used as a meat substitute, legumes must be supplemented with other products that will "complete" the protein. Rice, whole grains, wheat, some nuts, and seeds are rich in the two amino acids that legumes lack.

Some people find legumes difficult to digest, which leads to intestinal flatulence (gas). Lentils, split peas, and lima beans are the most easily digestible. Introduce legumes gradually into your diet so your intestines can adapt to them, and follow the cooking tips suggested in chapter 9.

Tofu, or bean curd, is one of the highest protein vegetable foods (only slightly low in one of the essential amino acids), and it has the added advantage of being very low in calories. Tofu is made by mixing soybean milk with a mineral stabilizing agent—the process is not unlike that used to make cheese. While tofu's taste and texture don't lend to its being a stand-alone food, it is often used to supplement other foods. Tofu has no taste of its own so it picks up the flavor of the

FRESH VEGETABLE SHOPPING GUIDE

Vegetable	Best Season	Nutrients	Vegetable	Best Season	Nutrients
artichoke	spring	fiber, potassium, folic acid	lettuce (romaine or other dark, leafy variety)	year-round	vitamins A and C, folic acid, iron, calcium
asparagus	spring	vitamins A and C, niacin, folic acid, potassium, iron			
beens (green)	late spring–summer	fiber, vitamin A, potassium; some protein, vitamin C, calcium	mushrooms	year-round	potassium, niacin, riboflavin
			onions	year-round	minor source of nutrients
beets	year-round	potassium, folic acid	peas (green)	spring–early summer	fiber, vitamin A, protein, potassium, B vitamins
broccoli	year-round	calcium, potassium, iron, vitamins A and C, fiber, folic acid, niacin	peppers (sweet)	year-round	vitamins A and C, fiber, potassium
Brussels sprouts	autumn–winter	fiber, vitamins A and C, folic acid, potassium, iron, protein	potatoes	year-round	protein, vitamins B and C, potassium
			spinach	year-round	iron, vitamin A, fiber, potassium; some vitamin C, protein
cabbage	year-round	vitamin C, fiber, potassium, folic acid			
			squash (summer)	year-round	fiber, potassium, vitamins A and C, niacin
carrots	year-round	vitamin A, potassium			
cauliflower	year-round	fiber, vitamin C, folic acid, potassium; some protein, iron	squash (winter)	year-round	fiber, vitamin A, niacin, potassium, iron, protein
celery	year-round	potassium	sweet potatoes	year-round	vitamin A; some protein, fiber
corn	late spring–summer	vitamin A (yellow), potassium, protein	tomatoes	late spring–summer	vitamin C, iron, protein
cucumbers	year-round	minor source of nutrients			
eggplant	year-round	potassium			
greens	year-round	vitamins A and C, fiber, iron, calcium, B vitamins			

BUY VEGETABLES AT THEIR BEST

When you examine vegetables in the produce department for freshness and quality, follow these guidelines:

Vegetable	Look For	Vegetable	Look For
artichokes	olive green, plump, tightly attached greens	mushrooms	tightly closed "veil" (underside); cream-colored, white, or light brown; no bruises
asparagus	firm spears, compact tips; avoid if yellowing or if tips are flaking	onions	dry and firm (not mushy), no soft spots or cut
beans (green)	firm, fresh and bright color; avoid limp or overbulging jackets	peas (green)	firm, crisp pods with bright green color; avoid wilted or unfilled pods
beets	deep purple-red color, firm, smooth		
broccoli	dark color, tightly compacted clusters of buds, firm (not thick) stalks	peppers (sweet)	bright color (red, green, or yellow), no soft spots, relatively heavy for size
cabbage	heavy, solid head; strong color (green or red) on outer leaves	potatoes	well-shaped, relatively smooth; no eyes, sprouts, soft spots, or bruises
carrots	strong orange color, healthy-looking greens		
cauliflower	white or creamy-white clusters; solid, firm heads; fresh green leaves	spinach	dark-green color, crisp, smells like earth (not sour)
celery	thick, crisp, healthy stalks; avoid limp, bruised, or cracked stalks	squash (summer)	heavy for size, strong color, noncoarse skin
corn	healthy green husks; golden, smooth silk ends	squash (winter)	heavy for size, tough rind, stems attached
eggplant	heavy for size, rich dark-purple color	sweet potatoes	even skin color, firm; avoid if bruised, discolored, or cut
greens	crisp green leaves, small stems		
lettuce (romaine or another dark, leafy variety)	bright color; crisp texture for romaine, otherwise tender; avoid brown-edged leaves and stems and brown ribs	tomatoes	heavy for size, plump, firm, strong color, fresh smell.

ingredients with which it is mixed, making it ideal for soups, casseroles, dips, and salads.

SHOPPING TIPS

▶ To insure freshness, look for legumes with a bright color. Faded color indicates that they've been in storage too long.

▶ Cracks, pinhole marks, and discolorations are signs that the legumes may be less than fresh and may even be decaying.

▶ Buy legumes that are uniform in size and shape. They'll cook more evenly.

▶ Inspect the bag legumes are sold in to be sure there are no cracks or tears. Exposure enhances decay.

▶ Tofu is best when it's purchased fresh out of a container of chilled water. You'll know it's fresh if it has a smooth texture and is odorless

Bread

NUTRITIONAL BENEFITS

Fiber-poor "white" bread is still the most common type sold in supermarkets (accounting for more than 60 percent of all bread sales). Whole

LEGUME SHOPPING GUIDE

Legume	Description	Common Uses
black beans	small, round, black	soups; main course with rice
black-eyed peas	small, round, off-white with small black "eye"	main course with rice
chick peas (garbanzos)	coarse, round, hard, tan	additions for salads and stews; base for Middle Eastern hummus
kidney beans	large, deep-red, kidney-shaped	chili, hearty soups, three-bean salad
lentils	small, round, flat, brown or red	soups, stews
lima beans	broad, flat, white	delicate flavor for soups and stews
pea (navy) beans	small, oval, white	soups, stews, baked beans
pinto beans	pink with brown dots	baked beans, soups, chili, salads, with rice
soybeans	small, round, hard, tan (highest protein content)	meat substitutions; ingredient in soups, salads, sauces, and casseroles

wheat, rye, and multigrain breads can be excellent sources of fiber. Bread that has been fortified with a variety of vitamins and minerals may still be low in fiber.

Wheat and whole-grain bread can be relatively good sources of fat-free protein, made complete by eating them in a meal with legumes.

NUTRITIONAL CAUTIONS

Almost without exception, white bread is low in fiber, since the refining process removes the bran (wheat's outer coating) and the germ (the kernel that is the seed of the new plant). As much as 90 percent of the fiber is lost with the removal of the germ and the bran.

SHOPPING TIPS

▶ Check the label to determine if you're getting a fiber-rich brand. If the bread contains 2 or more grams of fiber per slice, it's considered a good fiber source.

▶ Some brands are high on sodium. Check for levels above 700 milligrams per serving.

▶ Check the "sell by" date to be sure your choice is fresh.

BEST CHOICES

100 percent whole wheat

whole grain

multigrain

rye (check sodium)

oat

cracked wheat

stone ground

whole-wheat bagels

whole-wheat pita

whole-grain English muffins

corn tortillas

Cereal

NUTRITIONAL BENEFITS

Cereals can be one of our best sources of fiber, in addition to being fortified with a number of vitamins and minerals. The primary cereal grains in our diets are made from wheat, corn, oats, barley, rye, and rice. They contain approximately 70 to 80 percent complex carbohydrate (starch), 7 to

13 percent protein, and very little fat. The whole grain contains vitamins, especially B and E, and various minerals—plus whatever the manufacturer adds in fortification. (Some manufacturers will add nutrients not ordinarily found in cereals, including vitamins A, C, and D.)

Hot cereals, which are usually made from unrefined grains, are good sources of B vitamins, iron, zinc, and fiber.

Different fiber-containing cereals are composed of different parts of the cereal grain, making for variations in their nutritional content. Whole-grain cereals, for example, contain the fiber-rich bran portion of the grain as well as the germ, which contains vitamins and minerals. All-bran cereals, on the other hand, have the highest fiber concentration but lack the vitamin and mineral-packed germ and must depend largely on fortification.

NUTRITIONAL CAUTIONS

You may choose a fibrous, vitamin-and-mineral-packed cereal only to discover that it is heavily sugared and high in sodium. If you're trying to avoid sugar altogether, there are very few commercial brands that are totally sugar-free. But check the labels, because some use less sugar than others. (If you are in the habit of adding sugar to unsweetened cereals, you may find that some brands contain less than you might add but are quite satisfying.)

The fact that a cereal contains the entire RDA for certain vitamins and minerals does not necessarily guarantee that it is healthier than one that is less fortified. For one thing, chances are that you'll get these vitamins and minerals in other foods throughout the day, especially if you eat a variety. Also, the fortification lure can mask other problems with the cereal, such as a high sugar, sodium, or calorie count.

It is also important to realize that even high-fiber cereals do not supply all the fiber you need in a day. Moreover, it's best to get fiber from a variety of sources, including fruit, vegetables, beans, and whole-grain breads.

SHOPPING TIPS

▶ Watch out for granola-style cereals, which often contain fat because nuts and oils have been added. Many use palm or coconut oils, which are highly saturated.

▶ Stick to the information on the nutrition label for the facts about the cereal you're purchasing. Packaging terminology can be misleading. Remember: a claim that a product is sugar-free doesn't necessarily mean it contains no sweeteners.

▶ Check the serving size. For a dense cereal, such as granola, your 100-calorie serving may amount to only a couple of mouthfuls.

BEST CHOICES

whole-grain puffed wheat, corn, and rice
shredded wheat
whole-grain wheat, oat, and rice flakes
oatmeal
mixed-grain hot cereal

Pasta

NUTRITIONAL INFORMATION

Pasta is high in complex carbohydrates and can be a low-calorie, low-fat main course. It is high in protein and, when made from whole grains, it is a good source of fiber. Pasta is also a good source of the B vitamins and iron.

Since pasta is rarely eaten without some kind of sauce, the ultimate nutritional benefits usually depend on the topping. Vegetable-based sauces, like those made with tomatoes, green peppers, onions, and mushrooms, will enhance the final product. Cream-based sauces made with large amounts of butter and rich cheeses can turn your healthy pasta meal into one that is loaded with fat and calories.

FIBER CONTENT IN SOME POPULAR CEREALS

Cereal	Dietary Fiber (g)	Serving Amount (Cups)
Whole-grain cereal		
Nabisco Spoon Size Shredded Wheat	3.0	⅔
Kellogg's Nutri-Grain (Almond Raisin)	2.1	½
General Mills Total	2.0	1
General Mills Wheaties	2.0	1
Post Grape-Nuts Flakes	2.0	⅞
Quaker Old Fashioned Oats (cooked)	1.6	¾
Whole-grain cereal with added bran		
Post Natural Bran Flakes	5.0	⅔
Kellogg's Bran Flakes	4.0	⅔
Nabisco Shredded Wheat 'n Bran	4.0	⅔
Post Fruit & Fibre (all varieties)	4.0	½
Post Natural Raisin Bran	4.0	½
Kellogg's Fruitful Bran	3.1	½
Kellogg's Raisin Bran	2.9	½
All-bran cereal		
Kellogg's All-Bran with Extra Fiber	13.0	½
General Mills Fiber One	12.0	½
Nabisco 100% Bran	10.0	½
Kellogg's All-Bran	9.0	⅓
Kellogg's Bran Buds	8.0	⅓
Quaker Corn Bran	5.0	⅔

Rice

NUTRITIONAL INFORMATION

Like other grain-based products, rice is an excellent source of complex carbohydrates, protein, and, as long as the bran has not been removed, fiber. Polished, refined rice is the most common kind sold in America. While it is often fortified to replace vitamins lost in the refining process, this does nothing to replace the fiber that is lost. Instant rice has undergone even more refining, making it the least nutritious. Brown rice (long- or short-grained), on the other hand, is packed with fiber.

Soups

NUTRITIONAL BENEFITS

No soup is nutritionally perfect, no matter how bracing it is on a cold winter day. Americans love soup (we spend more than two billion dollars on it each year), but it should be considered one component in a meal, not an entire meal, since most soups are at least 90 percent water and do not contain enough nutrients to constitute a well-rounded meal. The most nutritious soups are the "chunky" styles, which are heartier and contain higher levels of protein. For example, a cup of Campbell's Chunky Chicken Noodle soup provides about 15 percent of the USRDA for protein, Vitamin A, and niacin. Progresso's Chicken Noodle is not actually labeled chunky, but it's on the hearty side, as are several other Progresso soups. An 8-ounce serving of Progresso chicken noodle soup contains 14 percent of the USRDA for protein, 42 percent for vitamin A, and 17 percent for niacin.

NUTRITIONAL CAUTIONS

Most canned or dried soups are high in sodium; the lowest level found in regular soups is around 600 milligrams. Unfortunately, some that are lowest in calories are also highest in sodium and fat. For example, Swanson's clear chicken broth, which contains only 33 calories in a 1-cup serving, has more than 1,000 milligrams of sodium and 60 percent of its calories from fat. The broth is also extremely low in protein, so it's not a particularly nourishing choice.

Creamy-style soups usually require the addition of milk, rather than water, which can inflate the calorie toll. Use low-fat or skim milk to reduce calories and fat.

Ramen, which are Oriental noodle soups, have grown in popularity and now constitute a hefty share of the market. These soups are often marketed as main courses, but unless you add protein (such as meat, fish, or tofu), Ramen doesn't contain enough nutrients to make a healthy meal. Ramen soups are also very high in sodium.

BEST CHOICES

If you usually buy soup to add to a meal that contains other sources of protein, your primary concern might be to limit sodium. Campbell's, Lipton, and Borden have lines of low-sodium soups, as do specialty manufacturers like Featherweight and Hain. These contain as little as 50 milligrams of sodium per portion. Even those, like Lipton Harvest Vegetable Cup-a-Soup, that contain more than 600 milligrams of sodium, are much lower than regular soups, which will often have more than 1,000 milligrams per portion.

If you're choosing soup as a primary meal component, look for heartier varieties, such as Campbell's Chunky Beef or Old-Fashioned Chicken, or Progresso Chicken Noodle or Lentil. Always read the labels, since terms can be deceiving. Lipton's Beefy Mushroom Soup Mix, for example, contains only a small amount of "beef powder," not chunks of beef, and only has 2 grams of protein.

Vegetable Oils and Margarines

NUTRITIONAL INFORMATION

All vegetable oils contain approximately the same number of calories (about 120 in a tablespoon), and they're all pure fat. But for the sake of their health, many Americans have increased their consumption of vegetable fats and oils (including margarine as a butter replacement), since animal fats are high in saturated fats.

One would think that all vegetable oils would be more or less equally healthy, but that's not the case. Coconut oil, palm oil, and palm kernel oil all contain high levels of saturated fat.

Common oils include:

Safflower oil: highest in polyunsaturated fats; used mainly in margarine, salad dressing, and mayonnaise

Sunflower oil: has a pleasant, slightly nutty taste; used in cooking oil, salad dressing, and margarine and for deep-frying

Corn oil: used for salad dressings, cooking oil, and margarine

Soybean oil: the most highly consumed vegetable oil in the United States and the rest of the world, although much of its use is commercial; often used in margarines and shortenings; at home, you can use it for cooking and salad dressings

Cottonseed oil: a preferred cooking oil (second most popular after soybean); used for cooking, salad oil, shortening, and margarine

Sesame oil: pleasant tasting and durable; used for salad dressing, cooking oil, and margarine

Peanut oil: peanuty taste and flavor; used for frying foods and salad dressings

Olive oil: a good source of monounsaturated fat, which appears to lower cholesterol; popular for salad dressings and cooking, but more expensive than most cooking oils; unrefined or "virgin" olive oil will be less processed and have a stronger flavor

Palm kernel oil: used frequently in margarine; high in saturated fat

Coconut oil: the highest in saturated fat; used in many snack and pastry foods

SHOPPING TIPS

▶ Just because a product advertises "100 percent vegetable oil," doesn't meant that one of the highly saturated oils won't be used. Also, don't be confused by products that advertise "no cholesterol": There is no cholesterol in any vegetable oil. However, bear in mind that saturated vegetable oils can have the same effect on cholesterol levels as animal fats.

▶ Hydrogenation is a process that solidifies oils, thus making them more saturated. Hydrogenated or partially hydrogenated oils are used in many processed products (including margarine).

▶ The best margarine choices are those that list a liquid oil as the first ingredient. These products will be less saturated.

▶ Palm and coconut oils—both high in saturated fat—are frequently used by manufacturers for packaged products.

Sugar

All sugars are created equal when it comes to nutrition—or rather, lack of nutrition. While recent studies show that sugar isn't the evil substance it's long been accused of being, neither does it add anything to the diet except calories. The more sugar in your diet, the less room there is for foods that supply essential nutrients. You will see sugar in various forms on the labels of products. Contrary to popular belief, among these varieties none are healthier than others.

Jams and Jellies

You'll find a wide variety of jams and jellies in the supermarket and, from a nutritional standpoint, these products are quite similar to one another. By law, anything called a jelly, jam, or preserve must be sweetened with sugar and contain 55 percent sugar by weight. When something other than sugar is used as a sweetener (like fruit juice), the product must be identified as a "spread" or "conserve." However, that doesn't necessarily make it lower in calories. For example, two teaspoons of Smucker's Simply Fruit red raspberry spread, which is sweetened with white grape juice, have 35 calories, the same number as are in two teaspoons of Smucker's red raspberry jam.

Fruit-sweetened spreads are also fairly equal in

vitamins. The small amount of juice used to sweeten spreads contains a negligible amount of essential nutrients. Most sweet spreads contain less than 2 percent of the USRDA for vitamins C and A.

If you're interested in cutting calories, you might want to try products like Smucker's "low sugar" spreads. These have half the sugar and also half the calories.

Juices and Juice Drinks

You may be uncertain about how to choose the healthiest drinks, especially since major companies, including Dole, Libby's, Minute Maid, Ocean Spray, and Welch's are continuing to roll out fruit-based drinks to suit every taste. Some of these beverages are made of juice, with no added sugar or water. Others are only part juice (sometime as little as 10 percent), with sugar and water as the main ingredients; they may not be good dietary additions.

These beverages are found in many parts of the store. They may be refrigerated alongside milk containers; bottled; boxed or canned in the dry-food aisle; or frozen. The first tip-off on what is in the container is whether the label calls it a juice, drink, or cocktail. Beverages labeled fruit "drink" or "cocktail" contain less than 100 percent juice.

Be sure to pay attention to the wording. Welch's, for example, make a blended juice drink that bears a label almost identical to its all-juice products. Instead of saying "100% Juice," these labels say "100% Natural." The words "fruit juice cocktail" appear in small print underneath the flavor. In other words, they are not 100 percent juice.

Only some fruit drink and cocktail labels supply the percentage of juice the product contains. But you can get a good idea by reading the ingredients list. Since ingredients must be listed in descending order by weight, drinks that list water and/or high fructose, corn syrup, or sugar before the juices have more water or sweeteners than juice. That's the case with both Capri-Sun Natural grape drink and Hi-C Double Fruit Cooler, which both list water and sugar as their first two ingredients.

Also be aware that not all juice-flavored sparkling waters and seltzers are a simple blend of water and juice. Flavored beverages like Anheuser-Busch's Zelter Seltzer and Original New York Seltzer are sweetened with sugar. Furthermore, the amount of juice in these drinks can be minuscule.

Condiments

The condiment aisle is full of products that add pizzazz to a meal. But beware that condiments are not always benign extras. Some contain large amounts of fat, calories, and/or sodium. For instance, each tablespoon of tartar sauce (mayonnaise with chopped pickles) adds 70 calories, almost all of it from fat. Plain mayonnaise, at 99 calories a tablespoon, is almost 100 percent fat. Soy sauce, on the other hand, is virtually fat-free, but just one tablespoon of the standard variety contains 1,029 milligrams of sodium. Ketchup is better in terms of sodium, with only 170 milligrams in a tablespoon. But since Americans pour 570 million bottles of ketchup a year onto everything from scrambled eggs to meat loaf, the sodium in ketchup is something to watch.

You don't have to give up your favorite condiments, but it is possible to use them more wisely. For instance, once in a while, in place of tartar sauce, purchase cocktail sauce, which is a low-fat mixture of ketchup, lemon juice, and horseradish. Chili sauce or salsa, used in Mexican dishes, is also low in fat and contains fewer than 20 calories per tablespoon. And mayonnaise can be "stretched" by mixing it with an equal amount of plain, low-fat yogurt. Imitation mayonnaise also cuts fats and calories.

Chutneys—low-calorie, low-sodium condi-

THE COMPOSITION OF POPULAR CONDIMENTS

Condiment (1 tbsp.)	Calories	Fat (g)	Sodium (mg)
chili sauce	16	trace	201
chutney, tomato	41	trace	34
cocktail sauce	20	trace	160
ketchup	16	0.1	170
mayonnaise	99	11	78
imitation mayonnaise	35	2.9	75
mustard	11	0.1	188
sweet-pickle relish	21	0.1	107
soy sauce	11	0	1,029
steak sauce	18	trace	149
sweet & sour sauce	32	trace	320
tartar sauce	75	8	182
teriyaki sauce	15	0	690
Worcestershire sauce	12	0	147

ments made with fruits and vegetables—are available in supermarkets and go well as relishes on many sandwiches. Mustard is also a good choice, with only 11 calories per tablespoon and only a trace of fat.

The new low-calorie or "light" mayonnaise products are created by adding water. The dilution gives them fewer calories and less fat per serving. Some brands are also low-sodium.

The above table shows how your favorite condiments stack up in terms of calories, fat, and sodium.

The supermarket offers an ever-increasing variety of foods that appeal to the nutritional and life-style needs of consumers. By keeping in mind these basic guidelines, you can enjoy the variety without suffering adverse nutritional consequences.

11

Learn the Language of Labels

Most packaged foods available in American supermarkets are labeled with a Nutrition Information Panel. If you know how to read this label, it can be a useful guide as you design a balanced, healthy diet.

The Food and Drug Administration (FDA) first established nutritional labeling guidelines for a wide variety of goods in 1938. In recent years, Nutrition Information Panels printed on the packaging of many products have supplied detailed information about a product's nutrient content. These panels reflect the growing consumer interest in nutrition and increased awareness within the food industry of that interest.

In its 1988 report, the National Academy of Science's Board on Agriculture applauded producers, processors, and retailers for growing more responsive to health trends. But the board urged further development of nutritional labels that allow consumers to make informed choices and recommended that manufacturers supply all the nutritional information desired, avoid misleading terms and descriptions, help consumers bridge the gap between information and application, and support their products with nutritionally helpful point-of-purchase materials. Current legislation now being considered would assure greater accuracy and clearer guidelines.

Reading the Nutrition Information Panel

Nutrition Information Panels have become relatively standardized, although some don't give cholesterol information, specify which type of carbohydrate (starch or sugar) the product contains, list fiber content, or identify the oils used. Legislation has been proposed that would make a listing of cholesterol information mandatory, and it may well be in effect by the time this book is published.

Generally, a Nutrition Information Panel includes the following information:

Serving size and number of servings in the package: Serving sizes vary from product to product, so if you're comparing the number of calories between two products, you should check the two serving sizes. You might also find that the manufacturer's idea of a serving is much less than you would normally eat: You may require one and a half servings or even two or three.

(The rest of the information on the nutrition panel applies to each serving.)

Calories: The number of calories per serving.

Protein: The amount of the product that is protein, usually stated in grams. (To translate protein grams into calories, multiply the number of grams by four.)

Carbohydrates: The amount of the product that is carbohydrate, usually stated in grams. The panel won't always tell how much of the carbohydrate content is starch and how much is sugar. (To translate carbohydrate grams into calories, multiply the number of grams by four.)

Fat: The amount of the product that is fat, usually stated in grams. Sometimes the panel will specify the type of fat that is used. If not, check the ingredient list to see which fats are listed. Each fat gram contains a higher number of calories than do carbohydrate and protein grams. (To translate fat grams into calories, multiply the number of grams by nine.)

USRDA for Nutrients: A suggested daily allowance for protein and certain vitamins and minerals, established by the Food and Drug Administration.

Every package is required by law to list each ingredient in order of its weight. However, the FDA uses "standards of identity" or basically accepted recipes for about 350 products. In other words, a product like mayonnaise doesn't have to list separately the ingredients that are always found in mayonnaise. If a manufacturer follows these recipes, only the additional ingredients must be listed. Most manufacturers voluntarily include an ingredients list for the products covered by the "standards of identity," but it's not required by law. Any food additives must be specified (unless they are part of a standardized recipe), but it's not required that the exact additive be listed (with the exception of the food dye FD & C Yellow No. 5).

Specific nutrition information must be included if the product is fortified with additional vitamins and minerals or if the package makes nutritional claims such as "high protein" or "low sodium."

One thing the label doesn't tell you is exactly how much of a certain ingredient is in the product. For example, you can tell by reading the ingredients list that your chicken noodle soup has chicken stock, noodles, chicken, and water, and these ingredients are listed in order by weight, but you can't tell the actual amounts or proportions of each ingredient.

Another thing a label doesn't always reveal is the type of fat used. Some products list "vegetable oil" and add in parentheses that the product "may contain one or more of the following: coconut, soybean, palm nut, or cottonseed." This practice allows the manufacturer the flexibility to use the oil that's least expensive at the time of production, but it leaves the consumer guessing about which oil the product contains. This factor is important since some oils are not as healthful as others. For example, since coconut oil and palm kernel oil are high in saturated fat, some people wish to avoid them.

Label Reading for Smart Shopping

How can you use the package label to help make better nutrition choices? That depends to a great extent on where your primary nutritional concerns lie. Remember that "good nutrition" does not exist in a vacuum: It presupposes an individual set of needs and goals. Most people who have nutritional priorities look for specific information when they shop. The following are several common nutritional concerns, with suggestions about what information you should look for on the label:

You want to lose weight: There's more to weight watching than calorie control. Total calories are important, of course, but check the label for fat content, too. Besides supplying more than twice the calories per gram (fat provides 9; protein and carbohydrates each provide 4), fat is even more "fattening" than the calorie content alone suggests because your body converts it to body

A Sample Nutrition Label

Wish-Bone Italian Reduced Calorie Dressing

Nutrition Information Per Serving:

serving size	½ fl. oz. (1 tbsp.)
servings per container	16
calories	6
protein, grams	0
carbohydrate, grams	1
fat, grams	0
cholesterol, milligrams *	0
(cholesterol/100 grams, mg)	0
sodium, milligrams	210

Percentage of U.S. Recommended Daily Allowances:
Contains less than 2% of the USRDA for protein, vitamin A, vitamin C, thiamine, riboflavin, niacin, calcium, and iron.

---

* Information on cholesterol content is provided for individuals who, on the advice of a physician, are modifying their dietary intake of cholesterol.

Calories Per Serving:

Wish-Bone Italian Reduced Calorie Dressing	6
Wish-Bone Italian Dressing	70

Ingredients: water, vinegar, sugar, salt, soybean oil; garlic *; xanthan gum for consistency; onion *; natural flavor; spice; red bell pepper *; calcium disodium EDTA to protect flavor; coloring including yellow 5.

---

* Dehydrated

The nutrition label for this reduced-calorie product provides information that is especially important for those who are restricting sodium intake. Just one serving (a tablespoon) contains more than 200 milligrams of sodium. Since many people douse their greens in dressing, they might be getting more than 500 milligrams per salad.

fat more efficiently than it converts carbohydrates and protein.

You might also check the fiber content. Since high-fiber foods are likely to fill you up faster, you might therefore consume fewer total calories. When fiber content is not listed on the nutrition label, check the ingredients list for high fiber foods.

You want to keep your fat intake under 30 percent. Many health organizations suggest that daily fat calories not exceed 30 percent of total calories. To calculate the percentage of fat calories in a food serving: multiply the number of fat grams by nine (the number of calories per gram), divide the number of fat calories by the number of total calories, and multiply the result by 100.

You're on a diet designed to lower choles-terol: Some products list the cholesterol content on the label. Even if you're an average person with no special health problems, the American Heart Association recommends that you consume no more than 300 milligrams of cholesterol per day. If the label doesn't list the cholesterol content, check the ingredients list for meat, eggs, or dairy products. There is no cholesterol in plant products; however, saturated fats are associated with high blood cholesterol, and some plant oils, specifically coconut and palm oils, are high in saturated fats. Also watch for hydrogenated vegetable oils, since hydrogenating (hardening) unsaturated fats can make them more saturated. It's important to check the ingredient list since some labels might read "cholesterol free," but still contain one of these oils.

You're watching your sodium intake: Look for the sodium content on the label; the National Academy of Sciences recommends that adults not exceed the range of 1,100 to 3,300 milligrams per day.

If the nutrition panel doesn't supply sodium content, check the ingredients list for salt, which is 40 percent sodium. Other ingredients that might be of concern when they're in high enough quantities are sodium nitrite (a curing agent in meats), sodium phosphate (an emulsifier found especially in processed cheese), sodium bicarbonate or baking soda, monosodium glutamate (MSG), and sodium bisulfite or sodium propionate (preservatives).

You're an adult woman: Menstruating women need more iron in their diets. Check the label for the USRDA for iron and also for vitamin C, which increases the absorption of iron. Good food sources for iron, besides certain animal foods, include beans, broccoli, spinach, and fortified grain products.

Women who don't get enough calcium in their diets may be at risk for developing osteoporosis (thinning bones) as they age. Look for foods that are high in calcium. If you're watching your weight, choose low-fat dairy products.

Health-Conscious Comparison Shopping

In addition to the nutritional agenda you bring with you to the supermarket, there are other values to consider. Consumers also look for particular tastes and textures. In the Food Marketing Institute's 1988 *Trends* report on consumer attitudes, "taste" ranked number one in food choice factors, with 88 percent of consumers saying it was "very important." "Product safety" was second, with 83 percent, and "nutrition" third, with 72 percent.

Understanding how to read a label will help you make choices that meet your nutritional needs, as well as allowing you to find foods that you enjoy. As you compare brands, you might find that some offer a better combination of taste and convenience for the same nutritional value. Focus first on the nutritional information, then weigh the other factors that are important to you. The following samples show how this might be done.

SAMPLE A: BUYING A HEART-HEALTHY MARGARINE OR SPREAD
Points to consider: (1) Look for a liquid vegetable oil as the first ingredient; (2) look for a higher percentage of polyunsaturated fat to saturated—a ratio of 2:1 is good; (3) choose tub margarine over stick—the former has less fat because it's made with water and because less saturated fat is needed for soft brands.

The best choice is a product like Promise that contains liquid vegetable oil as the first ingredient. Choose tub over stick for less saturated fat and fewer calories.

SAMPLE B: CHOOSING CHEESE
Cheeses are high in saturated fat. It takes 9 to 10 pints of milk to make one pound of most cheeses; thus, cheese is a concentrated source of all the nutrients milk contains, including fat. However,

COMPARISON OF THE NUTRITION PANELS FROM THREE BRANDS

Parkay (stick)

Serving size	1 tbsp.
Calories	100
Fat	11 g
Polyunsaturated	1 g
Saturated	2 g
Cholesterol	0 mg
Sodium	115 mg

Higher percentage of saturated fats to polyunsaturated fat

Ingredients: Partially hydrogenated and liquid vegetable oil, water, salt, whey . . .

First ingredient is not a liquid oil. Partially hydrogenated fats are more saturated.

Krona

Serving size	1 tbsp.
Calories	100
Fat	11 g
Cholesterol	15 mg
Sodium	90 mg

There is no breakdown of saturated to polyunsaturated fats. That's because the primary fat is beef oil, which is almost entirely saturated.

Vegetable oils do not contain cholesterol. This spread does because it contains beef oil.

The first ingredient is a highly saturated animal fat.

Ingredients: Beef oil, cottonseed oil, water, dried whey . . .

Promise (tub margarine)

Serving size	1 tbsp.
Calories	90
Fat	10 g
Polyunsaturated	5 g
Saturated	1 g
Cholesterol	0 mg
Sodium	90 mg

Fewer calories because this product contains more water than stick spreads.

High percentage of polyunsaturated fat.

Ingredients: Liquid sunflower oil, sweet dairy whey, partially hydrogenated soybean oil, water, salt, partially hydrogenated cottonseed oil . . .

First ingredient is less saturated liquid vegetable oil

---

some cheeses are naturally lower in fat than others.

Look at the nutrition panels on each of three cheeses to see now many grams of fat there are in each 1-ounce serving:

Cheddar	Parmesan	Low Moisture, Part-Skim Mozzarella
1 oz.	1 oz.	1 oz.
Fat: 9 g	Fat: 7 g	Fat: 4 g
Calories: 110	Calories: 110	Calories: 90

In this comparison, the low-moisture, part-skim mozzarella is lowest in fat, with less than half the fat of the rich cheddar. However, "part-skim" or "low-fat" cheeses are only *lower* in fat, not necessarily *low* in fat. This part-skim mozzarella gets 36 (4 grams times 9 calories per gram) of its 90 calories (or 40 percent) from fat. The health message here: Opt for cheeses with less fat per ounce, but remember that these foods are still high-fat choices and should be used sparingly.

SAMPLE C: READING BETWEEN THE LINES OF
THE INGREDIENTS LIST

QUAKER CHEWY GRANOLA BARS

Chocolate, Graham, & Marshmallow

Ingredients: Granola [rolled oats, brown sugar, . . .
honey], corn syrup, semisweet chocolate chips [sugar
. . .], crisp rice [rice, sugar, . . .], brown sugar, corn
syrup solids [sugar, corn syrup], . . . corn syrup, . . .
honey, . . . sorbitol

Although the ingredients are listed by weight,
with the highest weight or most-used ingredient
appearing first, it's possible to confuse the situation when ingredients are products or have ingredients of their own. A granola bar, for example,
may have chocolate chips, rice cereal, granola,
and many other items, each of which in turn may
contain an ingredients list. If you are wondering
how much sugar a granola bar contains, you need
to read the complete list. Indeed, sugar is likely
to turn up in many of the products (it appears in
12 different places in the sample above) and is
more than likely the prominent ingredient
overall.

Fortification—For Better or For Worse?

If you're conscious of adhering to the basic guidelines of the RDAs, you might wonder: "Should I
shop for *food* or for *nutrients?*" That's a pertinent
question in light of the fortification boom. You've
no doubt noticed that many products are "fortified" with vitamins and minerals, and the list is
growing. Even Kool-Aid and some sodas have
added vitamin C.

When foods were first fortified in the early
1940s, the intention was to correct specific deficiencies and to protect the public if food short-

ages arose because of World War II. Scientists
added iodine to salt to combat goiter. Food manufacturers were encouraged to put a number of B
vitamins into flour, bread, and ready-to-eat cereal
products to prevent deficiency diseases. And milk
was fortified with vitamin D to fight rickets, a condition that impairs bone formation. Because of
efforts such as these, most deficiency diseases in
the United States have been eradicated.

Fortification with vitamins and minerals has
been so successful, in fact, that in 1982 the American Medical Association (AMA) recommended
expanding the list of nutrients added to foods,
and has offered guidelines that both the National
Academy of Sciences and the Institute of Food
Technology have endorsed. The AMA's basic suggestion is that any nutrient added to food should
be one that a large group of people are not getting in sufficient amounts. In addition, the item
selected for fortification should be a staple food
for large segments of the population that is at risk.
Finally, adding a vitamin or mineral should neither cause harm nor result in a nutrient imbalance when the food it fortifies is part of the
regular diet.

Unfortunately, in today's competitive commercial environment, fortification often has more to
do with marketing than with nutrition, and the
outer limits of these guidelines are being
stretched. It is difficult to see a pressing need to
add B vitamins to soda pop, for example, considering that most Americans eat more than
enough foods that are rich in B vitamins. The fortification trend makes it easy for food marketers
to add particular nutrients to their products for
the purpose of making them more salable, not
necessarily better.

Are there any nutritional hazards to the fortification trend? Not directly, but the implications of
product marketing have federal agencies concerned. For example, a calcium-fortified orange
juice that is marketed as having the same amount
of calcium as milk may lead consumers to believe
that orange juice can replace milk. But if they
choose orange juice as a milk substitute, they will

shortchange themselves on a number of other important nutrients that milk provides, including protein, vitamins A and D, and riboflavin.

Furthermore, the abundance of "highly fortified" foods might be giving consumers the false impression that eating a few foods fortified with huge amounts of particular nutrients takes care of all their dietary needs. In fact, foods provide more than 40 essential nutrients, and even a heavily fortified product that supplies 100 percent of the USRDA for 10 or 12 vitamins and minerals cannot foot the entire nutrition bill. Moreover, eating a fortified food does not fully compensate for eating "empty" foods, items filled mainly with calories, sugar, and fat.

Your best defense is to eat a varied diet. Be attentive, but not tied, to the RDA guidelines. When you shop, focus on the Nutrition Information Panel and ingredients list, not the advertising claims. Never select a food based on its claimed percentage of USRDA for certain nutrients until you've looked to see what else the product contains.

Maneuver through the Marketing Hype

Food manufacturers have taken many positive steps toward improving the nutritional quality of products and supplying useful information to consumers. However, in today's competitive marketplace, some try to capture the edge with creative twists of label language and package design.

Even when consumers know that real nutrition information appears in only one place on the package (the Nutrition Information Panel and ingredients list), it's nearly impossible to put blinders on and ignore what the companies are saying. Realistically, most shoppers don't go right to the nutrition label without first picking up some clues about the product from the package design, illustration, or description. The key to suc-

cessfully maneuvering through the blaze of color and hype is to take it for what it is, while keeping one's eye on the true nutrition information.

Food manufacturers are required to tell the truth on labels, but they're not necessarily required to tell the whole truth, and there are countless ways to create misleading impressions.

It is rightly assumed that, all else being equal, consumers will be drawn to foods that boast "new," "fiber rich," "low sodium," "cholesterol free," "enriched," or "light." But often the products contain more (or less) than meets the eye. Consumers can be misled when a package focuses on an isolated positive characteristic ("High Fiber," "Low Fat") while ignoring mention of other contents, such as sugar or sodium, that might diminish the healthfulness of the product.

Many cereals feature a large "100%" on the front of the package, indicating that the product contains 100 percent of the USRDA for certain essential vitamins and minerals. These claims often mask other facts about the product, such as a high sugar content. Furthermore, there's little need to eat 100 percent of your nutrients in a serving of breakfast cereal, assuming you will be eating other nutritious meals during the course of the day. It's much better to get your daily nutrients by eating a variety of healthy foods.

Another misleading gimmick is to promote the absence of contents that don't exist in the product under any circumstances. For example, a corn-oil margarine label that states "no cholesterol" might lead shoppers to assume that there is cholesterol in competing brands of corn-oil margarine. In fact, corn oil doesn't contain cholesterol.

Manufacturers know that many impulse decisions are made in the supermarket aisle, particularly for brand selection. It stands to reason that customers will notice a bread or cereal with the word "Fiber" in the name. By the same token, "Honey Wheat" might sound like a more nutritious bread choice than "All Butter." When "Vita" appears as part of the product name, it creates an instant impression of good health. So does "Rich," as in "Fiber Rich" or "Calcium Rich." Other more subtle lures exist behind the words "country," "home," "fresh," "nature," and "old-fashioned."

Manufacturers are within their legal rights to promote products in the most aggressive way they can as long as they don't give blatantly false information. However, the tides might be turning as advocates of stricter advertising and labeling regulations become more vocal. Some of the issues now being hotly contested are:

▶ Should dairy-food manufacturers be required to mention high fat content when they advertise the calcium benefits of their products?

▶ If a company advertises that its product is low in fat, should it also have to mention negatives like a high sodium level?

▶ Should all products be required to display nutritional information? (Currently, only about half do.) And should the information be more explicit?

▶ Should companies be allowed to directly or indirectly allude to a connection between their product and the avoidance of cancer, heart disease, or any other illness?

It appears that more extensive labeling laws will be passed by Congress in the near future. But in the meantime, the FDA has proposed a rule that will allow manufacturers to make health claims about ingredients in their products. While they would also be required to list the substances that might compromise good nutrition, manufacturers would not be required to state warnings. Most health organizations, including the American Medical Association, the Academy of Medicine, and the American Institute of Clinical Nutrition have opposed the rule, stating that evidence linking diet and disease is still quite controversial and far too complex to be handled in this way.

While the debate rages on, consumers can act by becoming more informed about the meaning of the terms that appear on labels, and by using caution in responding to claims that certain products can decrease the risk of cancer or other diseases.

The FDA places restrictions on certain foods, and the U.S. Department of Agriculture (USDA) monitors poultry and meat products, but there are plenty of gaps. While the FDA requires that packages under its jurisdiction list ingredients in descending order according to the percentage of weight they contribute to the total, there is no requirement to list many of the additives available. Consequently, a "natural" product may be filled with artificial ingredients and the consumer has no way to know.

It is a further complication that at times the FDA and the U.S. Department of Agriculture seem to be working at cross purposes. For example, certain USDA standards for meat and poultry labels make it harder for consumers to judge the health value of nonmeat items. For example, the USDA requires that a meat or poultry product that is labeled "natural" contain no artificial colors, flavors, preservatives, or synthetic ingredients. However, the FDA has no standard for the use of the term "natural" in the foods it regulates, so baked goods, beverages, and other nonmeat and poultry products can claim to be "natural" without offering any evidence at all.

Until the federal standards for labeling become more complete, consumers are left to exercise as much caution as they can when they're shopping. Once again, it is important to read the nutrition panel and the ingredients list for true nutritional information.

A Glossary of Terms

The following are the most common descriptive terms found on labels and what they mean.

Low calorie. The standard requires that there be no more than 40 calories per serving and no

---

Protectors of Our Food

The Food and Drug Administration (FDA), with regional offices throughout the country, monitors the safety of all foods and beverages (including their packaging) with the exceptions of meat, poultry, and alcohol. That includes lobster and other seafood, fruits, vegetables, and even rubber nipples on baby bottles, since they come into contact with food.

The United States Department of Agriculture (USDA) monitors the safety of meats and poultry, as well as any products that contain more than 2 percent poultry and 3 percent meat by weight. Inspectors who work for a branch of the USDA called the Food Safety and Inspection Service examine meat and poultry at approximately 8,000 plants in the United States where slaughtering, processing, and packaging occur.

The Environmental Protection Agency (EPA) indirectly protects meats, produce, and processed foods by setting standards for the amount of pesticide residue allowed on raw and processed foods, including animal feed. (Both the FDA and the USDA help to make sure that these requirements are met.) The EPA also sets standards for the safety of drinking water and monitors the safety of tap water throughout the country. (The FDA monitors bottled water.)

The Bureau of Alcohol, Tobacco, and Firearms, which is a branch of the Treasury Department, is responsible for the safety of alcoholic beverages. It also works closely with the FDA and EPA on issues such as sulfites in the wine supply.

---

more than 0.4 calories per gram. Be careful to check the serving size to see that it's not too small to negate the low-calorie benefit. In other words, if a normal serving size is three or four times larger than the one given, you won't eat fewer calories when you eat this food.

Reduced calorie. A reduced-calorie food must have at least one-third fewer calories than the "regular" product and must include a comparison on its label. (Note how this appears on the Wish-Bone Italian Reduced Calorie Dressing sample label shown earlier in the chapter. For meat and poultry products, the standards are slightly different because they're regulated by the USDA: They must have a 25 percent reduction in calories. If a food is labeled "diet" or "dietetic" and it falls under the FDA jurisdiction, it must meet the standards for either low-calorie or reduced-calorie foods.

High (as in "high protein"). The food must have at least 10 percent more of the particular nutrient's USRDA than similar products.

Nothing artificial added. There are no artificial additives, such as preservatives, artificial colors and flavors, and nonnutritive sweeteners.

Low sodium. The food contains no more than 140 milligrams of sodium per serving. A product labeled "very low sodium" must have a maximum of 35 milligrams per serving.

Fortified/Enriched. For products labeled fortified, the manufacturers must have added 10 percent or more of the USRDA for the stated protein, vitamin, or mineral. (Fortifying a product doesn't necessarily make it nutritious, since it can still contain a heavy dose of sugar, sodium, or fat.)

Enriched foods are enhanced with nutrients that may have been lost during necessary processing or that were not present in the product to begin with.

Naturally flavored. The product's flavoring must be the essential oil, extract, or other derivative of a juice, herb, spice, root, or other natural source.

Naturally sweetened. The FDA has no regulation regarding this term, but many manufacturers use it to indicate that the product has been sweetened with fruit or juice rather than sugar. Check the list of ingredients.

Sugar free/Sugarless. The product cannot be sweetened with sucrose (table sugar). However, it may contain sweeteners that are just as high in calories as, and no more nutritious than, table sugar, such as honey, corn syrup, fructose, sorbitol, or manitol.

Light/Lite. Somewhat complicated, this guideline differs depending on the substance; the USDA has established guidelines for meat and poultry products only. When they're labeled "light," "lean," or "lower fat," they must have at least 25 percent less fat than similar products; sometimes "Light" on a meat label refers to a 25 percent reduction in sodium, breading, or calories (the label will tell you which). Note that these guidelines do not apply to frozen meat dishes.

For other products, there is no standard for "Light," or "Lite." It can mean anything, including a lighter color.

Natural. The USDA has established guidelines for meat and poultry products, but for other foods the term could mean anything. For meat and poultry, "natural" means that there are no artificial colors, flavors, preservatives, or synthetic ingredients.

No preservatives. Contrary to popular belief, the absence of preservatives is not always positive. Preservatives are a type of additive that can improve the quality of a product; they also protect foods against spoilage. In addition, the claim "no preservatives" can be misleading. Preservatives are only one kind of additive; the product might contain others, such as colors, flavors, and emulsifiers.

Unsalted/Salt free/No salt added. These terms mean only that no salt was added in processing. However, the food could contain high levels of sodium, either naturally or from added preservatives or other processes.

Prime/Choice/Select (gradings for beef). These grades assure that the meat has been graded at the slaughterhouse according to USDA guidelines. The official government graders assign these designations based on specific criteria, such as age and the degree of fat marbling. The beef with the most fat tends to be the most tender and, therefore, is the most likely to be labeled "Prime." The leanest meat is labeled "Select"; it was formerly labeled "Good."

Unfortunately, most retailers are not required to label meats according to the government's grading system, only to have the meat inspected. They don't have to identify the meat at all, which can leave customers confused.

12

Balancing Life-style and Nutrition

Must the pursuit of a nutritional eating style be a time-consuming and costly venture?

Not at all. It is possible for most Americans to balance the demands of their life-styles with healthy diets. This is good news for the post-World Wat II generation, whose way of life is vastly different from that of their parents.

Today, more than two-thirds of adult women are in the work force, making two-career families the norm. And Americans seem to be working harder than ever. According to a Lou Harris survey, today's worker spends more time on the job than he or she did in 1983, with less time devoted to leisure activities.

New technologies for food packaging and preparation and the increase in outlets for prepared food have expanded the role of convenience foods in the American diet. According to the 1988 *Trends* report of the Food Marketing Institute, 25 percent of consumers frequently purchase delicatessen or carry-out food items; 20 percent often purchase items from grocery salad bars; and 18 percent regularly buy food products designed specifically for microwave cooking.

Perhaps the greatest shift in American eating patterns is that many families no longer sit down to the table to share two or three "square" meals each day. In households where both adults work outside the home, breakfast is often a rushed affair, when it is not skipped altogether. (It is estimated that as many as 33 percent of Americans skip breakfast.) For lunch, there is the cafeteria, the "business lunch," the fast-food restaurant, or the quick cup of yogurt or sandwich at the desk. It is often just one of many hurried segments in a busy day. At school, the children are on their own; even if you've packed a nutritious lunch, it is not unheard of for a child to trade a piece of fruit for a bag of potato chips, or simply to discard portions of the lunch. For dinner, convenience cooking and restaurant meals are common; many families and couples manage relaxed, home-cooked dinners together only a couple of nights a week or on weekends.

Many people have abandoned three-meal-a-day patterns altogether. Data from the Continuing Survey on Food Intake conducted by the Department of Agriculture indicates that people are eating more frequently throughout the day, rather than confining themselves to set meals.

Healthy Eating for Active Americans

It may not always be clear how nutritional balance can be achieved when eat-and-run is the norm.

But, in spite of changing styles, people are more attentive to nutrition than ever; indeed, FMI's *Trends* report states that more than two-thirds of grocery shoppers select foods with nutrition in mind. Nevertheless, consumers often lack a practical understanding of how to incorporate nutritional concepts into convenience-oriented eating styles. For example, if you consume a number of small meals throughout the day (a practice sometimes called "grazing") rather than sitting down to full meals that include a balance of nutrients, how can you make certain that you're getting all the nourishment you need? Or if you eat three meals a day but their content varies widely depending on your schedule or other factors, what adjustments can you make to satisfy both your life-style and your dietary requirements?

The goal of your daily meal pattern, whatever it is, is to provide your body with its nutritional requirements. One meal per day, for example, is not a recommended way to eat, even if that meal is a very large one, containing a variety of nutrients. Eating at regularly scheduled periods throughout the day is a better way to keep your health and energy levels high, and six small well-balanced meals can be as good as three hearty ones.

Whatever your meal pattern, it's a good idea to examine the nutritional quality of your diet over a week's period. You can do this by keeping a precise diary of what you eat and comparing it with dietary guidelines to find out where you may be shortchanging yourself. This analysis will also tell you where you may be overdoing it on foods that are high in fat, sodium, and calories. Questions to ask about your week's food balance include:

Are you getting enough calories, but not too many? The best way to determine this is to weigh yourself and then to compare your weight with the recommended range for your height and age (see chart in chapter 22). Also be aware that other factors, such as the amount of exercise you do and certain illnesses, affect your calorie needs.

Of your daily calories, is the percentage of fat calories 30 percent or less? Foods that are low in fat will help you limit your caloric intake. (To calculate the number of fat calories, multiply each gram of fat times nine.)

Here's one simple way to balance your fat intake: If you plan to eat a high-fat lunch, such as a hamburger and fries, eat a light morning meal such as fruit and low-fat cottage cheese, and end the day with a lean meal of broiled fish, fresh vegetables, and brown rice.

Are you taking steps to reduce the amount of saturated fat in your diet? In addition to keeping your total fat calories at 30 percent or less of your daily intake, it is also advisable to limit the amount of saturated fat, which comes from animal products and from oils like coconut and palm. This is particularly important if you're trying to keep your blood cholesterol low.

Are you keeping your sodium intake in check? If you're a snacker, sodium could be a problem, since many popular snack foods are high in sodium. In addition, many convenience foods, including some dinners, contain high levels of sodium.

Are you eating a variety of foods throughout the week? The greater the variety, the better the chance that your diet contains the essential nutrients in adequate amounts. Balance your diet from the four basic food groups: milk, meat, fruits and vegetables, breads and cereals.

Are you eating calcium-rich foods each day? Government surveys show that most Americans, particularly women, don't meet their calcium needs, and low calcium diets may increase the risk of osteoporosis, or loss of bone mass. Good sources of calcium include milk, cheese, yogurt, sardines (unboned), and canned salmon (unboned). Broccoli, collards, and tofu are good supplementary sources. If you're concerned about your fat and calorie intake, use low-calorie dairy foods.

Are you eating enough fiber foods? According to the National Cancer Institute, most Americans fall short of the recommended levels of dietary fiber—about 20 to 30 grams per day. Water-insoluble fiber, or "roughage"—found in wheat bran, most vegetables, and whole-grain breads—is a digestive aid that promotes regularity. Certain soluble fibers—found in oats, dried beans, and some fruits and vegetables—seem to be a factor in lowering blood cholesterol.

Be a Healthy Vegetarian

Vegetarianism has gone mainstream. No longer is it the domain of the soyburger or the seaweed sandwich. The vegetarian trend, which is up 30 percent since 1970, has opened the way for a proliferation of vegetarian restaurants, convenience food products, and cookbooks that offer enticing meatless meals.

It is unlikely that the United States will become a vegetarian nation, but the trend has plenty to recommend it, since those who fill their plates with fruits, vegetables, and grains rather than with large quantities of animal foods place themselves at a lower risk for the most common American illnesses: heart disease, colon cancer, diabetes, hypertension, and obesity.

Some of the strongest evidence that a diet rich in plant foods and sparing of animal foods confers a variety of health benefits comes from observations of a group of Seventh Day Adventists, many of whom eat no animal flesh, although they may consume dairy products and eggs. Compared to those who eat the typical high-fat American diet, members of this sect who were tested had a dramatically lower rate of heart disease. One group of researchers in California found that the death rate from coronary disease in male members of this sect is as low as half of that found in the average California male. Undoubtedly, the fact that Seventh Day Adventists are also nonsmokers

contributes to the health picture, since smoking is one of the risk factors for heart disease. But diet apparently plays an integral role, since the rate of heart disease among Seventh Day Adventists who are not vegetarians was found to be three times higher than that of their vegetarian counterparts.

Their low-fat diets may also account for the fact that Seventh Day Adventists are only half as likely as other Americans to develop colon and rectal cancer. Their rate of cancer of the breast, prostate, pancreas, and ovaries is much smaller, too. Diets that favor fruits, vegetables, and grains, in addition to being low in cholesterol, are also high in fiber.

There are three kinds of vegetarian styles: Semivegetarians are those who dramatically cut back their meat, poultry, and fish intake, using them as sideline items rather than a main course. Lacto-ovo vegetarians don't eat animal flesh but consume dairy products such as eggs, cheese, and milk. Vegans consume no meat or dairy foods. Nutrition needs vary for each group.

Cutting Down on Meat

Many people have become semivegetarians because they've taken to heart the advice of organizations like the American Heart Association and the American Cancer Society to cut the fat in their diets.

Just changing the proportions of plant foods to animal foods in your diet will automatically lower your fat intake. For example, a traditional ten-ounce steak intended for one person can easily be turned into two five-ounce servings.

The "hole" that's left on the plate can be filled with a heftier salad, a large serving of a cooked vegetable like broccoli or spinach, or even a second baked potato or a second piece of corn on the cob. Indeed, cutting out that five ounces of steak will result in your consuming 120 fewer calories as fat. Even if you add two teaspoons of margarine to a potato or corn on the cob, it will put back only 70 calories of fat—most of it unsaturated.

Cutting down on or even cutting out meat does not have to mean risking deficiencies of essential nutrients. Even small quantities of meat added to the main course of a meal can supply the nutrients you need. And dairy foods and eggs are a good source of complete protein, so lacto-ovo vegetarians are not at risk for protein deficiency.

Keeping a Nutrient Balance for Strict Vegetarians

The strictest vegetarians—a small minority called vegans, who abstain from eating both meat and dairy products—need to pay closer attention than others to their intake of certain nutrients in order to avoid deficiencies. For them, managing a healthy diet involves some savvy about the science of nutrition. Diets that do not include any animal foods often lack calories, along with essential vitamins and minerals, and are usually inadequate for growing children or others with special nutritional needs.

Vegans need to be aware that the proteins in plant foods, particularly grains and legumes, are not "complete." That is, one or another plant food by itself cannot provide the body with all the amino acids, the building blocks of proteins humans require for building and maintaining body tissues. In order to be assured of getting complete proteins, vegans must combine certain imcomplete proteins in the same meal. Eating red beans with rice, for instance, turns two sources of incomplete protein into one complete source. Split pea soup and a slice of rye bread makes for another full complement. (See chapter 1 for more information about complete and incomplete protein sources.)

One nutrient vegans must consider more carefully than others is calcium, since dairy products are the best sources. It is hard to fulfill the dietary requirement for this nutrient from vegetables alone. Further, the calcium in plant foods may not be absorbed as readily as the calcium in animal foods. It's important to eat generous portions of calcium-containing vegetables. One large stalk of broccoli provides more than 10 percent of the recommended adult allowance. Collard greens and mustard greens supply appreciable levels, too. Small amounts of calcium can be found in other plant foods, but a diet dependent on plant foods for calcium is not likely to be adequate.

Vegans must be careful to look for sources of iron in their diet. Fortunately, a wide variety of plant foods are iron-rich. A cup of dried beans, peas, or lentils contains about five milligrams of iron, or just under one-third of the RDA of 15 milligrams for women, and half the RDA of 10 milligrams for men. But similar to calcium, the iron in plant foods is not well absorbed, something to consider in light of the fact that even many meat eaters lack iron in their diets. Making sure there's enough vitamin C in the diet will help, since vitamin C aids in the absorption of iron.

Vegans must pay particular attention to their intake of vitamin B-12 because that nutrient, without which pernicious anemia develops, is only available naturally in animal foods. One way to insure sufficient vitamin B-12 is to eat cereals that have been fortified with the vitamin. However, strict vegetarians should consult a knowledgeable physician about taking vitamin B-12 supplements or multi–vitamin/mineral supplements that contain B-12, since fortified cereals and soy foods often do not contain the nutrient.

The same doctor's visit should also include a discussion about whether supplements of vitamin D are necessary. People who do not drink milk may be at risk for a vitamin D deficiency since vitamin D fortified milk is about the only food that contains adequate amounts of the vitamin. It is true that exposure to the sun allows the body to synthesize vitamin D, but not everyone, especially those living in northern climates, gets the amount of sunlight necessary to make all of the vitamin D the body needs. Further, there is increasing evidence that with age our ability to synthesize and metabolize vitamin D is diminished.

Making Meals Appetizing

The American imagination, accustomed to creating meals around meat, may falter at the prospect of making low-meat or vegetarian meals appetizing and hearty. But many ethnic cuisines have discovered the secret to using meat as a condiment rather than a main course, or stretching small amounts of meat to go farther. A Chinese stir-fry, for example, can utilize thin strips of beef or chicken or go without the meat altogether and still make for a hearty dish. Traditional pasta sauces don't need meat as an ingredient, or can get by with small amounts.

Nutritious Nibbling

Consumers are snacking more than ever: Last year Americans spent $1.8 billion on potato chips and $9 billion on candy and gum. But snacking does not have to mean throwing nutritional caution to the wind. Snack foods high in calories, salt, sugar, and fat are available in abundance, but there are plenty of healthy options that you can buy or make yourself.

Unfortunately, palm kernel and coconut oil, two highly saturated vegetable fats, are often used in making a wide variety of snack foods, including crackers, chips, cookies, cake mixes, and granola bars. Palm oil, a highly saturated relative of palm kernel oil, is also used frequently in snack foods. So snacks made from "pure vegetable oil" don't necessarily reduce the amount of saturated fat in your diet. Check the label to be sure the oil used is the unsaturated variety, such as soybean or corn oil.

Snack foods are often salty, and since salt is nearly half sodium, it's best to watch snack items like chips, salted nuts, salty crackers, and salted pretzels.

Sugar-filled cookies, ice cream, and candy are often high in fat as well. For example, 72 of the 150 calories in a one-ounce Nestle Crunch Bar come from fat.

Can you avoid the calorie-fat-salt-sugar trap by purchasing "healthy" snacks? Health food stores offer plenty of foods like "natural" potato chips and "sugarless" candy bars. But, upon close inspection, you might find that these potato chips are fried in fat and laden with salt, just like supermarket brands. Granted, the potatoes in the "natural" brand may be fried in a less saturated oil, like safflower oil. But saturated or not, a one-ounce, 150-calorie bag of potato chips still contains 60 percent fat calories, which hardly qualifies it as a "health food."

One health food store markets a high-fiber candy bar, but the nutrition claims are misleading. While the little bar does contain 5 grams of dietary fiber, fat makes up more than 35 percent of its calories. In fact, ounce for ounce, it has more fat than a Milky Way bar! Worse still, the candy's "nectar vanilla yogurt coating" is made with palm kernel oil. The candy bar also contains less than 7 percent of the USRDA for all the vitamins and minerals listed on its label. It's not that health food stores don't carry any nutritious snack. Just be sure to read the label before you buy.

Snacking can actually be a way to round out your meal plan, adding nutrients that you may not be getting enough of elsewhere in the day. Remember, a snack doesn't have to consist of a prepackaged food. The only requirement is that it be quick, convenient, satisfying, and, of course, healthy. Here are some ideas for nutritious nibbling:

Popcorn: What could be more all-American? And it's fast, fun, and good for you, too. If you make it in a hot-air popper, a cup of popcorn has only 27 calories. If you don't have a hot-air popper, you can pop a half cup of kernels in as little as a tablespoon of oil, which adds only 11 calories per cup of popped popcorn. Microwave varieties differ widely in the amount of fat and sodium, but many are relatively high in fat. However, check the packages of some of the new low-fat brands that manufacturers like Orville Redenbacher are producing.

Graham crackers and milk: An old-fashioned afternoon snack that is still a good bet. Two graham crackers have only about 70 calories, and a glass of (1%) low-fat milk has about 100. Although the graham crackers add little nutritional value, this snack is an enjoyable way to help meet your daily calcium requirement.

Fruit: Buy "convenience fruits" that are easy to carry in a briefcase or lunch bag. These include apples, peaches, oranges, pears, nectarines, and plums. Snack-size cans of unsweetened applesauce or fruit juice are a good bet, as are miniature boxes of raisins.

Vegetables and dip: Because they are high in fiber, vegetables are filling, as well as being a source of vitamins and minerals. Enjoy them alone or add low-fat cottage cheese stuffing or low-fat yogurt dip. A serving of low-fat yogurt has less than 150 calories. To make a tasty vegetable dip, stir in such seasonings as dill, caraway seeds, chili powder, mint, paprika, mustard powder, garlic, or pepper. Good vegetables for dipping include celery sticks, carrot sticks, cucumber slices, mushrooms, radishes, cherry tomatoes, broccoli or cauliflower florets, green or red peppers, and asparagus spears.

Fruit and yogurt: Make your own fruit yogurt, adding bananas, diced apples, peaches, berries, and other favorites to low-fat, plain yogurt. This fresh snack will taste great, and it's much better than commercial fruit yogurts, which can have as many as 250 calories per serving and more sugar than fruit. Top your creation with cinnamon or even mix in a teaspoon of sugar, which has only 16 calories.

Fast and Frozen—
The Right Choices

Americans spend nearly $14 billion every year on frozen dinners, and health-conscious consumers are finding that they don't have to sacrifice nutrition when they shop the frozen-food section. A wide variety of "diet" dinners are available, featuring portion and calorie control, low fat and cholesterol, and low sodium.

How can you take advantage of the convenience benefits of frozen dinners and still eat healthily? In an evaluation of more than 450 frozen dinners (see Appendix C) Tufts found 33 dishes that we could "highly recommend" on the basis of our nutritional criteria, and 70 others that fell only slightly short of the standards. Our guidelines included:

▶ A maximum of 30 percent of calories from fat, the recommended level for an American-style diet

▶ No more than 800 milligrams of sodium— about one third of the upper daily limit the National Academy of Sciences deems healthful

▶ At least one-third of the USRDA for protein —a minimum of 15 grams

▶ No more than 300 calories per serving, a comfortable level for weight watchers that also allows "room" for the addition of side dishes that round out the meal's nutritional value

▶ A net weight of nine ounces or more

Even a frozen meal that meets all of these requirements might be somewhat low in one or another essential vitamin or mineral, particularly vitamins A and C. Also, most frozen dinners do not provide the level of calcium recommended for keeping bones healthy. To make up for the lack of calcium, include one or two of these items in your daily menu: a cup of skim or low-fat (1%) milk, 1½ ounces of low-fat hard cheese, a cup of yogurt, 2 cups of broccoli, or 4½ ounces of salmon or sardines with bones.

An unknown in many frozen dinners is the cholesterol content, since many manufacturers do not include this information on the label.

If you enjoy the convenience of popping a frozen dinner into the oven or microwave but are not satisfied with commercial products, you can make your own nutritious frozen dinners. Home-made frozen dinners give you the advantage of controlling the ingredients used. By choosing fresh and low-fat foods, the home cook can elim-inate the extra fat content of many commercial dinners. And by using lively herbs and spices in-stead of extra salt, the amount of sodium normally found in these dinners can be cut substantially.

People who prepare frozen dinners in their own kitchens also have the option of increasing the fiber content by choosing whole grains as well as including vegetables rich in vitamins A and C, nutrients that are sometimes lacking in commer-cial dinners. Making your own frozen dinners brings substantial benefits to your pocketbook, too. While commercial dinners may be affordable for a single person or a couple, the cost of feeding a larger family this way could become prohibitive.

In addition to being relatively inexpensive to prepare, frozen dinners don't require much in the way of special equipment. All you need to buy are some freezer bags and/or freezer wrap, wire twisters, small aluminum tins, microwave contain-ers (if you'll be cooking with a microwave), strong tape, and a marking pencil to label each package with the name of the food, the portion-size, and the date it was frozen. With these items on hand, and after a well-planned shopping trip, you will be ready to put together, with very little effort, dinners that you and your family or friends can enjoy later with a minimum of preparation.

The following suggestions will guide you in preparing and storing your own nutritious frozen dinners:

▶ Set your freezer at 0°F to insure optimal quality of frozen foods. Freezer thermometers are sold in housewares and hardware stores.

▶ Avoid putting too many hot dinners into your freezer at once. Cool them for five to ten minutes first so the freezer temperature will not rise.

▶ Before freezing vegetables, blanch them (placing them for one minute in water that has come to a rolling boil and then plunging them into cold water) to destroy enzymes that can in-terfere with their texture, color, and flavor. With the exception of salad greens (tomatoes, celery, cucumbers, radishes, and potatoes, which lose their texture during freezing) most vegetables freeze well.

▶ Slightly undercooking dishes before freez-ing will prevent overcooking when you reheat.

▶ To slash fat from stews and soups, refrigerate them after cooking, skim the fat, then freeze.

▶ Use arrowroot or cornstarch rather than flour to thicken sauces. They'll be less likely to separate when frozen.

▶ Be creative with your use of freezer contain-ers. For example aluminum tart shells can be used for individual pot pies, and muffin tins can hold mini–meat loaves and vegetable purees.

▶ Do not place aluminum foil directly over dinners that contain tomatoes and fruit juices. The acidity can eat through the foil, causing pits in the wrapping and eventual "freezer burn." Instead, use plastic containers or wrap.

▶ Since liquids expand when frozen, make sure to allow about a half inch or more of head space to prevent containers that have sauces or other liquids from bulging or bursting.

▶ If you prepare food in a casserole dish that you don't want to keep in the freezer, line the dish with freezer foil that covers the bottom and sides and also expands outside of the casserole. When the dinner has finished cooking, take the foil ends, lift the food out and wrap it separately or place it in a different container.

▶ Stock your freezer with a few frozen dinner "staples." Homemade chicken stock stored in ice cube trays, for example, is an invaluable ingredi-ent to have on hand. Fresh herbs, whole-grain bread crumbs, and grated cheese can be frozen and sprinkled directly onto dinners as they finish reheating.

▶ For extra convenience in preparing quick side dishes, you can freeze fresh-sliced or chopped vegetables in such products as Baggies Extra Protection Freezer Bags, which can go straight from the freezer into boiling water. Fill each bag with a single serving. When you're ready to use one, just take it from the freezer and cook it right in the bag. As an alternative, prepare chopped vegetables as side dishes to go with your homemade frozen entrees.

▶ To freeze fresh fruits, simply place whole fruits, such as berries, in a single layer on a cookie sheet and freeze. Once fully frozen, the fruits can be placed in a container without sticking together. Fruits that are susceptible to browning, such as sliced apples, pears, and peaches, should be sprinkled with lemon juice and ascorbic acid powder (vitamin C) before freezing to prevent discoloration.

▶ Since certain spices, including oregano, thyme, and parsley, often intensify in flavor during freezing, you might choose to slightly under-season dishes in which you use them. You can always add more seasoning later if it's needed.

▶ For dinners that will be reheated by microwaving, cover containers with plastic wrap rather than foil before freezing so the dish can be placed directly into the microwave.

To assure that the dinners are properly stored, defrosted, and reheated, follow these guidelines:

▶ Store your meals in aluminum foil or in plastic containers that specify "freezer-proof" or "freezer safe" on the label. These products are specially designed to prevent moisture loss. You can also reuse containers and microwave trays saved from store-bought frozen dinners as long as you clean them thoroughly.

▶ Try to get rid of as much air as possible from plastic freezer bags by pressing it out with your palms before sealing. This will help foods stay fresh.

▶ Never thaw frozen dinners on the kitchen counter. The longer food sits at room temperature, the greater the chance it will become a breeding ground for bacteria. It's best to thaw foods in the refrigerator overnight.

▶ If you forget to defrost a frozen dinner in advance, place the sealed container in cold water, changing the water approximately every 30 minutes.

Make the Most of Microwave Magic

With the advent of the microwave oven, the true promise of convenience cooking has been realized. Now the most complex dishes can be served up in minutes, and the tedium of pot scrubbing is virtually eliminated. Even children can use the microwave to fix quick snacks.

If consumers found this space-age cooking machine intimidating at first, they nevertheless have embraced it with enthusiasm. Today, as many as 70 percent of American households have a microwave in the kitchen, outnumbering households with toaster ovens, VCRs, food processors, and even dishwashers. Food manufacturers, happy to oblige the demand, have made increasing numbers of microwaveable products, which now account for nearly 20 percent of all supermarket items purchased.

Still, consumers have some lingering questions about the safety of microwave ovens, the quality and taste of foods cooked in them, and the nutritional benefits of microwaving.

Setting Fears to Rest

Safety concerns occasionally nag even the most knowledgeable microwave owners. People have sometimes associated microwaves with nuclear radiation, but the two are vastly different. Microwaves are just that: *waves*. They are similar to

Try These Healthy Homemade Frozen Meals

Parmesan Chicken with Herbed Barley

10 servings. Nutrition information per serving: cholesterol, 81 mg; sodium, 172 mg; protein, 35 g; calories, 287; calories from fat, 19 percent

For the Chicken:
¾ cup finely ground whole-wheat bread crumbs
½ cup grated parmesan cheese
1 tbsp. dried basil
⅓ cup skim or low-fat (1%) milk
2 lb. boneless, skinless chicken breasts

For the Herbed Barley:
1 8-oz. can low-sodium chicken broth
½ cup chopped onion
2 tbsp. safflower oil
⅓ cup chopped green pepper
3 cups pearl barley
¼ tsp. each: salt and black pepper
pinch of tumeric (optional)

Instructions:

To prepare chicken, combine bread crumbs, parmesan cheese, and basil in a bowl. Dip chicken breasts one at a time into milk and then roll in parmesan mixture, shaking off excess. Cook on foil-covered baking sheet coated with nonstick spray at 350° F for 10 minutes. Wrap each breast in heavy-duty freezer foil. Label and freeze.

To make herbed barley, sauté onion in oil in a medium-sized saucepan for about 3 minutes or until translucent. Add green pepper and cook for an additional 3 minutes. Add chicken broth and bring to a boil. Add barley and spices. Lower heat and simmer, covered, for about 45 minutes. Divide the mixture into 10 individual freezer containers.

To prepare from frozen, place foil-covered breast(s) on a baking sheet and heat in the oven at 375° F for 30 minutes or until heated thoroughly. To heat barley, bake at 375° F for 45 minutes. Serve with shredded raw cabbage and carrots, along with steamed asparagus.

Cincinnati Chili

12 servings. Nutrition information per serving: cholesterol, 53 mg; sodium, 356 mg; protein, 21 g; calories, 240; calories from fat, 30 percent

2 lb. lean ground beef
4 bay leaves
1 cup chopped onion
3 finely chopped medium garlic cloves
1½ tsp. cinnamon
1 tbsp. allspice
4 tbsp. vinegar
1 tsp. crushed red pepper

1 tbsp. chili powder
2 tsp. cumin
½ tsp. oregano
2 tsp. sugar
1 6-oz. can tomato paste
5 cups water
2 15-oz. cans kidney beans, drained
4 cups cooked vermicelli

Instructions:

Place a nonstick skillet over medium heat and add ground beef when skillet is hot. Cook over low heat until the beef is brown. Drain fat from pan. Add remaining ingredients, except kidney beans, and bring them to a boil. Simmer, uncovered, for about 1½ hours, skimming fat from the surface as necessary. Remove bay leaves. Add kidney beans. Simmer 30 minutes more.

Divide chili into 12 individual freezer containers. Cover and label.

To heat from frozen, bake at 375° F for 40 minutes or until thoroughly heated. Serve with slice of whole-grain bread and a spinach-mushroom salad.

radio waves that are in the air at all times, the difference being that radio waves are broadcast over a distance, while the microwave "broadcasting" is self-contained, inside the oven. The electromagnetic rays in ovens cause the molecules in food to vibrate, and this vibration creates the heat necessary to turn an item from cold to hot or from raw to ready-to-eat. The microwaves do not actually touch most of the food they cook. They penetrate only its surface, three-quarters of an inch to an inch and a half deep. As the vibrating molecules near the surface agitate the deeper molecules, they create the friction required to heat the food all the way through.

While it's true that too much exposure to any kind of radiation can be dangerous (the way an overdose of ultraviolet light causes sunburn), the safeguards built into microwave ovens make it virtually impossible for any harm to come from them as long as they are in good working order. The leakage limits set by the Food and Drug Administration (FDA) are substantially below acknowledged danger levels. Even if the leakage was to reach the maximum level set by the FDA, moving only a couple of inches back from the oven dramatically decreases radiation exposure. Indeed, a person standing 20 inches away from a microwave that has any leakage will receive just one-hundredth the exposure of someone standing two inches away.

The construction of microwave oven doors provides another safeguard. No microwaves can be generated while the door is open: By law, two interlock switches must be activated for operation. The door is sealed to keep the microwaves inside the oven, and the viewing window contains a metallic screen that reflects microwaves back into the appliance and prevents their escape into the kitchen.

Once the food is cooked, it is not "full of microwaves." They dissipate once they've completed their job.

Attention to these safety basics will virtually eliminate any risk:

▶ Never tamper with the safety interlocks or allow residue to collect on the sealing surfaces of the doors.

▶ Do not operate the oven if the door or viewing window is bent, cracked, loose, or damaged in any way.

▶ Don't operate the oven without food or liquid in it, as this could result in damage to the magnetron tube or energy-absorbing glass tray. Leave a small cup of water in the oven to absorb energy in case the oven is turned on accidentally.

▶ avoid using metallic materials in your oven unless they're specifically noted to be safe. Metal reflects microwave energy away from the food and can disrupt the operation and damage the oven. Read the owner's manual to find out which materials are safe.

▶ Fires can start when food is overcooked. Be sure to experiment with cooking times in advance.

▶ Care should be used with combustible products. Eggs cooked in the shell may burst; popcorn cooked without a microwave popping accessory can explode. Airtight bags should be punctured before heating.

▶ If materials inside the oven catch fire, don't open the door. Turn the oven off and disconnect the power.

▶ Always read the owner's manual thoroughly before using the microwave oven for the first time.

Nutritional Bonuses

Not only are microwave ovens perfectly safe, they also offer nutritional benefits that cannot be attained by traditional means. The fast-heating feature prevents the loss of nutrients that can be caused by overcooking. And since microwaves require little or no water to cook foods, vitamins are not lost into the water.

A number of vitamins, including vitamin C, rapidly break down when they're exposed to heat, dissolving in the cooking water. With shorter cooking times, more vitamin C is retained.

To demonstrate the point, Gertrude Armbruster, Ph.D., a professor in the Division of Nutritional Sciences at Cornell University, tested fruits and vegetables cooked both in the microwave and by traditional means of boiling and baking. She found that 23 of 24 varieties of produce—ranging from apples to turnips—came out of the microwave with more vitamin C. For example, an apple baked in a conventional oven for 30 minutes is left with only 7 of its original 15 milligrams of vitamin C; microwaving the apple takes less than four minutes and preserves all 15.

Other water-soluble and heat-sensitive vitamins are "saved" by the microwave. The B vitamins thiamin, riboflavin, folic acid, and B-6 are preserved in foods at full strength.

The microwave can be a big help in cutting back on salt and sugar, too. Since it enhances the natural flavors in food, there's less temptation to reach for the salt shaker or the sugar bowl.

The microwave is literally a "lean machine." Since foods cook in their own moisture, no additional fats or oils are needed for cooking. Vegeta-

ble, fish, and poultry dishes steamed or poached in the microwave are light, healthy, and delicious.

Some people might consider the effect on bacon safety as another nutritional bonus of microwaves. Conventional high-temperature frying converts nitrates used for curing bacon into nitrosamines, which have caused cancer in laboratory animals. But in the microwave, the equivalent frying temperatures are reached only in the last seconds of cooking, not enough time to trigger the reaction.

Still Working on Taste and Texture

If there are limitations to the wonders of microwave technology they exist in the way food tastes, how it looks, and its texture. The fast-cooking feature of the microwave oven renders it less effective for foods that require gradual cooking or dry heat. The microwave's moist heat steams rather than bakes food; it can't crisp a pot roast, fry meats, or get a rise out of bread dough.

Some forecasters predict that public taste may adjust to the microwave's limits by undergoing an evolution; in other words, ten years hence, we may no longer find a browned cake top normal or a crackling potato skin desirable. We'll chew rather than crunch our pizza crust, cut grilled cheese sandwiches with a knife and fork, admire the consistency of limp French fries, and accept a gray tint to our pot roasts.

More likely, the technology will rise to the demands of tradition. Food engineers are working hard to develop taste and texture-enhancing methods that will combat many of the microwave's perceived limitations. Precooked, presealed meats—already browned and ready to reheat—might provide one solution. And while most of the dough-based items now prepared for microwaves—like pizza, waffles, and sandwiches—lack a flakey home-baked texture, the invention of new cooking ingredients and utensils could change that. Multipurpose equipment is being introduced that takes the full range of cooking needs into consideration. The two-in-one microwave convection combination is a single unit that can be used as both a microwave and a regular convection oven, coordinating cooking between the two. For example, with a roast baking in a conventional oven, the microwave element can be programmed to switch on when it's time to steam the vegetables.

For the most part, it's best to use the microwave for cooking tasks it does best: producing rich, moist casserole dishes; steaming fresh, crisp vegetables; making creamy thick soups and puddings; producing tender, flavorful steamed chicken and fish; defrosting foods; and reheating leftovers quickly.

Ten Tips for Microwaving

New owners find that there's an adjustment period involved in learning to make the most of a microwave oven. Individual microwaves differ in small ways. For example, finding the precise cooking time for various dishes is a trial-and-error process. Once mastered, a microwave has great versatility, and it can't be beat for convenience. These tips will help make microwave cooking simpler and more nutritious.

Remove food from the oven a little before it is done: Even after the oven has shut off, food keeps cooking for a while since the molecules near the food's surface continue to agitate those deeper down. If you fail to account for this, food will overcook and you'll lose some of the nutritional benefits. For example, a frozen dish may not look ready when it first comes out, but let it stand for five minutes and you'll see a difference. It can always go back in the oven if it needs more cooking after that.

Cover dishes to promote steaming: A cover will help promote steaming and shorten the cooking time by sealing in the heat. Any food you would cook covered in a conventional oven—casseroles, vegetable dishes—should be covered in the microwave.

Don't cook large items: The microwave is probably not the best vehicle for your Thanksgiving turkey. Large items don't work well because the microwave energy is too close to the item to cook it evenly. If possible, cut up pieces of meat before cooking—cubes of beef will work better than a whole roast.

Use dishes that promote evenness in cooking: Wide, shallow dishes work better than deep and narrow ones. Uniformity of shape is also enhanced by the use of a round dish rather than a rectangular or square one. If you must use a dish with corners, cover them with aluminum foil at first since food cooks faster at corners and foil will keep out the microwaves. (It's okay to use a little aluminum foil in the microwave, but be sure to keep it away from the oven walls.)

Microwaves make great baking aids: Even if you're baking in a conventional oven, the microwave can cut the preparation time substantially. Butter, margarine, and chocolate melt quickly and more evenly than on a stove top; milk heats up and water boils within seconds.

Check the liquid level of leftovers before reheating: Some dishes may absorb all the liquid the first time around, and a dab of butter or a couple of tablespoons of water should be added before reheating.

Heat baby bottles on the stove: Don't use the microwave for heating up bottles of baby's milk. Since the exterior of the bottle remains cool, it is harder to judge the heat of the milk, and infants have been scalded as a result of it being too hot.

Experiment with cooking levels: Practice cooking or reheating foods at various levels to find what works best. Try not to reheat foods at 100 percent heating capacity. Turn your microwave to 50 percent for the first few minutes, and up to 100 percent only during the last minute or two.

Cook foods in advance and freeze: Save time by preparing and freezing favorite dishes in advance. If you slightly undercook them the first time around, reheating will take nothing away from the flavor or texture.

Learn the secrets of browning: Contrary to popular belief, there are ways meat can be browned in the microwave. Trim as much fat off as possible, since fat attracts and absorbs the microwave energy. (Remember, oil isn't needed for cooking in the microwave the way it is in a conventional oven.) The absence of excess fat allows more heat to get to the meat, and any fat in the meat will then begin to brown. There are also a number of commercial products that enhance the flavor and add the rich brown coloring we're used to in meat.

13

Insure Your Food's Safety

When some states banned apples from the public schools in early 1989 after hearing reports that the pesticide daminozide (marketed under the trade name Alar) might cause cancer, the dramatic event once again focused public attention on the safety of the American food supply. More than ever, people are concerned about the pesticides being used on our fruits and vegetables, the contaminants that enter the water from toxic waste dumping, oil spills, and other hazards, and the bacteria that might be infecting common foods, such as eggs. To what extent is public concern warranted?

The Bacterial Invasion Can Be Halted

As many as 80 million Americans suffer from some form of food poisoning each year, experiencing problems that range from mild cramps and diarrhea to severe nausea, diarrhea, and dehydration. While few die as a result, small children and the elderly are particularly vulnerable.

The growing problem of food contamination is an issue that industry and government must reckon with. Most of our food supply, including meat, poultry, fish, dairy products, fruits, and veg-

etables, is capable of being contaminated with one of several bacteria. However, in spite of this seemingly grim picture, control over microbiological risk is mostly in the hands of individual homemakers and consumers. According to the Centers for Disease Control, up to 85 percent of the incidences of food poisoning could be avoided if people followed basic health and safety guidelines in the preparation, storage, and serving of foods.

The bacteria that cause food poisoning are invisible. You cannot see, taste, or smell them. They attach themselves to dust particles, cling to the skins of fruits and vegetables, linger on peoples' hands and in their noses, and reside in the intestines of animals.

Although there are many varieties of bacteria, four are most familiar to Americans: salmonella, *Staphyloccus aureus (S. aureus), Clostridium perfringens (C. perfringens), and Clostridium botulinum (botulism).*

Salmonella

Salmonella is the most common bacteria, responsible for about half of all food poisoning. It is generally found in raw animal foods, such as meat, eggs, and poultry. Lately, salmonella has been turning up with increasing frequency in slaughtered chickens. The symptoms of salmonella poisoning, which include nausea, diarrhea, and fever, occur within 12 to 48 hours of ingesting the contaminated food. Not everyone who eats contaminated food gets sick—the problem seems to occur most frequently in young children, the elderly, and the infirm—but, even in mildly infected people, the unpleasant symptoms can linger for a few days.

The federal government and the food industry are engaged in efforts to reduce the incidence of salmonella poisoning. In the meantime, you can avoid it by following these guidelines:

▶ Rinse meat and poultry with cold water before cooking to rinse away some of the bacteria.

▶ Cook poultry until there is no pink meat. If you use a meat thermometer, check to see that the meat reaches an internal temperature of 180° to 185° F. Make sure to insert the thermometer into the thickest part of the chicken—the thigh, away from the bone—to get the most accurate reading.

▶ Keep utensils and cutting boards used to prepare meat and poultry separate from those used to prepare fruit and vegetables. For example, if you prepare a mixed chicken and vegetable dish, use a separate knife and cutting board for the chicken and the vegetables.

▶ Be sure to thoroughly wash all the utensils you use to prepare raw meat and poultry with hot, soapy water (dishwasher water is hot enough).

▶ For extra protection, keep wood cutting boards clean by washing them every few days with a diluted bleach-and-water solution. The bleach should kill any bacteria.

S. aureus

The microorganism *S. aureus* is responsible for a little more than 25 percent of all food-borne illnesses. It is carried in the noses and throats of most people. That's why sneezing or coughing on

food—especially a protein-containing food like meat, or pudding—can contaminate it. Symptoms include mild diarrhea, sometimes accompanied by nausea and vomiting.

It is not the bacterium itself that brings on the symptoms, but the toxins (poisons) it produces. Even though cooking kills the bacteria, it does not destroy the toxins. You can cut down on the effects of *S. aureus* by following these guidelines:

▶ Never leave yet-to-be-cooked or already cooked foods at room temperature for long periods of time. A lukewarm temperature of 40° to 140° F (not piping hot but not as cold as a refrigerator) allows bacteria to grow rapidly and thereby produce more toxins.

▶ Thaw frozen foods in the refrigerator, not on the counter, to prevent them from getting too warm.

▶ Keep foods hot on the stove or in the oven until you are ready to serve them. Even a dish as seemingly harmless as a rice casserole can produce enough toxins to be potentially dangerous if it is left out at room temperature for more than two hours.

▶ Refrigerate leftovers as soon as possible.

C. perfringens

Sometimes called the "cafeteria germ," this bacteria accounts for about one in ten reported cases of food poisoning. It usually occurs in settings where large batches of meat, turkey, and other foods are cooked. Like *S. aureus,* it produces toxins, or spores, that are resistant to the heat of cooking. It causes a mild illness of short duration (12 to 24 hours) and is rarely serious enough to warrant medical treatment.

Precautions to be taken are similar to those listed for *S. aureus.*

▶ Don't leave food out at room temperature for longer than 2 hours.

► When cooking large batches of food, such as stew, divide the leftovers into small batches so that, once in the refrigerator, they will quickly cool to temperatures that limit the growth of bacteria.

Botulism

Botulism is the most severe food-borne illness, but it is also the most rare; there are fewer than 100 cases reported during a year in the entire country. One familiar telltale sign of the presence of bacteria that leads to botulism is a bulging can. The toxin responsible for the bulging is produced by the bacterium *Clostridium botulinum,* commonly found in soil, water, and manure. Besides bulging, also watch out for cracked jars and loose lids.

Occasionally, isolated incidents of botulism have been attributed to foods that are not in damaged containers. In one such case, a restaurant allowed a batch of sautéed onions to be kept throughout the day at temperatures slightly lower than 140° F, within the range at which bacteria thrive. Over the course of several hours, large enough quantities of the toxin were produced to make several people very ill. If the onions had been refrigerated and reheated in small batches as needed, the incident could have been prevented.

Symptoms of botulism can range from double vision and difficulty in breathing to, in the most severe cases, death.

Other Bacteria

Thanks to improved detection methods, food safety experts are now able to identify other microorganisms in our food supply. One, *Campylobacter (C. jejuni),* is widely recognized as a source of illness in cattle, but has rarely been identified as harmful to humans. *C. jejuni* is present in the intestinal tract of healthy cattle and can taint meat and poultry during the slaughtering process. However, heat destroys this bacterium, so you can easily eliminate the danger by thoroughly cooking raw meat and poultry. To assure the safety of hamburger and other kinds of beef, be sure that the meat is brown or at least brownish-pink in the center before you eat it. Does this mean you shouldn't eat rare meat? Rare beef, cooked to an internal temperature of only 140° F, may still contain some bacteria. Although it probably won't cause any illness, it is nevertheless more likely to result in adverse reactions than meat that is well-done.

Another newly identified cause of human illness is *Listeria monocytogenes.* In the past identified only with animal disease, it is now known to bring on flu-like symptoms in people. In severe cases, it can cause meningitis, a life-threatening inflammation of the membranes that encircle the brain and spinal cord. Pregnant women, infants, and the elderly seem to be at the greatest risk.

Proper cooking can also destroy *Listeria.* But in some cases it is present in foods that do not require cooking, such as some dairy products. At present, the best defense, in addition to cooking foods properly, is to avoid raw or unpasteurized milk products.

Raw Fish Alert

Americans have always eaten certain seafoods raw, but in recent years sporadic reports of illness associated with raw clams and oysters have given rise to concerns. Health hazards, while not common, do exist from parasites that imbed themselves in fish.

Anisaki is a tightly coiled, clear, worm-like parasite (about one-half to three-quarters of an inch in length) that imbeds itself in salmon, herring, and other fish. Symptoms of illness caused by ingestion of the worm are a combination of intestinal problems that include diarrhea and abdominal pain. However, incidents of illness are rare in the United States.

If you are concerned about eating raw fish, you might want to substitute vegetable sushi for the kind that contains raw fish, although a well-

▶ NUTRITION QUIZ ◀

Can You Pick a Good Egg?

Salmonella poisoning has occurred from eating eggs. Do you know a good egg from a bad egg? Do you know the best way to store your eggs before and after cooking? Can you tell if an egg is fresh and safe to eat? Take this quiz and find out.

1. How many minutes does it take to be certain an egg is hard-cooked?
   (a) 7   (b) 15   (c) 20

2. Dyeing Easter eggs
   (a) makes them spoil more quickly   (b) poses a risk because of hazardous food dyes   (c) is a harmless tradition

3. A raw egg is "bad" if it has
   (a) a blood spot   (b) a dark ring around the yolk after it is cooked   (c) a cracked shell.

4. Which type of egg keeps longest?
   (a) fertilized   (b) unfertilized   (c) whether or not an egg is fertilized has nothing to do with how long it will keep

5. Raw eggs will remain fresh in the refrigerator
   (a) in a paper bag   (b) in the box they came in   (c) in the refrigerator's built-in egg tray

6. A sure sign that an egg has lost some of its freshness is that
   (a) the white is thick and cloudy   (b) the white is runny and clear   (c) the white separates easily from the yolk

ANSWERS

1. Seven minutes is the recommended time to be sure the egg is cooked but not over-cooked. To prevent cracking and toughness, place uncooked eggs in a pan of cold water, then bring them to a boil over high heat. After cooking, remove eggs from the burner and let them sit, covered, for 15 minutes, then rinse them in cold water.

2. (c) There is no reason to worry about the safety of packaged dyes used to color eggs. However, you do have to be careful not to leave the eggs at room temperature for too long. Easter egg hunts are fun, but be sure to hide the eggs right before the hunt and refrigerate them immediately after.

3. (c) If a shell cracks in the supermarket or on the way home, it is best to throw the egg away because it may become contaminated with salmonella or other bacteria before it is refrigerated. If you crack an egg in your kitchen and immediately refrigerate it, it should be safe.

Blood spots and dark rings are harmless. A blood spot is simply the result of a blood vessel rupture on the egg's surface. The ring results from an interaction between the iron and sulfur naturally present in eggs.

4. **(b)** The unfertilized eggs typically sold in the supermarket are likely to keep longer than the fertilized eggs sold in certain health food stores. Once an egg is fertilized, the yolk can start to develop, leading to quicker deterioration. Contrary to what health food proponents claim, fertilized eggs offer no additional health benefits.

5. It's best to store eggs in the covered containers in which they are bought because they readily lose moisture and absorb odor from other foods. For best taste and freshness, eggs should be used within two to three weeks after you bring them home.

6. **(b)** As an egg ages, it gives off carbon dioxide, causing the white to spread and turn clear.

trained sushi chef can spot the translucent worm, as can most other people once they know what to look for. It might be more risky to eat raw clams and oysters. (To make sure clams are bacteria-free, steam them from four to six minutes. The one minute of cooking needed to open the shell is not enough to kill bacteria.)

Dining Out Defensively

When you're away from home, what can you do to protect yourself from food poisoning? Evaluate a restaurant's overall health by checking these details:

▶ Are the dishes and utensils clean?

▶ Is food (for example, desserts) displayed uncovered?

▶ Are the hot foods served to you really hot?

▶ How are the tables cleaned? Are fresh rags used for each table?

▶ Do employees appear clean and neatly dressed? Do you notice that they smoke in the kitchen or nibble at food while they're cooking?

▶ Are the bathrooms clean? Do they have sanitary soap and towel dispensers?

Of course you can never be 100 percent certain of food that you eat in a restaurant. But if you're concerned about food safety, you should never eat in an establishment that doesn't make cleanliness a priority.

Guidelines for Globetrotters

For people traveling overseas, bacterial infections are one of the greatest nutritional impediments. Unfortunately, there's no surefire way to prevent traveler's diarrhea, which infects an estimated 3 million Americans a year with symptoms that include abdominal cramps, nausea, bloating, fever and malaise. But the risks can be substantially decreased by paying attention to what you eat and where you eat it.

First of all, use common sense. In most industrialized countries you need only to use the same precautions that you use when dining out at home. No matter where you are, if you have any questions about the food or water, do not consume it. In those instances, your health and comfort take precedence over everything—including the sensitivities of your host.

In locations where you have reason to believe that sanitation is a problem (and this information is readily available to travelers), completely avoid eating raw or undercooked meat and seafood. Raw vegetables and fruit should also be avoided, unless they can be peeled first. Tap water, ice made from tap water, and unpasteurized dairy products should also be avoided. (Safe, bottled water is almost universally available.) All of these have a comparatively high chance of being infected with diarrhea-causing bacteria. In addition, it is best not to drink more coffee, tea, or alcohol than usual, since large amounts of these can bring on diarrhea.

Food safety is also influenced by how clean food is kept during preparation and the way it is cooked. Dishes bought from street vendors are the most likely to be contaminated. Restaurants vary in their sanitary conditions. The finer ones that have good reputations and are listed in travel guides are most likely to be careful about using high standards of food safety. But it is best to be on guard. Consider also the way food is prepared. Some chefs season foods with spices or other ingredients which may cause severe, though short-lived, reactions. Others do not regularly change oil used for deep-fat frying, so that foods are cooked in rancid fat, which is very irritating to the intestines. The taste of rancidity is sometimes masked by the spices.

High-risk countries for traveler's diarrhea include the developing countries of Latin America, Africa, the Middle East, and Asia. Among the intermediate-risk destinations are most of the southern European nations and some of the Caribbean islands. Those traveling to northern Europe, Japan, Australia, and New Zealand are least likely to be affected.

If traveler's diarrhea does strike, it's usually within a week of arrival in a foreign country, and it rarely lasts longer than three or four days. Many travelers wait it out without taking any special measures other than increasing fluid intake to avoid becoming dehydrated. However, before leaving the United States, you can obtain a prescription drug from your physician (Lomotil or Imodium) that will slow down intestinal motility and cut down on the number of trips you make to the bathroom. But avoid taking antimicrobial drugs to prevent diarrhea, since these medications can bring on side effects such as allergic reactions, skin rashes, and blood disorders.

If you come down with the "runs," it is important to maintain your body's fluid and electrolyte needs by consuming caffeine-free soft drinks, salted crackers, and fruit juices that come in cans or that you know have been made with clean water and peeled fruits. Stay away from dairy products, alcohol, and beverages with caffeine. Although some people think the bacteria in yogurt can help treat this condition, there is no evidence that it works.

Since the water in the United States is treated with chlorine, we rarely encounter many of the microorganisms found in the water of some foreign countries. For this reason, many Americans suffer intestinal problems from drinking the water. Locations that are of particular concern include South and Central America, Asia, the Middle East, Africa, and some parts of the Caribbean.

In developing countries, travelers should usually not feel safe drinking the tap water in large hotels. Wherever you are, be sure to ask if the hotel has a water purification system.

Bottled water can be used for drinking and for brushing your teeth. Carbonated water may be the safest, since carbonation appears to kill some of the microorganisms. Be sure that the bottles have been properly sealed.

When dining out, it is safe to drink liquids that require boiling water—such as coffee and tea—since boiling kills bacteria. Bottled drinks such as beer, soda, and juices are also safe. But avoid mixed drinks or drinks served with ice cubes.

In developing countries and rural areas where milk is not pasteurized, all noncanned and dehydrated milk and dairy products should be avoided. Contaminated milk products can cause severe intestinal ailments. If necessary, unpasteurized milk can be made safe by boiling, but this is impractical for most travelers.

If you're "roughing it"—hiking or backpacking through undeveloped areas—there are water-purifying tablets available (Halzone or Potable-Aqua) in sporting goods stores and pharmacies. If electricity is available, you can purify your water by boiling it on an electric hot plate—if you have one. Remember that outside the United States almost all countries use equipment that takes 220 volts.

Storing Foods for Taste and Safety

Although no rigid standards have been established as a result of scientific tests, we recommend that you follow these guidelines for food storage to promote safety and maintain quality. To help yourself keep track, date all packages before storing them.

In the freezer at 0°, these foods will last:

▶ Fresh chickens (whole or in parts): 10 months

▶ Beef roasts: 6–12 months (the larger the roast, the longer it will store)

▶ Lamb and veal: 6–9 months

▶ Pork: 3–6 months

▶ Lean fish: 6 months (examples: sole, haddock, and flounder)

▶ Fatty fish: 2–3 months (examples: salmon, mackerel, and bluefish)

▶ Baked bread and rolls: 3–6 months (frosted: 2 months)

▶ Frozen juice: 12 months

▶ Frozen vegetables: 8 months (unless otherwise dated)

▶ Hard cheese: 6–8 weeks

▶ Soft cheese: 3 months

▶ Main-dish casseroles or other precooked dishes: 3 months

▶ Butter: 6–9 months

In the refrigerator at 40°, these foods will last:

▶ Ground meat: 2–3 days

▶ Steaks and chops: 2–3 days

▶ Opened baby food: 2 days

▶ Eggs: 2–3 weeks

▶ Margarine: 4–6 months

▶ Butter (sweet): 2 weeks (a little longer if lightly salted)

On the shelf at 70°, these foods will last:

▶ Salad oils (opened): 1 year (longer in the refrigerator)

▶ Flour: 6–8 months (if kept in a dry container)

▶ Dry cereals (opened): 2–3 months

▶ Dry cereals (unopened): 12 months

Food Safety on Land and Sea

The environment has become one of the principal topics of public debate in the United States and other industrialized countries. To what extent do we need to be concerned about the influence of pollution on the food we eat and the water we drink?

Polluted Fishing: Is There Cause for Alarm?

There has been concern among environmentalists for some time about pollution in the bodies

► NUTRITION QUIZ ◄

How Safe Is Your Kitchen?

You may know that raw pork is not safe, or that a bulging can spells trouble. But how aware are you of the safety of other items in your kitchen? Take this quiz to find out.

Is it safe or risky to eat . . .

1. Hot dogs that have been stored in an unopened package in the refrigerator for 10 days?
   Safe _____ Risky _____

2. A bruised or moldy piece of fruit?
   Safe _____ Risky _____

3. Frozen ham that was thawed on the counter?
   Safe _____ Risky _____

4. An opened jar of mayonnaise that has been in the refrigerator for six months?
   Safe _____ Risky _____

5. A baked potato left out on the counter from the night before?
   Safe _____ Risky _____

6. Meat loaf that's pink in the middle after cooking?
   Safe _____ Risky _____

7. Raw ground beef that turns brown after a day or two of refrigeration?
   Safe _____ Risky _____

8. An uncooked potato with a greenish cast?
   Safe _____ Risky _____

9. Lettuce or other produce moistened by poultry drippings in a grocery bag?
   Safe _____ Risky _____

10. Steak that was thawed in the refrigerator and then refrozen?
    Safe _____ Risky _____

11. Cooked shrimp that was never "deveined"?
    Safe _____ Risky _____

12. Mustard or ketchup with a black, crusty ring around the rim of the jar?
    Safe _____ Risky _____

13. Moldy or shriveled peanuts?
    Safe _____ Risky _____

ANSWERS

1. (Safe) Hot dogs that come in vacuum-sealed packages can be kept in the refrigerator for up to two weeks. Once opened, you can keep them for about seven days, carefully wrapped in plastic.

2. (Safe)—if it's just bruised; but possibly risky if the bruised portion has become moldy. Some molds can produce harmful toxins, and it's not yet clear whether fruit molds are among them. The best bet is to cut away the moldy section, which should also remove any toxins that might be present.

3. (Risky) Many people think that they can take chances with ham because it has been smoked and salted. But these processes don't make the meat immune to bacterial contamination, especially since a number of manufacturers are lowering the salt content of cured meats. As with any meat, the safest way to thaw ham is in the refrigerator.

4. (Safe) It's a misconception that foods prepared with mayonnaise may go bad sooner. In fact, its high acid and salt content may actually inhibit bacterial growth somewhat. You can keep an opened jar of mayonnaise in the refrigerator for up to a year, provided you don't let it sit at room temperature for extended periods.

5. (Risky) We usually don't think of potatoes as a likely source of food poisoning, but there have been reports of deadly botulism in people who ate foil-wrapped baked potatoes left at room temperature for a day or more, even when they were reheated. Leftovers of most foods should be promptly refrigerated.

6. (Risky) Ground meat undergoes a great deal of handling, compared to other forms. This increases the likelihood of bacterial contamination. For this reason, the USDA suggests cooking meat loaf until it is brown or at least brownish-pink in the center. An even better guide is to cook it to an internal temperature of 170° F, checking with a thermometer, particularly if the meat loaf contains pork.

7. (Safe) Whether it's brown or pink has to do with the amount of oxygen with which it has come into contact. As a general rule, however, don't keep raw ground beef in the refrigerator longer than two days, and don't use it under any circumstances if it doesn't smell right or was left unrefrigerated for any length of time.

8. (Risky) Green-skinned potatoes contain a chemical called solanine, which can cause gastrointestinal illness. You can use green potatoes if you peel them well and remove a layer of flesh underneath the skin.

9. (Risky) Uncooked poultry juices may contain harmful bacteria that could lead to trouble when they get into foods that are eaten raw. If the produce is really saturated, you'd better not use it. But if contact was minimal, you can remove outer sections or rinse and peel.

10. (Safe)—especially if some ice crystals remain. Make sure to thaw the frozen meat in the refrigerator the second time around. Be aware, too, that refreezing might

(continued)

How Safe Is Your Kitchen? (*cont.*)

cause flavor and texture deterioration. You might get better flavor and texture if you cook the meat the first time it is thawed, then refreeze it.

11. **(Safe)** You can eat shrimp that hasn't been deveined as long as you cook it. The black line running down the back is actually the intestines of the shrimp, which are more susceptible to contamination.

12. **(Safe)** The ring is the result of an interaction of the contents with air, not a sign of spoilage. Simply wipe it off and use the remaining contents.

13. **(Risky)** When you crack open peanut shells only to find sickly-looking nuts, don't eat them. The types of mold that grow on nuts (as well as on grains) can produce aflatoxins, some of which are very potent carcinogens.

of water that give us our fish supply. But when beaches up and down the East Coast were closed because of medical waste washing up on shore, the scare hit home for many people. To what extent can we trust that the fish we eat are safe from the effects of industrial pollution and other man-made pollutants? And how can our waters be better protected from indiscriminate illegal dumping of dangerous substances?

It is true that the fish and shellfish we eat has been somewhat compromised by the dumping of industrial and sewage waste into harbors, lakes, and rivers, and by such problems as "red tide," which results in a poison getting into the shellfish we eat.

However, most of the fish we buy is caught offshore or deep at sea where the waters are significantly cleaner. Fish contamination is much more likely to be a problem in sheltered bays, harbors, and recreational freshwater lakes and streams that are near industrial sources of pollution. In addition, most of the problems connected with bacterial contamination are limited to mollusks and shellfish, and these can be avoided with adequate cooking.

Even the industrial waste chemicals polychlorinated biphenyls (PCBs), which are most likely to be concentrated in large, fatty fish, may not be as great a problem as some people think. In an analysis of 1,200 bluefish (considered to be one of the fish most susceptible to contamination because it is fatty) caught off the coast from Massachusetts to North Carolina, all samples under 20 inches in length were within the two-parts-per-million limit set for PCBs by the federal government. Although some of the larger fish exceeded the limit, the National Oceanic Atmospheric Administration, which conducted the study, believes it may pose a problem only for recreational fishermen and their families who eat the fish day after day, year after year. In the summer of 1989, the National Wildlife Federation, the nation's largest conservation organization, issued a report on toxic chemicals that were present in Lake Michigan's fish supply because of industrial contaminants. The report stated that eating these fish posed a greater cancer risk than had been previously acknowledged. Since sport fishing is a $4.2 billion-a-year industry in this area, the report came under sharp attack from state health and fisheries officials, who suggested the danger was overstated. The heat of controversies like this one make it hard for consumers and fishermen to judge the extent to which they should be concerned. However, if you fish and are not aware of advisory warnings regarding certain species in your area, call your state's wildlife association or department of health to see if any cautions have been issued.

There are no mandatory federal inspection programs for fish, but the government does watch the fish supply. For example, the FDA monitors swordfish because it is one of the species that is most likely to be contaminated with mercury. If the mercury level is found to be above acceptable limits, regulatory action is taken to prevent the fish from reaching your table. More recent studies have focused on the potential danger of airborne pollutants, which sometimes travel great distances before falling into the water. Congress is currently reviewing legislation that would require the EPA to study the effects of airborne toxic chemicals on the Great Lakes.

You can exercise appropriate caution by taking the following measures:

▶ Buy your fish at reputable outlets. Even though the "catch of the day" a local fisherman may be selling off the back of his truck might seem appealing, it's best to avoid fish whose origin is uncertain. You might pay more at the fish store or supermarket, but the extra protection is probably worth it.

▶ Once home, keep fish chilled in the refrigerator prior to cooking to retard the growth of bacteria.

▶ When preparing fish for cooking, cut away the skin and dark-colored flesh of fatty fish to eliminate the chance of contamination from PCBs.

▶ Grill or broil fatty fish in ways that allow the drippings to run off.

Can We Safely Drink the Water?

Some experts believe the safety of our drinking water may be the most important public health issue of the next decade—especially the safety of our groundwater, which is the large reservoir lying beneath the earth's surface that supplies half the drinking water flowing through our faucets. One reason for the heightened concern is that

industrial chemicals have been discovered in about 20 percent of the country's public water systems, and many of these chemicals have not been rigorously tested to see if they are reaching homes in levels that may be toxic. To help deal with the problem, Congress has voted to impose a stricter schedule on the Environmental Protection Agency (EPA), the arm of the government that has been setting maximum levels of contaminants since the Safe Drinking Water Act was put into effect in 1974. The EPA must set maximum permissible levels for 61 additional substances by 1989, 25 more by 1991, and 25 more each year from 1992 through 1994.

Aside from industrial pollutants, environmentalists are concerned about the levels of lead in our water supplies. Indeed, the EPA has recently estimated that 42 million Americans may be drinking water that exceeds a proposed safe level (20 parts per billion) of lead, a metal that can damage the nervous system in infants and children and worsen high blood pressure in adults.

Fortunately, lead in drinking water is a problem you can do something about without waiting for someone to take action from the outside. Here are the practical ways you can act to protect your own water.

First, check your plumbing. Copper pipes may contain some lead solder at their joints. Older homes sometimes have lead pipes.

To find out whether any lead is actually leaching into the water that runs through the pipes, have your water tested, either by the local water utility or by a private laboratory. If the lab determines that a significant amount of lead is getting into your drinking water, consider installing a water purification system.

In the interim, use the cold water tap for making coffee and for cooking, since lead leaches more easily into hot water than cold. You can also let your water run for a few minutes before using it, since water that has been sitting still in pipes will contain more lead. Of course, these are emergency measures that should not be relied upon for any substantial length of time.

Buying bottled water is an expensive alternative —more than 625 times the cost of tap water!— and it isn't necessarily the answer to all the problems associated with tap water. Legally, bottled water does not have to be any freer from contaminants than water from a faucet, aside from meeting regulations that apply to the sanitary bottling of a beverage. And since some bottled water comes from municipal water supplies rather than privately owned and protected springs and wells, do not assume it is any cleaner than the water from your kitchen sink.

If you want your tap water analyzed, the EPA will refer you to the certified laboratories in your area. Call toll-free: 1-800-426-4791. If you decide to install a water filter but aren't sure how to choose one that is reliable, the EPA recommends that you contact the National Sanitation Foundation at P.O. Box 1468, Ann Arbor, Michigan, 48106.

The Pesticide Problem

In recent years, the federal government has stepped up its efforts to control the levels of harmful pesticides used to protect our fruit, vegetable, and grain supply from insects. One, ethylene dibromide (EDB), a highly effective insect killer, was taken off the market in 1984 after many studies showed that it caused cancer and genetic mutations in animals.

But a public outcry has accompanied evidence that the Environmental Protection Agency (EPA) is moving far too slowly in its review of pesticides. Even with EDB, there have been complaints that the EPA did not act for several years after the danger became evident. Furthermore, hardly any imported fruits and vegetables from countries that do not share the United States ban are tested for the pesticide. Responding to the outcry, the House of Representatives passed legislation in 1988 that set a nine-year deadline for retesting 600 active ingredients that are used in nearly 50,000 commercial pesticides.

The status of daminozide, a pesticide used primarily to keep apples firm and red (marketed under the trade name Alar), is an example of how slowly the EPA has moved. Studies showing that daminozide caused cancer in laboratory animals were emerging during the mid-1970s, and the EPA began testing the pesticide in 1977. After eight years, the agency's pesticide office finally recommended a ban of Alar. But the EPA's science advisory board determined that the studies were not adequate to warrant a ban, and Alar was left on the market pending further tests. Although the controversy led many manufacturers and suppliers to discontinue its use, it was hard for consumers (that is, those who were even aware of the situation back then) to know when their apples, apple juice, and other apple products had been sprayed with the chemical.

The daminozide battle heated up again in 1989 after the National Resources Defense Council (NRDC), a New York-based environmental group, published a study titled "Intolerable Risk: Pesticides in Our Children's Food." Authors of the study argued that children consume larger quantities of certain fruits and vegetables (and therefore pesticides) than adults. For example, fruit comprises an estimated 34 percent of the diet of preschoolers, as opposed to 20 percent of adult diets. In particular, the study cited the potential danger from Alar, noting that the typical child consumes seven times as many apples and seven times as much applesauce as adults. The EPA announced in February that it would again try to ban daminozide. But meanwhile, many schools were pulling apples from the menu and many parents were eliminating them from the family diet.

To some extent, the public has overracted to the Alar revelations. The EPA estimates that Alar is only used on a very small percent of the total crop, and while there might be a minute risk for some, it is questionable whether eliminating apples, which are an important source of dietary fiber, is a healthier course of action.

To keep the pesticide issue in perspective, it must be noted that the overall cancer death rate during the 1950s through the 1970s, the decades during which the use of pesticides increased dramatically, rose only slightly. While the use of pesticides must be monitored carefully, in some respects the public outcry has distracted us from the more significant and personally controllable factors related to cancer, such as cigarette smoking and a diet high in saturated fat and low in fiber.

14

Winning at
Restaurant Roulette

Today, dining out has become commonplace, with more than 66 million Americans consuming at least one meal outside the home every day. According to the National Restaurant Association (NRA), restaurant traffic has more than doubled since the 1950s, when restaurant meals were reserved for special occasions.

Dietary control is harder to manage when someone else is doing the cooking, but eating out doesn't have to mean sacrificing nutrition. In fact, evidence points to a trend toward healthier dining. A 1986 study conducted by Gallup for the NRA showed that 23 percent of customers use less salt or no salt when dining out, 15 percent avoid fried foods; and 20 percent avoid fats. Four out of ten reported altering their dining out habits in one of these ways. When asked which of a list of various foods they were likely to try at a restaurant, responses included lean meat (64 percent), broiled/baked fish or seafood (63 percent), poultry without skin (47 percent), and food cooked without salt (36 percent). Restaurant managers questioned by Gallup mentioned more requests for lean meats, foods prepared without sauces and butter, and foods cooked without salt.

Furthermore, Consumer Reports on Eating Share Trends (CREST) Household Reports shows that changes in menus during the past five years have shifted in the direction of nonfried fish, main dish salads, rice, fruit, chicken, and low-fat Asian foods.

About two-thirds of restaurants today will serve salad dressing on the side, cook with unsaturated fat, broil or bake instead of fry, and alter foods upon customer request. Food service establishments are making more of an effort than ever to meet the demand for healthier restaurant fare. The NRA has published a booklet that outlines recommendations for cooking food more nutritionally and has made it available to both member and nonmember restaurants.

Become a Healthy Gourmet

Even when your restaurant choice is a last-minute impulse and you can't check the menu in advance, it's possible to make nutritional decisions in most restaurants, if you know what to look for.

The cardinal rule of dining out is: Ask questions. Keep a written or mental list of queries and don't be timid about getting the information you need from your waiter before you order. Some of the primary questions nutrition-conscious diners might ask include:

What type of fat is used in preparation? Saturated fats, such as butter, cream, and beef fats, are often used in cooking. These can increase blood cholesterol levels. Better choices are foods prepared with unsaturated fats derived from plant sources like corn, safflower, and sesame.

Are high-sodium ingredients used? Ask if salt is added in preparation. Smoked, cured, or canned meats and fish tend to be high in sodium, as do canned, powdered, and dried stocks often used in preparation and for sauces and gravies.

Which cuts of meat are used? Lean cuts of meat (with a minimum amount of marbling) contain less fat. The best cuts are loin, round, flank, shoulder, and leg. Also, when you order ground beef, ask for extra-lean hamburger or ground round. The light meat on poultry has less fat.

What types of liquids, fats, and thickening agents are used in sauces? Some sauces are reduced from vegetable or chicken broth by cooking the broth long enough for the water to evaporate. These are preferable to sauces made from cream or fat.

What cooking methods are used? The best preparation methods for meat, fish, and poultry are baking, broiling, grilling, poaching, roasting, and boiling. For vegetables, the best methods are microwaving, steaming, and stir-frying.

Make Wise Selections from the Menu

Learn to find the healthiest options on the menu. And don't hesitate to ask for substitutions. Three out of five restaurant managers surveyed by the NRA have expressed the willingness to make substitutions in ingredients and preparation when they are requested by customers. This new flexibility can make dining out a more pleasurable experience.

Use the guidelines on p. 162 when you order.

Take Advantage of "Light" Trends

One new trend in light dining has emerged in the form of "grazing," a practice that is best accomplished in groups. Grazers, who might eat up to six small meals per day can order appetizers or share main course orders in a family-style manner, rather than ordering a full meal consisting of appetizer, salad, main course, and dessert for each person. The end result can be a lighter meal since there's more control over portion sizes and more variety. Grazing also allows you to taste fattening favorites without filling your plate with them.

Certain cuisines naturally lend themselves to grazing: Spanish restaurants feature *tapas,* small, snack-sized portions of main-course selections; both Ethiopian and Indian cuisines offer feasts of finger food for nibbling; Chinese hot and cold appetizers give plenty of variety; and most Italian restaurants feature hearty antipasta and appetizer-size pasta dishes.

Main-course salads represent another health-related trend, although there are plenty of nutritional land mines hidden in the average salad bar. Diners who head for the salad bar instead of ordering a hamburger or meat dish might be surprised if they added up the calorie toll. A recent Mississippi State University study that compared salad bar meals with regular cafeteria hot meals found that the average salad contained 1,000 calories, compared to only 900 for the hot meal.

Today's salad bars are soup-to-nuts affairs. Many offer cheeses, breads, soups, desserts, and side dishes of macaroni, potato, and pasta salads—not to mention bacon bits, croutons, olives, and heavy cream dressings. If you pay attention to what you're putting on your plate at the salad bar, you can have a satisfying meal without adding extra calories and fat.

The samples on p. 164 show two salads built from the same salad bar. Salad Plate #1 has 880 calories, is high in saturated fat contributed by the coleslaw, cheese, macaroni salad, and dressing.

DINING OUT NUTRITIONALLY

Choose These Foods . . .	Instead of These . . .	Choose These Foods . . .	Instead of These . . .
Appetizers		**Vegetables and Grains**	
Fruits and juices, vegetables and juices, low-fat dip made from yogurt or cottage cheese	Hard cheeses, cheese dips, chips, nachos	All (except avocado) fresh, frozen, or canned; seasoned with herbs, spices, or citrus fruits	Vegetables covered with sauces or butter; avocado (except sparingly)
Relish trays with raw vegetables such as carrot and celery sticks, cherry tomatoes, and cauliflower floretes	Breaded or fried vegetables	Brown, white, or wild rice; noodles, bulgur; couscous; buckwheat; macaroni	Fried rice; egg noodles
Broth and vegetable-based soups, and consommé with the fat removed	Traditional cream soups, chowders, soups with cheese	Breads: brown, white, wheat, rye, pumpernickel, French, pita, Italian, and raisin; dinner and hard rolls	Biscuits, cheese breads, croissants, popovers, brioche, fried bread, egg bread
Steamed shrimp and scallops; skewered grilled chicken	Breaded or fried fish, shellfish, or chicken; pâté; mousse	**Desserts**	
Salads		Fresh, frozen, canned, or dried fruit; sherbet, fruit ice, sorbet, ice milk, fruit whip, pudding made with skim milk, angel food cake, frozen yogurt	Ice cream, pies, pastries, frosted cakes, whipped cream, custard, flan
Vegetable, fruit, or gelatin salads	Salads with bacon, eggs, cheeses, cold cuts, sour cream, or nuts		
Dressings (request that it be served on the side): reduced-calorie, oil and vinegar	Roquefort, blue cheese, and other creamy dressings	If you're particularly concerned about reducing sodium, follow these guidelines:	
Entrees		Fresh or frozen meats, fish, poultry, and shellfish	Cured, salted, or smoked meats (corned beef, ham, bacon, sausage, cold cuts, frankfurters); canned meats or fish
Beef: "Select" cuts: flank steak. Loin: tenderloin and sirloin steaks, sirloin tips. Round: top and bottom round steaks, eye of round roasts and steaks, rump roast, round tip roast and steak, ground round; lean veal	"Prime" cuts: marbled, fatty meats such as corned beef, ground beef, brisket, ground chuck; rib roasts and steaks, porterhouse and T-bone, organ meats	Fresh, frozen, or low-sodium vegetables	Canned vegetables, sauerkraut, pickles, olives, vegetables in brine
		Whole-grain or white breads, rolls, unsalted crackers, biscuits, muffins, and pastry	Saltines, salted snacks (pretzels, chips)

Choose These Foods . . .	Instead of These . . .	Choose These Foods . . .	Instead of These . . .
Pork: shoulder steak, blade chops, loin roast and chops, tenderloin leg (fresh ham)	Ribs, sausage, bacon, salt pork, ground pork	Unsalted homemade soups and stocks, and low-sodium canned soups and bases	Canned or dried soups and stocks
Poultry (with skin removed): chicken, all cuts; turkey, all cuts; cornish game hen; capon; pheasant	Goose, duck	Seasonings: fresh or dried spices and herbs, horseradish, aromatic bitters, extracts, Tabasco, vinegar, dried mustard	Salt, seasoned or flavored salt, MSG, chili sauce, soy sauce, meat tenderizers, capers
Fish: all types of plain, fresh, or frozen; canned fish packed in water	Breaded or fried fish, canned fish in oil, caviar		
Eggs: whites only	Whole eggs or egg yolks		
Pastas with low-fat sauce (like vegetable sauces or those made with skim milk and thickened with arrrowroot or cornstarch)	Traditional sauces made with cream, butter, or eggs (such as velout, hollandaise, and white sauces		

These ingredients plus the egg also make it high in cholesterol. More than one-half of the calories are accounted for by nonvegetable items.

Plate #2 has only 300 calories and very little fat, contributed by the grated cheese, which is also a source of "complete" protein. The reduction in calories was achieved by eliminating bacon bits, croutons, egg, coleslaw, macaroni salad, and potato salad, and substituting a low-calorie, low-fat dressing.

Other variations of Salad Plate #2 could be put together by making the following choices:

Substitute low-fat cottage cheese for grated cheese

Top the salad with bean sprouts

Add kidney beans, in moderation (stay away from three-bean salad, which is high in fat and sodium)

Add plain, water-packed tuna

Add two whole-wheat crackers or breadsticks

Add a fresh fruit salad or an apple, orange, banana, or half of melon

Use a dressing of vinegar and a little olive or vegetable oil

Delight in the Ethnic Cornucopia

One of the great pleasures of dining out is the chance to sample a wide variety of the world's best cuisines. Ethnic dining has gained in popularity in recent years. According to an NRA study of consumer preferences, Americans patronize Italian, Chinese, and Mexican restaurants regularly, although they sample an even wider variety of ethnic cuisines.

From a nutritional standpoint, dining in ethnic

SALAD BAR COMPARISONS

Salad Plate #1: ¼ cup sliced beets, ½ cup broccoli, ¼ cup shredded carrots, ¼ cup grated cheese, ¼ cup Chinese noodles, ½ cup coleslaw, 2 tbsp. diced egg, 2 tbsp. potato salad, 2 tbsp. macaroni salad, 3 slices tomato, 5 slices cucumber, ¼ cup mushrooms, ¼ cup green peas, 2 tbsp. chopped green pepper, 1 cup lettuce, 1 tsp. bacon bits, 1 tsp. sunflower seeds, 2 tbsp. croutons, 2 tbsp. Thousand Island dressing.

Total Calories: 880

Salad Plate #2: ¼ cup sliced beets, ½ cup broccoli, ¼ cup shredded carrot, 2 tbsp. grated cheese, 3 slices tomato, 5 slices cucumber, ¼ cup sliced mushrooms, ¼ cup green peas, ¼ cup sliced green pepper, 1 cup lettuce, 2 tbsp. Low-Cal Italian dressing.

Total Calories: 300

restaurants can be confusing, especially if you're testing a new cuisine. Lack of familiarity with language, terminology, and the ingredients of dishes can leave you guessing.

Happily, you can enjoy healthy and delicious meals no matter which type of cuisine you are eating, if you know what to look for. The following guidelines for seven popular ethnic cuisines demonstrate that a variety of good choices are available.

Italian

Southern Italian dishes, cooked with olive oil instead of butter, are better choices than northern Italian. And there is a rich variety of hearty vegetable and bean dishes. Pay attention to the descriptions: *Crema* or *Fritto*-style is heavy cuisine, usually cooked with butter or lard; *Pomodora* indicates a light preparation.

Enjoy!	*Go Easy*
Pasta with meatless marinara or pesto	Veal in cream sauce
Boneless chicken breast with tomato-mushroom sauce	Fettuccine Alfredo
	Meatballs
	Gnocchi
Sautéed shrimp in white wine wauce	Lasagna
Pizza with cheese and vegetable toppings	Cannelloni
	Garlic bread
Eggplant *Pomodora* style	Pizza with sausage and pepperoni toppings
Green salad with oil and vinegar dressing	*Crema* or *Fritto* style
	Cannoli or other cream pastries
Fresh fruit dessert	
Italian ice	

Mexican

Mexican cuisine offers many dishes that are high in complex carbohydrates. If you limit grated cheese and try to avoid Americanized fare such as tortilla chips fried in lard, and heavy sour cream, you can make a healthy feast of Mexican food. Guacamole, a favorite topping made from avocado, is high in fat, although it's unsaturated. Eat it sparingly. Take advantage of the many seasonings that give Mexican food its special flavor: *salsa,* made of chopped tomato, onion, and chile, and spices, is a favorite. If you like to make your own *fajitas,* choose chicken instead of beef, and keep them light by avoiding sour cream, grated cheese, and guacamole toppings.

Enjoy!	*Go Easy*
Chicken taco or tostada	Sour cream taco or burrito
Corn tortilla	Beef and bean burrito with cheese
Chicken or bean burrito	

Fish or chicken marinated in lime juice

Chicken fajitas

Shredded lettuce and tomatoes

Rice

Soft shell taco

Salsa

Nachos

Refried beans

Beef and cheese enchilada

Guacamole

Tortilla chips

Chimichangas

Frozen margaritas and pina coladas

French

Like Italian food, French cuisine varies in style depending on the region. Provençale and Riviera-style cooking favors olive oil rather than butter or lard, and features fish and vegetable dishes. If you choose your restaurant correctly, you won't be tempted by heavy pork and goose dishes or elaborate cream sauces. *Haute cuisine* and *cuisine bourgeoise* both indicate the use of butter, cream, pork lard, goose fat, and eggs. If you order salad nicoise, you might request the dressing on the side, and avoid eating the olives when calories are a consideration. *Cuisine minceur* literally means "cuisine of slimness."

Enjoy!	*Go Easy*
Poached fish	Quiche
Salad nicoise	Duck or goose
Bouillabaisse	Meat or fish in béarnaise or hollandaise sauce
Chicken in wine sauce	
French bread	Pâté
Endive and watercress salad	Fondue or crepes
Fresh or poached fruit	Brioche, croissants, eclairs, and other pastry

Chinese

Chinese cooking's reliance on vegetables, rice, and noodles makes it a naturally healthy cuisine. Pork is the primary meat used in Chinese dishes, followed by poultry and duck. Many vegetables

and meat dishes are stir-fried or steamed; avoid those that are deep fried. Also stay away from heavy sauces like lobster sauce or sweet and sour sauce. Sodium can be a problem if monosodium glutamate (MSG) is added in the cooking. You might want to request that food be prepared without it. Soy sauce is also sodium-heavy, with 800 milligrams of sodium in a tablespoon.

Enjoy!	*Go Easy*
Stir-fried vegetables	Sweet and sour pork
Stir-fried fish or chicken	Fried rice
	Spareribs
Broccoli chicken	Egg rolls
Vegetable dishes with mushrooms, broccoli, water chestnuts, bamboo shoots, bok choy, squash, snow peas, lotus root, and mushrooms	Egg Fu Yung
	Pork or beef dumplings
	Seafood with lobster sauce
	Pressed duck

Indian

Indian cuisine employs a creative use of unusual spices and seasonings to produce wonderful flavors without paying nutritional costs. Perhaps the most problematic aspect of Indian cooking is the use of highly saturated *ghee* (clarified butter) and coconut oil in food preparation. Shredded coconut and coconut milk are also added to some dishes. Stick with the nonfried foods and abundant vegetable and bean dishes.

Enjoy!	*Go Easy*
Tandoori chicken	Deep fried meat, fish, or vegetable pastries
Chicken marinated in yogurt	
Vegetable or fish curry	Fried breads
	Coconut soup or dressing
Vegetables or salad with yogurt dressing	Lamb dishes

Enjoy!
Lentil beans, chick
  peas, tomatoes,
  onions, cucumbers

Go Easy
Rice or cheese
  pudding
Honeyed pastries

Japanese

Japanese cuisine is basically low in fat, stressing soybean-based foods, small quantities of fish and meat, and rice and noodles. Traditional sauces contain no oil: Teriyaki sauce is a mixture of soy sauce, sake, and sugar; mixo is a paste made of fermented soy beans, rice mold, and salt. Strong spices—green mustard and ginger—heighten the flavors. The primary foods to avoid are pickled, smoked, and salted dishes and sauces that have a high sodium content. Surimi (fake crab) is also high in sodium. You should also avoid deep-fried dishes like tempura. If you're concerned about eating raw fish, order sushi made with vegetables or cooked crab or shrimp.

Enjoy!
Sushi (except surimi
  and salmon caviar)
Sashimi
Chicken teriyaki
Broiled fish or
  chicken over rice
Sukiyaki
Japanese vegetables
Tofu and other
  soybean dishes
Rice and noodles
Miso soup
Rice crackers

Go Easy
Tempura and other
  deep-fried dishes
Smoked or pickled
  fish
Pan-fried pork
Fried dumplings
Breaded meat, fish,
  and chicken
Surimi (white fish
  with crab) and
  ikura (salmon
  caviar)
Salted fish
Soy sauce

Southern and Cajun-Style

Southern and Cajun-style dining has increased in popularity. There are many good dishes available, but watch for the preponderance of fried and richly sauced dishes. Sample the tasty and nutritious vegetables—like okra, black-eyed peas, sweet potatoes, and greens—but be alert to the cooking oils used, which are often grease, lard, and fatback. Replace traditional Southern fried chicken with a Cajun dish: Blackened fish is usually cooked with less oil.

Enjoy!
Seafood gumbo
Blackened fish and
  chicken
Grilled seafood
Rice and pinto beans
Vegetables: okra,
  greens, black-eyed
  peas, sweet
  potatoes
Corn bread
Shrimp or crab boil

Go Easy
Fried fish and
  chicken
Crab cakes
Hush puppies
Gravy
Jambalaya
Honeyed dressings
Corn or fish chowder
"Mudpies" and other
  rich desserts

Health Tips for Diners

Make your restaurant meal a healthy pleasure by following these basic guidelines:

▶ Contact the restaurant in advance to find out if it offers entrees that are steamed, broiled, baked, or poached without sauces. Ask if special requests are honored, such as serving sauces on the side or not adding salt or MSG in the preparation of dishes.

▶ As a general guideline, a restaurant meal should be in the 500 to 800 calorie range, with 30 percent or fewer of the calories in fat. Cut down on or avoid rich cream sauces, condiments, butter on bread, and cheese sauces.

▶ Learn to recognize the language of menus. Descriptions like "garden fresh," "broiled," "steamed," and "cooked in its own juices" indicate low-fat preparation; "pickled," "smoked," and "cured" indicate high sodium content; "butter sauce," "pan fried," "sautéed," "rich," and "crispy" indicate high fat content.

▶ Don't hesitate to consult with the waiter on preparation methods and ingredients used in the dishes.

▶ Trim the visible fat off meat or ask for "lean" cuts, if they're available.

Request dishes cooked in vegetable oils such as corn, soybean, or safflower, instead of butter. These oils contain no cholesterol.

▶ Select vegetable dishes that have been minimally cooked. Overcooking depletes them of vitamins.

▶ If you have an appetizer, choose raw vegetables, melon, a seafood cocktail with sauce on the side, a small green or endive salad, or fresh cold or hot asparagus with vinaigrette dressing.

▶ At dessert time, look for fruit, fruit ices, or sherbets. If you must have a rich dessert, order one serving to share between two people.

▶ Alcoholic beverages add empty calories to your total. Stick to a glass of wine with dinner, a wine spritzer (half wine and half sparkling water) or a nonalcoholic glass of soda water with a twist of lime. Avoid after-dinner liqueurs and drinks that use high-calorie mixers.

If you would like to find restaurants in your area that serve low-fat meals, the American Heart Association's regional offices print lists. For information, contact your local chapter.

Find the Fast-Food Balance

Of the 66 million Americans who consume at least one meal a day away from home, 33 percent choose fast-food restaurants. The availability of fast, filling, and inexpensive food has been a boon to the American life-style. Today more than 55,000 fast-food restaurants service a demanding public with an expanding range of selections. But these meals are not always nutritious. According to the

New England Journal of Medicine, the typical fast food meal derives between 40 and 55 percent of its calories from fat. Sometimes diversification makes a direct appeal to nutrition-conscious customers, as in the addition of salad bars and the inclusion of baked potatoes and broiled entrees. Unfortunately, many of the intended benefits are compromised by calorie-and-fat-laden extras. For example, a plain baked potato is an excellent nutritional choice; even the addition of a pat of margarine won't hurt. But potatoes are often topped with bacon and cheese, a Stroganoff mixture, sour cream, and chili and cheese, along with other high-fat and high-calorie foods. For example, the Wendy's Baked Potato with Bacon and Cheese has 570 calories (more than the Double Hamburger), and 47 percent of the calories come from fat.

In recent years, fast-food chains have expanded to include breakfast. Consumer purchases of take-out breakfast items like McDonald's Egg McMuffin or Biscuit with Sausage, Burger King's Croissan'-wich, Wendy's omelets, and Carl Jr.'s Sunrise Sandwich are on the rise. Some choices are better than others; the worst are usually the combination sandwiches. For example, the McDonald's meal of an English muffin with butter, scrambled eggs, and six ounces of orange juice has 40 percent less fat and fewer calories than the Sausage Egg Mc-Muffin.

Fast-food chains spend a total of nearly $1 billion a year in television advertising. The commercial lure is strong: convenience, economy, flavor, and variety. More recently, chains have incorporated nutrition as a theme in their advertising, featuring sizzling beef patties, farm fresh eggs, and whole potatoes—the "nutritious natural ingredients" used in a fast-food meal. Of course, by the time a potato is peeled, chopped, and fried in a mixture of vegetable shortening and beef tallow, it bears little resemblance to the original.

Since fast-food restaurants appeal to the life-style requirements of so many consumers, the question becomes how to make healthier choices. Indeed, there are a number of ways to find a balanced, reasonably nutritious meal in a fast-food restaurant. Follow these guidelines when you dine:

ENTREES

▶ Choose plain hamburgers or cheeseburgers instead of those that contain a "special sauce."

▶ "Junior" burgers and sandwiches are smaller and contain fewer calories.

▶ Don't be misled into thinking that fish or chicken sandwiches are better than burgers. The fish and chicken are often breaded and then fried in fat. For example, the McDonald's Filet-O-Fish has 435 calories, and 53 percent of them are from fat. Some restaurants, like Arthur Treacher's, offer broiled fish and shrimp, which are good choices, but diners should go easy on the tartar sauce.

▶ Occasional indulgence is okay if you watch the total calorie intake. If you must have a Burger King Whopper (626 calories), skip the French fries (227 calories) and vanilla milkshake (321 calories).

▶ Pizza is one of the best fast-food nutrition values, if you use the right toppings. Choose vegetable toppings like mushrooms, onions, and green peppers. Avoid extra cheese, olives, pepperoni, sausage, and anchovies.

BREAKFAST

▶ Avoid sandwiches that combine a cheese, egg, and/or meat filling with a muffin, croissant, or biscuit; it's hard to find one that doesn't top the fat chart.

▶ Hotcakes and French toast with syrup are reasonable choices if you don't use butter.

▶ Scrambled eggs or omelets are occasionally okay, but don't order them with sausage, bacon, or ham on the side.

SIDE DISHES

▶ Many fast-food restaurants have salad bars. Use the suggestions cited earlier in this chapter to keep your salad low in fat and calories.

▶ A plain, baked potato is a good choice, even with a pat of butter or margarine. These are available at Arby's, Roy Rogers, and Wendy's. Avoid the elaborate toppings. Kentucky Fried Chicken also serves mashed potatoes and corn on the cob. McDonalds is test marketing celery and carrot sticks.

DRINKS

▶ A typical 10-ounce milkshake has between 300 and 400 calories, and about as much sugar as a can of soda. A shake isn't bad (especially as a combination drink/dessert), but be on the alert for chains that offer larger shakes or malts. For example, Dairy Queen's chocolate shake is 20 fluid ounces and nearly 1,000 calories.

▶ Whole milk is usually the only kind on the menu, but ask if low-fat or skim milk is available.

▶ To round out your fast-food meal, add low-fat or skim milk or orange juice.

▶ If there's a salad bar, avoid bacon bits, cheddar cheese, olives, croutons, coleslaw, macaroni salad, potato salad, and nondiet dressing.

▶ For dessert, take fresh fruit from home.

▶ Take out your fast-food meal and serve it at home with salad, vegetables, and fruit.

FAST-FOOD SANDWICH SAVVY

Note: While the sandwiches listed on the right constitute "better choices," some of them still contain more than 30 percent fat calories. Figures for all items are based on the most current information available at the time of publication.

Skip These High-Fat and High-Calorie Sandwiches	These are Better Choices	Skip These High-Fat and High-Calorie Sandwiches	These are Better Choices
Arby's		**Hardees**	

Chicken Club Sandwich
    Calories: 621
    Fat: 46%
	Junior Roast Beef
	    Sandwich
	    Calories: 218
	    Fat: 33%
		Bacon Cheeseburger
		    Calories: 556
		    Fat: 53%
			Cheeseburger
			    Calories: 309
			    Fat: 37%

Burger King		**Jack-in-the-Box**	

Double Beef Whopper with
    Cheese
    Calories: 970
    Fat: 59%
	Hamburger
	    Calories: 275
	    Fat: 39%
		Bacon Cheeseburger
		    Supreme
		    Calories: 724
		    Fat: 57%
			Club Pita
			    Calories: 284
			    Fat: 27%

Carl Jr.'s		**McDonald's**	

Super Star Hamburger
    Calories: 780
    Fat: 58%
	California Roast Beef
	    Sandwich
	    Calories: 300
	    Fat: 21%
		Mc D.L.T
		    Calories: 680
		    Fat: 58%
			Hamburger
			    Calories: 263
			    Fat: 39%

Dairy Queen		**Wendy's**	

Triple Hamburger with
    Cheese
    Calories: 820
    Fat: 55%
	Single Hamburger
	    Calories: 360
	    Fat: 40%
		Triple Cheeseburger
		    Calories: 1,040
		    Fat: 59%
			Chicken Sandwich,
			    Multi-Grain Bun
			    Calories: 320
			    Fat: 28%

Domino's Pizza			

16" Pepperoni Pizza
    (2 slices)
    Calories: 440
    Fat: 29%
	16" Cheese Pizza
	    (2 slices)
	    Calories: 340
	    Fat: 16%		

PART THREE

Nutritional Life-Cycles

Every human being travels a cycle in life, from birth to growth to maturity to death. Each stage of the cycle is unique, marked by a new series of physiological changes, some of them dramatic.

In America, enamored as we are with the idea of lasting youth, we have tended to ignore the cyclical nature of human life. That tendency may partially account for the high incidence of heart disease and the other diet-related ills that plague us. Wanting only to focus on youth, we've been impatient with the concept of disease prevention, which mandates that we care for ourselves today to ward off the possibility of illness in the future.

But we are starting to come around. With advances in scientific knowledge regarding the prevention of cardiovascular disease and a whole host of other diseases, we are growing more aware that good health is something we build over a lifetime. It's not possible to reach a healthy old age through a last-ditch effort in the later stages of the cycle when the risks are skyrocketing.

This section addresses three specific populations whose nutritional concerns can be considered "special." Much of the advice in this book easily applies to most people, but children, women of childbearing age (including pregnant women), and the elderly face unique circumstances and needs. Some of the issues addressed in this section include:

▶ What should new parents know about starting their baby off on the right foot nutritionally? Is breast feeding substantially preferable to bottle feeding? When baby is ready for solid foods, how can parents avoid nutrient deficiencies and make the best choices from among commercial baby products? What are the special nutritional issues for children during the first two years of life?

Certain nutritional practices for infants present a clear example of how "common wisdom" for older children and adults can actually endanger a baby's health. In this section you'll see, for example, how well-meaning parents who put their infants on low-fat diets may be creating serious health problems for them.

▶ As they grow, children need a good balance of nutrients for the development of bone, muscle, and tissue. But as they pass into the toddler stage and beyond, children become conscious of their autonomy, and they can be very stubborn about their likes and dislikes when it comes to food. What are parents to do when faced with finicky eaters? How important is it that children eat certain foods? What can be done to neutralize the "sugar monster"? How can you avoid daily battles over food and still be sure your child gets the nutrients that he or she needs?

▶ Many parents throw up their hands in despair over the eating habits of their teenagers. They can seem like bottomless pits of hunger, and they often rely on fast-foods and snacks to fill the pit. During these years, parents exert less daily control over diet. How can a little nutritional know-how and planning help you create better nutritional options for your teenagers?

▶ Sometimes parents are confronted with "weighty issues" when it comes to their child's diet and health. How do you know if your child's weight should be of concern, or if he or she is just going through normal hormonal changes? Many parents overreact to a child's weight gain and try to force rigid restrictions. There is hard evidence that this approach almost always backfires. So what do you do if your child's doctor agrees that there's an obesity problem?

And what if the reverse is true? How can you recognize the beginnings of a severe eating disorder like anorexia nervosa before it has progressed to the danger point? What are the steps you can take to get proper care for a child who is "starving"?

▶ Adult women have special nutritional needs, particularly as they apply to pregnancy and lactation. As the RDAs stipulate, pregnant and lactating women need more of most essential nutrients. But what does this mean in terms of the nuts-and-bolts of daily eating? How can the mother-to-be and the breast-feeding mother plan diets that enhance health for both woman and child?

▶ Women also need special consideration during their menstruating years. Iron may become depleted during menstruation and need to be replaced. In addition, many women suffer a condition known as Premenstrual Syndrome (PMS) that involves symptoms ranging from mild to severe. Can nutrition make a difference? We'll look at the current expert wisdom on this subject.

▶ Tufts has devoted much attention to issues related to diet and aging. Since 1982 it has operated the USDA Human Nutritional Research Center on Aging. The center has led the field in research related to the nutrient needs during the aging process. Although the RDAs list general guidelines for adult men and women 51 years and older, we have learned that special considerations must be applied to senior citizens. Tufts has led the way in encouraging the RDA committee to establish a new category for adults who are 69 years of age or older.

For example, seniors often have trouble maintaining appropriate levels of certain nutrients, such as vitamin D. As people age, their "thirst signals" weaken, and many seniors don't drink enough liquids and suffer from dehydration. Another concern relates to the way medications interact with the foods seniors eat.

Life-style changes common among seniors can influence diet. They may lack the physical stamina to prepare balanced meals or the information or money to purchase the right foods. Widowed seniors, unaccustomed to cooking for one, often ignore their nutritional needs.

We believe that once people begin to consider good nutrition a part of their life-style in every stage of life, many of the nutritional problems that plague various populations will be diminished.

15

The Well-Nourished Child

Today's parents have access to more nutritional information than the parents of any other generation. But this knowledge can seem like a mixed blessing as they struggle to understand the complex and often conflicting advice they hear from dozens of sources. Parents also have to confront new dilemmas that have emerged out of the times we live in, such as worries over the safety of our nation's food supply, the growing crisis of obesity in children, and the changes in family styles that have led to fewer meals being prepared at home and less control over what their children eat.

Nutrition is a factor in many of the decisions parents make in raising their children, from the moment of birth to the time they leave home.

A Healthy Beginning for Baby

All new parents are intensely interested in making decisions that will start their baby off on a long and healthy life.

The first nutritional question, usually raised before the baby is born, is whether or not to breast-feed. For many people, it seems perfectly logical that a mother's breast milk, the "natural" form of nutrition for a baby, would be the best possible choice. Is this true?

In the mid-1970s, the American Academy of Pediatrics described mother's milk as "the best food for every newborn infant." That endorsement has received the support of the surgeon general and of the vast majority of nutritionists. Fortunately, for mothers who are unable to breast-feed, the formulas on the market duplicate breast milk to the extent that your child won't suffer ill health. But breast milk is considered the food of choice for infants.

Recently, researchers from Yale University reevaluated some of the original studies that identified protective antibodies in breast milk and reported a number of flaws in the methodology. However, medical experts believe that there is no serious reason to question the potential protective aspects of breast-feeding for infants.

The most important benefit of breast milk is that it is believed to carry, from mother to infant, immunity against several kinds of infection. In addition, colostrum, the premilk substance secreted during the first few days of breast-feeding, supplies even higher levels of antibodies. Research conducted over a period of 30 years provides evidence that mother's milk is a prime infection fighter.

An additional benefit of breast-feeding is that it may offer protection for the mother. Research indicates that a woman who breast-feeds her child,

175

even for only a few months, may be protecting herself against breast cancer. Scientists at the Fred Hutchinson Cancer Research Center in Seattle, Washington, found that women who breast-feed have as little as half the risk of developing breast cancer as those who have never breast-fed. The protective effect seems to extend from the time a woman starts breast-feeding until menopause. The reason behind this phenomenon is not fully understood, but it could be related to hormonal changes that occur during nursing. Another possibility is that breast-feeding might bring about some (as yet undiscovered) positive changes in the breast tissue.

Delay the Start of Cow's Milk

Rapid growth during the first two years of life makes very young children particularly dependent on nutrient-dense foods, which contribute to the growth of cells and development of muscle and tissue.

How can you be sure your baby is getting enough iron? Perhaps the most common mistake parents make is to replace vitamin-and-mineral rich breast milk or iron-fortified formula with regular cow's milk too soon. While cow's milk is a good source of nutrients that children need as they grow, it is a relatively poor source of iron. It contains less than a milligram of iron per quart and, of that, only about 2 to 10 percent is absorbed. Even if a six to twelve month old drinks the typical amount of one quart a day, he or she is still at least 14 milligrams shy of the RDA's 15 milligrams.

Delay the use of cow's milk until your baby is at least six months old, and when you do use it, supplement it with iron-rich solid foods. The best source is iron-fortified infant cereal that you mix with a liquid. Four tablespoons of dry cereal will provide almost five milligrams of iron. Fruits, vegetables, and their juices that are rich in vitamin C, when fed at the same time, will enhance iron absorption.

Picking the Best Baby Food

Baby-food manufacturers have gone to a great deal of trouble in recent years to send a nutrition-conscious message to consumers. In the past, baby food was criticized for containing too much salt and sugar. Manufacturers tended to make it taste the way Mom would like it, so that when she sampled it, she would think it tasted good. But babies don't need strong flavors since their taste buds are more acute, and many of today's baby-food selections reflect this understanding. It is possible, for example, to find many simple foods in jars, such as peas that have been pureed with water and don't contain a lot of "extras."

The key to finding the best baby food is to look beyond labels that read "no added salt, no artificial flavors or preservatives" to find out what else is inside the jar. To be sure, many parents prefer that their babies' food contains no added sugar, salt, or starch fillers whatsoever. If that's your concern, give labels a closer examination to insure that you're getting what you really want.

In most cases, the less sugar, corn syrup, starch, modified food starch, and added flour, the more nutrients you get for the calories. The problem isn't that these ingredients are harmful to your baby; it's more a matter of not "spending" calories on extra ingredients that are not nourishing.

Consider baby fruits, which can be good sources of vitamin C or A. The fine print on the ingredients label will show that plain fruits, such as baby pears, applesauce, or strained bananas, have no sweeteners added. However, fruits thickened with tapioca invariably have added sugar or corn syrup. While there is no evidence that small amounts of these sweeteners are harmful as long as a baby's teeth are kept clean, the sugary thickener takes up space in the jar that could be given to the fruits themselves. Also, be aware that the presence of fillers may dilute a food's vitamin and mineral value.

In general, we recommend that you limit the use of fruit "cobblers," "desserts," and "supremes" because they are typically high in sugar and therefore contain more empty calories.

Check for the protein content of baby meats. The highest protein baby foods are strained and junior meats and poultry that list broth or water as the only added ingredient. A three-and-a-half-ounce jar may provide up to 80 percent of the USRDA for protein. On the other hand, meat and vegetable combination dinners are not necessarily a high source of protein. A seven-and-a-half ounce jar of a vegetable-beef combination may have more vegetables than beef, and contain only 20 percent of the USRDA for protein. Few babies have a hearty enough appetite to eat the whole jar, in any case. Also be aware that the heavier, stew-type dinners for toddlers tend to be low in protein and very high in salt.

You may rely upon the popular instant baby cereals for their fortified iron content, particularly desirable if your baby is not on iron-fortified formula. But check the label because some brands have added sugar.

And this might surprise you: Although foods that are low in fat and cholesterol are often recommended as wise choices for older children and adults, this advice does not hold true for children under the age of two years old. For them, limiting foods that contain fat and cholesterol could spell trouble. Skimming the fat (and therefore calories) from a baby's diet could stunt his or her growth. Severely limiting an infant's dietary cholesterol could deprive the baby of the cholesterol he or she needs to form body cells, including those of the nervous system.

Doctors at North Shore Hospital in Manhasset, New York, have seen first-hand what diets low in fat, cholesterol, and calories can do to infants. Children were admitted to the hospital's research center with severe growth problems that, according to doctors, were related to their having been fed overly strict diets. Well-meaning mothers and fathers, concerned that their babies would become overweight, deliberately watered down their formula. In several cases, parents also cut back on snacks or fat in meals eaten by babies on solid foods. The end result was that babies were shortchanged on calories and their growth was poor.

Get Your Kids to Eat Right

If you're a parent, you may wonder why it's such a struggle to get your kids to eat a nutritious variety of foods. One good reason, of course, is that kids have minds of their own, and sometimes it takes Herculean strength to change those minds.

Most people get overly obsessed with their young children's eating habits. It's a rare parent who hasn't called the pediatrician to complain that "Billy won't eat anything but bread and jam" or "I'm worried about Susan—she eats like a bird." These small battles of will are usually short-lived, and your child's temporary eating quirks are unlikely to cause permanent harm. Cajoling, threatening, or bribing will only make things worse. In truth, American children, even when they're being finicky, have sufficient variety in their diets that they get enough of the nutrients they need.

The best way to teach your child to eat well is to maintain a relaxed attitude about food, avoiding fanaticism. Stay informed about the range of nutrients your growing child needs, and incorporate these foods into your family's daily diet, without making an issue of it.

It's a good idea to involve children in their own nutrition. Most respond better when they are included in the planning. They don't respond to abstract concepts such as "This is good for you" or "Eat your beans so you can grow up healthy and strong." Children will respond better if you take a more relaxed approach and don't try to make every meal a life-and-death nutritional battle. Let them help design the weekly menu and shopping list, gently educating them about simple nutrition concepts as you go along.

Children are creatures of habit, and the best way to guarantee that their habits are healthy ones is to keep eating periods structured. Mealtimes should be set for regular hours so you can keep track of what your child is eating. Be sure to schedule snack times, especially for small children, their energy needs are high, but their stomachs cannot hold a lot of food at one time.

If your child refuses to eat a certain food, don't force the issue. Simply try again a few days later, serving a small portion of it. Studies show that the more a child is exposed to a food, the more likely it is that he or she will eventually taste it, and maybe even enjoy it. You may have to try as many as 10 or 15 times, but your child should eventually come around. Even if it doesn't work, it's not the end of the world. Essential nutrients are available in enough foods that a child's refusal to eat one or two of them won't cause a nutritional deficit.

Which Foods Do Children Need?

A growing child's body demands lots of nutrients to support the creation of new tissue. Basically, that means eating enough from each of the four basic food groups. The average daily diet for a child under 12 should include:

▶ Three servings from the milk group: milk, yogurt, cheese, cottage cheese, and ice cream

▶ Two servings from the meat group: meat, poultry, and fish. High-protein meat substitutes might include soy products and peanut butter

▶ Four servings from the vegetable/fruit group: all vegetables and fruits, including at least one good source of vitamin C and one deep-yellow or dark-green vegetable

▶ Four servings from the bread and cereal group: bread, cereal, pasta, and rice

Remember that a child-size serving is usually smaller than an adult serving. Parents often worry that their children are not eating enough, but a young child does not require much quantity.

While children are growing, their appetites may be unpredictable. On some days thay may be ravenous, especially if they've been very active. On other days, they may seem to pick at their food.

As a general rule, consider an average child's serving to be one tablespoon for each year. For example, the average adult serving of a cooked vegetable is around one-half cup. For a three year old, it's three tablespoons or slightly less than one-fourth cup. A five year old would eat a little more than one-fourth cup.

Since children need to pack more nutrients into fewer daily calories, there isn't much room in their diet for junk food. Sugary snacks and drinks take away from the foods they need and should be limited to small 'treats" two or three times a week.

Pack a Healthy Bag Lunch

Once your child walks out the door in the morning, nutrition control is out of your hands. Although you may send your child off with a nutrient-packed lunch, once he or she is out the door those nutrients might end up any number of places other than your child's body: lunch items might get traded with a friend, the bag might be forgotten on the bus, or the most nutritious items might be dumped in the garbage.

The best way to insure that your child eats the lunch you prepare is to make it taste good. This is another place it might help to involve your child in the planning and shopping. Start with lists of foods in the basic food groups, including as many different choices as possible. Then use your imagination to make the bag lunch fun to open.

HAPPY, HEALTHY LUNCH TIPS

▶ Many kids like peanut-butter sandwiches, but you can jazz up the old standby with different toppings besides jellies. To a peanut-butter sandwich on whole-grain bread, add sliced banana, raisins, dates, or apple butter.

▶ Pep up chicken and tuna salad by adding almond slivers, sesame seeds, raisins, apple pieces, or seasonings such as curry powder.

▶ Make your own healthy, low-sodium lunch meats by cooking lean roast beef and chicken or turkey breast and slicing them thinly.

▶ If you do purchase lunch meats, choose the lean brands of roast beef, ham, turkey, and chicken. Unfortunately, most packaged lunch meats are high in sodium, but you can cut fat substantially by choosing one of the leaner, low-fat brands. Some tips: choose turkey bologna instead of beef bologna, turkey pastrami instead of beef pastrami, and turkey salami instead of hard salami.

▶ Pack snack-size applesauce or raisins. Or supply a tasty homemade side dish in a serving-size plastic container. Mix plain yogurt with raisins, apples, or berries, and add a dash of sugar and cinnamon. Or make your own trail mix with unsalted nuts, seeds, and raisins. Homemade carrot, zucchini, or banana bread makes a great dessert.

KEEP LUNCHES SAFE

▶ Freeze or refrigerate sandwiches the night before and pack them frozen so they won't be warm and soggy by lunchtime. Wrap tomato and lettuce separately so your child can add them right before eating. (You might also want to use frozen gel packs to keep foods cold.)

▶ Don't save paper bags for packing lunches. Used bags can pass insects or bacteria from other foods. Never use a bag that's wet or stained.

▶ Wash lunch boxes daily, and once a week scrub them with baking soda.

▶ Be sure that everything that touches food is kept clean. Wash all utensils, cutting boards, and counter tops thoroughly before preparing each portion of the meal.

Improve Your School's Lunch Program

Government-sponsored school lunch programs still have a way to go to be acceptable. Although the U.S. Department of Agriculture (USDA) has started supplying schools with more nutritious foods (adding fish, pasta, and fresh produce; packing fruits in natural juice or light syrup; limiting fats and oils used in processing to vegetable oils), there are still plenty of high-fat government surplus foods of lesser nutritional value on the average school lunch menu.

Indeed, cost-saving maneuvers may be undercutting your child's nutrition. The USDA supplies high-fat cheese free because it is available on the surplus basis. And it donates ground beef that has more fat than the lean ground beef you can purchase in the supermarket. Last year, the department donated 75 million pounds of butter and 50 million pounds of frozen whole eggs to the National School Lunch Program.

Perhaps most disturbing, in 1986 milk producers won the battle to get Congress to require that schools serve whole milk, making low-fat milk optional. Also, although a ban on selling junk foods on school grounds was instituted in 1980, lobbyists for the Nationaol Soft Drink Association managed to have it overturned.

On the positive side, the USDA published a new cafeteria cookbook in late 1988 (the first update since 1971) that includes some moderation in the use of sugar, salt, and fat in food preparation.

Parental pressure and community action have worked in some parts of the country to get schools to improve the nutritional quality of lunches. If you are concerned about this issue, you should contact your local board of education and parent groups.

Is Your Child a Cookie Monster Captive?

The cookie jar has been the bane of many a mother's existence. Many children consider cookies a favorite snack, dessert, and comfort food. In fact,

Americans love cookies, consuming more than 2 billion pounds of them each year. Supermarkets devote entire aisles to an increasing number of hard-to-resist cookies.

Should they be resisted? Should you simply ban the "monster" from your home? Probably not. A better alternative is to know how to choose the cookies that are lowest in sugar and calories, and then limit their consumption. And, as we have stated before, indulging in a small treat two or three times a week will do your child little harm.

Most cookies are made from three primary ingredients: sugar, flour, and shortening (in effect, fat). The differences among cookies result from differences in the ratios of these three components to one another, and whether other ingredients, such as chocolate chips or fillings, have been added. For exampple, a half-ounce Chips Deluxe cookie by Keebler has about 90 calories, 40 percent of which come from fat, while a Nabisco Almost Home oatmeal raisin cookie has just 65 calories, only 35 percent from fat.

As a general rule, the softer the cookie, the higher the fat content; it's extra fat that helps soften the texture of baked goods. Also, pay attention to cookie weights. There's no difference in calories between a Nabisco Mallomar and a Pepperidge Farm Chocolate Chunk Pecan cookie, but you get a little less cookie for the calories with the latter—two fifths of an ounce as opposed to half an ounce. You also get a few more fat calories.

Some of the lower-calorie, lower-fat selections include Nabisco's Nilla Wafers, Old Fashion Ginger Snaps, Honey Maid Graham Crackers, and Fig Newtons. Each of these contains less than 30 percent fat calories, and all but the Fig Newton have no more than 30 calories per cookie.

Nutrition Aid for Parents

You can help your child eat well by following these simple, no-stress guidelines:

▶ Establish set meal and snack times. Children who are allowed to help themselves to snacks when they feel like it may not have enough appetite to eat the nutritious foods that are served at the table.

▶ Make meals tantalizing by serving a variety of foods with different colors and textures. If children refuse to eat certain foods, look for others that offer the same nutrients. For example, the vitamin A precursor beta-carotene in dark-green, leafy vegetables can also be found in cantaloupe, apricots, and sweet potatoes.

▶ Include children in food choices. If you have served something several times that they won't eat, ask what they don't like about it. You might find that it's a simple thing to change. Children who turn up their noses at cooked carrots may be perfectly happy to crunch away on the raw variety.

▶ Allow for childrens' idiosyncrasies. For instance, children may refuse to eat if foods on the plate touch one another. Or they may dislike foods that are certain colors. Don't force the issue. Serve meals on a plate that has dividers. Try to mix new or objectionable foods with favorite foods to make them seem different.

▶ Give lots of time at meals. Children need more time to eat than adults. Never criticize children for dawdling over their food. Let them eat at their own pace.

▶ Keep meal times free of disruption. Meals are not the time to scold children or give them the third degree about school performance. It is impossible to enjoy food and digest it properly when one is in a harsh and stressful setting.

▶ Invite your children to participate in meal preparation. If they are involved in the process, they are likely to become more interested in the foods themselves. For example, if you let children create their own salads or "build" their own tacos, they'll feel that the food "belongs" to them, that it wasn't forced on them.

▶ Avoid creating the impression that there are "good" foods and "bad" foods. Rather, concentrate on communicating positive messages about food. For example, instead of saying, "Cookies are bad for you," tell your children, "Cookies are fun to have for a Saturday treat, but they're not for every day."

Keep Your Child Heart-Healthy

High blood cholesterol and the risk for heart disease have usually been associated with the adult population. But new studies show that heart disease may begin early in life. Indeed, current statistics show that an estimated 30 to 40 percent of children in families with a history of heart disease

CALORIE AND FAT CONTENT OF BEST-SELLING COOKIES

	Weight per cookie (oz.)	Calories	Fat (%)		Weight per cookie (oz.)	Calories	Fat (%)
Regular-Style				Gingerman	¼	33	36
				Milano	⅖	43	49
				Lido	⅗	90	55
Keebler							
Chips Deluxe	½	90	40				
Old Fashion Oatmeal	⅗	80	34				
Pecan Sandies	⅗	80	56	**Keebler**			
				Soft Batch Chocolate			
				Chip	½	80	45
Nabisco				Soft Batch Oatmeal			
Barnum's Animal				Raisin	½	70	39
Crackers	⅟₁₁	12	28				
Biscos Sugar Wafers	⅛	19	42				
Chips Ahoy!				**Archway**			
Chocolate Chip	⅓	47	44	**Homestyle ***			
Fig Newtons	½	50	18	Chocolate Chip			
Honey Maid				Round	1	120	40
Grahams	¼	30	15	Date Filled Oatmeal	1	104	30
Lorna Doones	¼	35	46	Molasses	1	111	24
Mallomars	½	65	42	Peanut Butter	1	122	48
Nilla Wafers	⅟₇	19	28				
Old Fashion Ginger							
Snaps	¼	30	23	**Nabisco, Almost**			
Oreo Chocolate				**Home**			
Sandwich	⅓	22	27	Dutch Apple Fruit			
				Sticks	⅔	70	13
Pepperidge Farm				Oatmeal Raisin	½	65	35
Chocolate Chunk				Peanut Butter Fudge	½	70	45
Pecan	⅖	65	48	Real Chocolate Chip	½	65	35

* Figures may vary slightly from state to state, since the cookie batches in different Archway factories may inadvertently differ a bit from the standard recipes.

have high blood cholesterol, and up to 80 percent of them will carry it into adulthood.

In one study, researchers observed the children of the Louisiana city Bogalusa, using techniques similar to those that are used with adults. The researchers interviewed thousands of children about their parents' habits and health, analyzed their blood, measured their blood pressure, and assessed their diets. Tests showed high cholesterol levels in the blood of many of the children. In addition, autopsies performed on 88 children who had died in accidents or from illnesses showed that almost 40 percent of them had the first signs of heart disease—fibrous plaque or fatty deposits in the walls of blood vessels.

The first step in lowering the risk of heart disease is to reduce the intake of dietary fat. But pediatric health professionals have traditionally been reluctant to impose strict guidelines on children, since they are growing rapidly and need vast nutritional resources to lay the foundation for brain, bone, and muscle.

Health experts unanimously agree that no dietary restrictions related to heart disease should be imposed on children younger than age two. But older children can benefit from a reduction in dietary fat, especially considering that American children consume an average of 37 percent of their diets as fat. The changes do not have to be dramatic; small adjustments in the way food is prepared can make a big difference. For example, begin trimming all visible fat from meats, avoid processed luncheon meats, and broil rather than fry chicken.

The American Academy of Pediatrics has issued a statement recommending routine cholesterol screening for all children in families where there is a history of heart disease.

Keep Your Teens on Track

If your child has not developed sensible eating habits by the time he or she reaches the teen years, you may feel it's useless to even try. Your teenager's diet is more or less out of your control, and it may seem that a typical menu for your teen is made up of hamburgers, french fries, sodas, ice cream, and other fatty or high-calorie foods.

Teenagers, especially boys, can appear to be bottomless pits of hunger. Unfortunately, they're not always very concerned about what they're eating.

As a recent Gallup Poll demonstrated, today's teens are aware of the fundamentals of good eating and are especially conscious of high publicized issues like the dangers of cholesterol and the need for adequate amounts of calcium. But their actual eating behavior seems at odds with their nutritional knowledge. For example, while 87 percent of those surveyed said they put a lot of effort into a good diet, 79 percent listed hamburgers, cheeseburgers, pizza, and luncheon meats as preferred foods.

Part of the problem seems to be an absence of practical knowledge. While most teens surveyed were very aware of the dangers of cholesterol, many didn't know that certain foods (specifically eggs and ice cream) contribute significant amounts of it.

You can't completely control your teenager's diet, and badgering certainly won't help. What you can do is encourage good eating at home. Schedule regular family meals and let your teens know you expect them to be present. Keep healthy snack foods handy—such as fruit, raw vegetables, and yogurt—so that refrigerator raids are good for them. Healthy snacks can also include moderate amounts of dried fruit and nuts, popcorn, and even oatmeal and raisin cookies and milk, or a slice of plain pizza. Instead of store-bought sodas, make your own fruit drinks, combining real fruit juices with seltzer. If you suspect that your teenager is indulging in sugar and salt-laden snacks outside the home (and he or she probably is), there's no need to keep those items in your home. It won't hurt your teen to indulge occasionally in fast-food meals, but if you provide a balance at home, you can better assure that the full range of nutrients are being consumed.

It helps to know which nutrients are particularly important for teens and to recognize the key distinctions between male and female dietary needs. For example, even though your teenage boy may consume many "junk" foods, that doesn't necessarily mean he isn't getting enough of the nutrients he needs. Indeed, teenage boys eat so much of all kinds of food that their diets usually end up meeting their needs. Boys continue to grow until about age nineteen, so an active boy of fifteen, at the peak of his growth period, may need as many as 4,000 calories a day to maintain body weight.

It's different with girls, who stop growing at around age fifteen. A sedentary sixteen-year-old girl who has stopped growing may have to consume fewer than 2,000 calories per day to avoid being overweight. She has less leeway in eating empty calories. Calories she consumed from "junk" become calories taken away from the foods that supply the nutrients she needs.

Be aware of the special needs of teenagers:

▶ Teenagers need calcium in large quantities. In fact, during the teen years (11 through 18), the RDA for this nutrient increases by 50 percent, from 800 to 1,200 milligrams per day, a rise that is not hard to understand when you consider that a full 45 percent of the adult skeletal mass is formed during the teen years. Because of this increased need, teenagers should consume four servings from the milk group each day.

Researchers have found that teenage girls and young women who drink milk with their meals have significantly denser bones when they reach middle age and are presumably more resistant to osteoporosis.

▶ Teens need plenty of iron, found in red meats, poultry, and fish, as well as in nuts and seeds. The RDA for iron increases by 80 percent from the elementary school years to the teenage years, rising from 10 milligrams to 15. Girls need extra iron to replace the iron they lose during the menstrual flow. Boys need more iron because the large increase in their tissue mass is accompanied by a rise in their levels of iron-containing hemoglobin.

▶ Keep in mind that at the start of the teen years, the RDAs for all nutrients rise to at least adult levels. To meet their dietary needs, teenagers are advised to consume four or more servings each day from the milk group, the vegetable/fruit group, and the bread/cereal group; and three or more servings from the meat group.

Every parent of teenagers knows that you have less control over their diets. But, in addition to having healthy foods around the house, you can be an educational force in your teen's life. Once again, if you avoid the "good/bad" distinctions about food and stress the point that there are more nutritional alternatives for every low-nutrient food, you'll be contributing practical data that will help your teen make better choices on his or her own.

Weighty Issues

The two most common dietary problems that afflict youth are obesity among children of all ages and anorexia nervosa (a syndrome of self-imposed starvation), usually seen in girls after the onset of puberty.

If you are concerned that your child's eating habits and weight gain or loss are causing problems, your first step is to get them a thorough health examination. There are any number of factors that might cause changes in appetite and weight, and the doctor should rule these out before you look for nutritional solutions.

You should also be aware that psychological factors can contribute to extreme eating behaviors, and your child's medical treatment may need to be supplemented by some form of psychological counseling.

Most important, remember that if your child

has an eating disorder, criticism will not help. To constantly nag a child about eating, in an effort to convince him or her to "shape up," is rarely, if ever, effective.

Obesity: A Crisis for Our Youth

American children are getting too big for their britches—literally. According to William H. Dietz, Jr., M.D., Ph.D., of the Tufts New England Medical Center, as many as 11 million of our country's children between the ages of six and seventeen may be overweight.

Tests for obesity are performed by measuring fat deposits in the body. Researchers define an obese child as one for whom the measurement of fat on his upper arm is greater than that of 84 percent of the thousands of children measured in a National Health Examination Survey in the early 1960s. A "superobese" child, by the researchers' standards, has a greater percentage of fat on his upper arm than 94 percent of the children measured. (Fat is more loosely attached on the back of the upper arm—between the shoulder and the elbow—and is therefore easier to measure. In addition, measurements of the fat on the upper arm provide clues about total body fat.)

Along with this increase in fat has come a rise in the number of children with high blood pressure, one of the major risk factors for heart disease. Obesity also puts children at greater risk for respiratory disease, diabetes, and a number of orthopedic disorders, as well as psychological and social problems.

A contributing factor to obesity is the overall decline in physical exercise among American youth. Part of the problem is the inadequate physical education programs in the schools. In 1988, Illinois was the only state to require physical fitness instruction from kindergarten through high school. Several states have no physical fitness requirements in the schools. According to Guy Reiff, Ph.D., professor of physical education at the University of Michigan and head of a fitness project involving 40,000 children, the average elementary

school schedules only 25 minutes of physical activity per week. "Contrast that with studies that show our youngsters watch TV 24 to 27 hours per week," said Reiff. "We have generations of youngsters who are getting fatter, not exercising, whose diets are very poor. We are raising a nation of butterballs."

Findings by the U.S. Public Health Service indicate that when schools do offer physical activity, they often concentrate more on performance and skill than they do on health and fitness. Putting the focus in the wrong place can cause children who are not natural athletes to grow frustrated and develop a dislike for physical activity. Good aerobic exercise—the kind that burns fat and may protect against heart disease—can be accomplished by anyone. Skill is not the issue; movement is.

If you think your child has a weight problem, have him or her checked by a doctor before trying to devise a weight loss diet of your own. Many health professionals question the wisdom of weight loss diets for children. It has been suggested that creating an obsessive atmosphere of denial might backfire later by leading to eating disorders. And not all apparent weight problems are what they seem to be. For example, it is normal for children's weight to fluctuate as they grow; don't overreact to a little plumpness, especially during puberty.

Also, before deciding that your child is overweight, examine your own attitudes about weight and diet. Americans have a thin-body bias that is at times unhealthy. When you communicate the thinness obsession to your children, you may be setting them up for a lifetime of dieting problems and even more severe eating disorders.

A case in point is a study reported by investigators at the University of California, San Francisco, which revealed that 81 percent of the nine-year-old girls surveyed were already dissatisfied with their weight and were dieting. This extreme reaction on the part of such young children is almost certainly due to the reinforcement of the American ideal that one cannot be too thin. It's a sad testimony to our values that we would set our children up in such a way. Many of these girls will, no doubt, have eating problems all of their lives; some may develop severe eating disorders such as anorexia nervosa and bulimia (a disorder characterized by frequent binging and purging).

In light of these cautions, if you and your doctor agree that your child needs to get fit, design a regimen that is practical and nonrigid, and one that stresses increased activity over decreased food. Here are some guidelines:

▶ Gradually incorporate good nutritional techniques into your cooking. Making moderate changes will benefit the entire family while it teaches your child good eating habits in a flexible, nonmoralistic way.

▶ Treat your overweight child just like everyone else in the family with respect to food. For example, if you want to serve him or her fruit for dessert, don't serve cake to the other family members.

▶ Encourage your child to be active. Current figures issued by the President's Council of Physical Fitness and Sports show that two-thirds of our youth between the ages of six and seventeen couldn't pass a basic fitness test. Regular exercise is the best way to promote fitness, and some studies indicate that it can be a more significant factor in preventing obesity than diet. Once again, get the entire family involved in active sports, walking, swimming, and other forms of exercise. You will all benefit.

▶ Serve occasional treats at the family meal; don't ban high calorie foods altogether. If your child feels deprived, he or she will want to eat more. Place the emphasis on controlling portions, rather than on avoiding favorite foods.

▶ Look for ways you can send positive messages of support and encouragement to your child. Nagging, even with subtle looks and comments, won't motivate a child to eat more wisely. If you let your child know that your love for him

or her is not tied to weight, your child will be more relaxed and open to making changes.

▶ Emphasize fitness over weight. Don't be "pound foolish." People tend to put too much value on what the scale says and not enough value on how they look and feel.

Teens Who Starve

You also have reason to be concerned if your child is not eating enough. Here, we do not refer to the occasional bouts of finicky eating that all children go through, but to young people (often preteen or teenage girls) who are suffering from the disease of anorexia nervosa.

Anorexia frequently starts near the time of puberty, when a young woman is undergoing a great many physical and psychological changes. As her body becomes more "womanly," she may experience embarrassment or fear and try to downplay the changes by staying thin. Or she may simply believe that she is getting fat. She becomes obsessed with diet and exercise in an effort to reach a thin ideal. (Another disease, bulimia, which involves a binge-purge response to eating, is also frequently the result of a weight obsession. However, bulimia occurs more often in young adult women than in young girls.)

Anorexia nervosa is a serious disease. Anorexics lose the ability to view themselves objectively. A girl who has reduced her weight to as little as 70 pounds might still regard herself as fat, even though she is literally starving herself to death. And a lengthy period of severe nutrient deficiency can have irreversible effects. The muscle waste eventually affects the heart, and even some girls who have been treated and started eating again have died from the disease. One of the most famous cases is singer Karen Carpenter, who suffered heart failure several months after she had started eating normally.

If you suspect that your child might be suffering from anorexia, do not try to reason with her or force her to eat. She'll find ways to thwart your efforts. She needs immediate attention.

What are the early signs that your child may have a problem? These are the most common:

▶ Changes in eating behavior, such as alternating between binging and starving, obsession with dieting, frequent loss of appetite.

▶ Frequent weighing, inappropriate concern about losing weight, overexercising, use of diuretics or laxatives.

▶ Constipation, dry skin and hair, skin rashes, and sluggishness.

▶ Gradual but constant weight loss or the appearance of weight loss. (Anorexics can be wily; they may carry heavy objects in their pockets when being weighed to convince you that they've gained weight.)

▶ Depressed behavior, withdrawal or extreme sullenness, accompanied by any of the above symptoms.

If your teenager shows these signs, do not take a wait-and-see attitude. The consequences of anorexia nervosa are so severe that it's better to overreact than to underreact. Take your child to a medical doctor, not a psychologist. The physical disease must be treated first. Your doctor can recommend therapists who specialize in counseling anorexics. (For more details about anorexia nervosa and bulimia, refer to chapter 22 or contact one of the organizations that addresses these conditions listed in The Nutrition Hotline at the back of this book.)

16

Women and Nutrition: The Childbearing Years

Whether a woman bears children or not, from the time she reaches puberty until the onset of menopause, her body is constantly preparing to do so. The role women play in the propagation (and therefore survival) of the human race makes them very special in their nutritional needs.

Many of the nutritional concerns that women have are in some way linked to their childbearing cycle. Even osteoporosis, which becomes a problem for many women when they have passed the childbearing years, is associated with a decreased production of the hormone estrogen, which aids the metabolism of calcium.

Here, we focus specifically on several key nutritional issues that women have during their childbearing years: The influence of a woman's general, pre-pregnancy health on her ability to conceive and bear a healthy child; the management of a successful pregnancy; and the avoidance of ongoing problems, specifically Premenstrual Syndrome, that can plague her throughout her childbearing years.

The Nutritional Key to Childbearing

It was not until the 1930s that serious research was started on maternal and child nutrition, with practitioners voicing the view that the mother's diet could substantially influence the birth weight and health of her baby. In 1946, the National Academy of Sciences appointed a Committee on Maternal Nutrition and child Feeding. The committee's 1950 report, *Maternal Nutrition as it Relates to Child Health—An Interpretive Review,* served as the basic guideline on the subject for many years. Maternal and infant nutrition was a major focus of the 1969 White House Conference on Food, Nutrition, and Health, directed by Dr. Jean Mayer, now president of Tufts University. The conference panel on Pregnant and Nursing Women and Young Infants clearly identified a sound diet as a necessary factor in the birth of healthy infants. The panel concluded that good nutrition throughout the mother's life was the best way to promote infant health. During the following years, more specific guidelines were developed for the nutritional needs of pregnant women and infants.

In 1979, *The Surgeon General's Report on Health Promotion and Disease Prevention* defined some broad goals for pregnancy and infant health to be achieved by 1990. These goals included a reduction in infant mortality, education of pregnant women about nutritional requirements and the dangers of alcohol, and an increase in the number of mothers choosing to breast-feed their babies. The 1988 *Surgeon General's Report on Nutrition and Health* includes a chapter updating nutritional recommendations for mothers and children. Its guidelines reflect the most current research available from medical scientists and nutrition experts on how a woman might manage her own and her child's health by paying attention to healthy eating, starting with the period before she becomes pregnant.

Before Pregnancy

If you are a healthy woman of average weight with no preexisting medical condition, the best way to prepare for pregnancy is to eat a balanced diet, using the RDA guidelines for your age group. However, if you are either dramatically underweight or obese, you should address this condition before becoming pregnant.

When it comes to pregnancy, it is possible to be too thin, since the fat stores in the hips and thighs are needed to nourish the fetus in the later months of pregnancy and for breast milk. It is ironic that the American ideal, which during the past twenty years has increasingly moved away from the "womanly" figure, is really at odds with the biological wisdom of giving women more generous hips and thighs. A woman with too little body fat—for example, an anorexic—would have a difficult time bearing a healthy child of normal birth weight. For this reason, women's bodies sometimes intervene to make it more unlikely that they will become pregnant. That is why menstrual periods sometimes cease in anorexic women or in women who diet and exercise too heavily. The same phenomenon occurs in conditions of famine, when women become less likely to conceive. Their bodies "recognize" that the famine condition makes it impossible to support the growth of a normal fetus, or to produce the milk a newborn baby needs to survive.

Obesity can also lead to problems in pregnancy. It is linked with an increased risk of complications to the mother, including hypertensive disorders, gestational diabetes, toxemia, urinary tract infections, and the need for cesarean deliveries. An obese woman—that is, one who is 30 percent or more above her normal weight—should plan to reduce her weight gradually before becoming pregnant, since weight loss during pregnancy has been associated with low birth weight. Studies have shown that when weight is not gained during pregnancy, even in obese women, infants suffer low birth weight. For example, one study showed that out of a group of pregnant, overweight women, infants born to those who gained the least weight had double the infant mortality rate of babies born to mothers who had higher gain.

Adolescent pregnancies pose greater risks for both the mothers and their infants. According to the American Academy of Pediatrics Committee on Nutrition, mothers who are 15 years old or younger (approximately 60,000 every year in the United States) have increased rates of pregnancy-induced hypertension and premature delivery. They are also more likely to deliver infants with low birth weights and have higher rates of fetal loss and infant mortality.

Weight Gain During Pregnancy

In recent years, nutrition and medical experts have revised their estimates of how much weight a woman should gain during pregnancy. Once, it was believed that weight gain should not exceed 18 pounds and was better if kept between 10 and 15 pounds. Today, most obstetricians believe that a weight gain between 22 and 27 pounds is acceptable. However, some research is currently being conducted at Tufts to see if an even greater weight gain might be advisable.

Further, most experts believe that the pattern of weight gain during pregnancy is as important as the total amount. Although each woman will have her own pattern, the goal should be a slow, steady gain. So, for instance, if you gain a large amount one month, you should not panic and start to cut back on your intake. The main thing to watch out for is sudden, unexplained jump in weight, which could be the result of fluid retention, a sign of toxemia and a serious problem if not treated promptly.

Should a woman who is carrying twins eat (and gain) twice as much? Although very little research has been conducted on the needs of a mother carrying twins, a study done at Grady Memorial Hospital in Atlanta showed that out of 137 twin pregnancies, the healthiest babies were born to mothers who gained about 41 pounds during the typical 36-week pregnancy term. Sherri Carlton, M.Sc., R.D., who led the study team, believes that tall or thin women who are expecting twins should gain somewhat more than that. She also says that the need for folic acid and protein appears to be greater for twin pregnancies, although the exact increment is not yet known.

Where does the additional weight go? Many women are surprised after delivery to discover how little of their added weight actually goes into the weight of the baby. For example, a woman who gains 27 pounds during pregnancy will usually find that the added weight breaks down this way: 7½ pounds is baby; 3 pounds is the increase in the size of the breasts and uterus; 9 pounds is contributed by a combination of the placenta, amniotic fluid, extra blood volume, and other fluids; and 7½ pounds is body fat, usually in the hips and thighs, as a reserve for the mother who breastfeeds.

Keeping Fit During Pregnancy

It is best to consult with your physician before planning an exercise regimen for your pregnancy since women with certain health risks or medical conditions may be advised not to exercise. However, the American College of Obstetricians and Gynecologists has recommended a number of exercises suitable for pregnant women, including walking, swimming, stationary cycling, and modified forms of low-impact aerobic exercises, dancing, and calisthenics. When exercising, be sure that your heart rate does not exceed 140 beats a

minute, and do not engage in strenuous activity for more than 15 minutes at a time.

It is also recommended that pregnant women practice deep-breathing exercises and gentle stretching, which will help during the delivery process.

Precautionary Measures

Health researchers are in agreement that alcohol consumption during pregnancy can adversely affect fetal development. The condition called Fetal Alcohol Syndrome was first discovered in the early 1970s among infants whose mothers were chronic alcoholics. The effects of the syndrome were severe, including abnormalities of the eyes, nose, heart, and central nervous system. Further, these infants suffered the pains of alcohol withdrawal and normally showed impaired mental and physical development, even after rehabilitation.

Although the minimum level of alcohol that can lead to Fetal Alcohol Syndrome is not yet known, some studies have shown that as little as a drink or two a day might lead to spontaneous abortion, premature detachment of the placenta, or infants born with low birth weights. While other studies contradict these claims, the surgeon general recommended in his 1988 report that, to be on the safe side, pregnant women should avoid alcohol completely.

Caffeine is another substance that pregnant women should view with caution, although studies on humans have yet to prove a firm link between caffeine consumption and impaired fetal development. The most well-known and controversial study on the subject was conducted with pregnant rats who, when given large amounts of caffeine, showed impaired development of fetuses. However, the study has been criticized because the amounts of caffeine fed to the rats were considered to be unnaturally high.

To date, studies on humans have not proved conclusive. One study of 20,000 pregnant women showed that coffee drinking has little or no effect on fetal health. However, another study of 5,200 women reported lower birth weights in babies born to women who consumed five or more cups of coffee a day.

Even though researchers have not yet reached a firm understanding of the effects of caffeine on pregnancy, it can be argued that, because the caffeine does pass on to the fetus through the placenta, limiting your consumption is probably a good idea during pregnancy. In fact, the Food and Drug Administration has advised cutting back on caffeine as a precautionary measure.

Gestational Diabetes— A Special Concern

Gestational diabetes, a special form of the disease, occurs in between 1 to 2 percent of all pregnancies. It appears between the sixth and seventh months, when the mother's pancreas cannot meet the demands of the pregnancy. The condition is most common among women who have family histories of diabetes, who have previously given birth to babies weighing more than 10 pounds, or who have a condition of "sugar in the urine" during pregnancy. Insulin resistance (a drop in the efficiency with which insulin is utilized) is linked both to the rising levels of several hormones and to increased weight.

Gestational diabetes can cause health problems both for the mother and the baby. The pregnant woman suffers an increased risk of hypertension. And, since infants of mothers with gestational diabetes tend to be large, they are more likely to be delivered by cesarean section. Infants suffer an increased chance of respiratory-distress syndrome, and they are more likely to be hypoglycemic.

The best way to decrease the risk of developing gestational diabetes is to be aware of the factors that might put you at risk: (1) a family history of diabetes of any type; (2) a prior personal experience of diabetes of any type, especially during previous pregnancies; and (3) previously giving birth to a baby weighing 10 pounds or more. If

these risk factors apply, be sure to alert your doctor so you can work together to counteract the risks during your pregnancy.

Even if no risk factors exist, the American Diabetes Association recommends that all women be checked for abnormal glucose tolerance between the sixth and seventh months of pregnancy. The test involves drinking a single dose of a glucose solution, after which blood-sugar levels are measured. If the levels remain abnormally high, further testing is required.

Often gestational diabetes can be successfully treated by making changes in the diet. The goal is to normalize blood sugar and, for some women, this can be accomplished by simply cutting down on sweets or spreading calories evenly throughout the day. Only in severe cases are insulin injections required.

Gestational diabetes usually disappears after pregnancy, although women who have had the condition are at a higher risk for developing adult-onset diabetes, particularly if they are obese.

Cravings and Other Food Dilemmas

Most people take it for granted that pregnant women will have strange cravings, although they probably think these cravings are "all in the head." In fact, there are two common types of cravings that affect pregnant women.

The first and most common craving is the proverbial "ice cream and pickles" syndrome, where women desire unusual amounts of certain foods, or offbeat combinations of foods, such as salty foods along with sweets. These women commonly feel an aversion to some foods: in particular, coffee, tea, alcohol, and meat. Usually these cravings seem to have nothing to do with nutritional needs.

A second type of craving is more rare. Known as "pica," this craving involves a strong desire to eat nonfood items such as cornstarch, laundry starch, or clay. Although such cravings have been described since biblical times, they remain a tantalizing mystery. We do know that pica is most common among pregnant women who suffer from iron deficiency anemia. How this craving might be linked to the need for the mineral is not fully understood.

Another factor of concern for pregnant women who are interested in meeting their nutritional needs is the onset of "morning sickness," or bouts of nausea, which can occur at any time during the day. Half of all pregnant women are afflicted by this ailment, usually between the second and fourth months of pregnancy. Although it is not known exactly what causes the nausea, it is believed by some to be linked with a drop in blood sugar. Many women experience it most intensely upon waking; for them, it helps to eat a couple of dry crackers right away. It also helps to eat small meals throughout the day and never allow yourself to get too hungry, and to drink liquids separately instead of with meals.

Pregnant women also complain of other digestive maladies, such as heartburn and constipation. It is best to take care of these problems by concentrating on a high-fiber diet and by eliminating spicy, greasy, or rich foods.

Growing a Healthy Child

During pregnancy, it is most important to be sure that you are eating a well-balanced diet, in accordance with the Recommended Dietary Allowances for pregnant women. Even if you are consuming adequate calories, your diet must reflect the proper nutrient balance or it could severely affect the health of your baby. Consider that during the approximately nine months of pregnancy, a baby's bone structure and tissue development are taking place.

Although there are difficulties in quantifying the effects of pregnancy and lactation on nutritional requirements for calories and individual nutrients, it is accepted by all knowledgeable people that pregnant and breast-feeding women have additional nutritional needs. Not only must the women meet their own needs, they also must meet those of their infants during fetal growth

and early infancy. Pregnancy and lactation may affect the nutrient requirements of women by altering their physiological and metabolic states.

To ensure that pregnant and lactating women receive sufficient nutrients, the RDA values have been increased for them (see chapter 7). For example, the RDA for protein is increased 65 percent, and those for vitamin D and folacin are 100 percent higher.

Dietary Guidelines: Getting Enough Nutrients

PROTEIN
Protein needs during pregnancy and breast-feeding (lactation) are substantially higher than normal. To supply enough protein, eat an additional 1 to 2 ounces of any of these foods 3 or 4 times each day: meat, poultry, fish, or cheese.

VITAMIN C
One cup of orange juice, broccoli, red or green pepper, grapefruit juice, strawberries, brussels sprouts, cauliflower, dark greens, or one orange will each come close to meeting the RDA for pregnancy.

THIAMIN, NIACIN, AND RIBOFLAVIN
Four or more daily servings or enriched or whole-grain breads, cereals, rice, crackers, or pasta will meet the requirement for pregnant women. Lactating women should add one serving.

VITAMIN B-6
Good sources include liver, light-meat chicken, bananas, and navy beans. A 3-ounce serving of each provides close to 20 percent of the RDA for pregnant and lactating women. Other good sources include tuna, halibut, avocados, peanuts, beef, and salmon.

FOLIC ACID (FOLACIN)
To help meet the doubled RDA for pregnancy, eat at least one to two cups a day of these folacin-rich vegetables: spinach, turnip greens, endive, dark-

green lettuce, asparagus, okra, broccoli, parsnips, cauliflower, peas, brussels sprouts, or cabbage. Lactating women's needs are closer to the average for nonpregnant women—only 100 μg more per day. But it is a good idea to include one of these foods in the diet each day while breast-feeding.

CALCIUM

About four servings of milk products are recommended for each day. A serving is an 8-ounce glass of low-fat or whole milk or buttermilk, 1 cup of yogurt, 1½ ounces of hard or American cheese, 2 cups of cottage cheese, 1½ cups of ice cream or ice milk, 8 ounces of tufu that was made from a calcium coagulant such as calcium sulfate, 2 cups of broccoli, or 4 ounces of salmon (with soft bones).

ZINC AND IRON

Even if you're taking an iron supplement, you should not ignore good sources in food, in part because most are also high in zinc. Both iron and zinc are available in animal foods, including red meats, organ meats, seafood (especially shellfish), and poultry. Fortified breads and cereals, as well as nuts and legumes, may carry extra iron, but rarely zinc. Milk is a good source of zinc, but not of iron.

Are Dietary Supplements Needed?

Many obstetricians routinely recommend prenatal multi–vitamin/mineral supplements to their pregnant patients as a safety precaution, just in case they're not getting adequate nutrients in their diets. But other physicians disagree, feeling that multi–vitamin/mineral supplements are unnecessary.

The only nutrient that virtually all physicians think is necessary as a supplement during pregnancy is iron. Because a large percentage of what is ingested isn't absorbed, anywhere from 30 to 60 milligrams of iron are suggested to assure that women absorb the 3.5 milligrams they need. Until recently, there was little information on the avail-

ability of iron to the body when it was given in the form of prenatal multi–vitamin/mineral supplements, which typically contain about 60 milligrams of iron, along with many other vitamins and minerals. But when a number of their pregnant patients developed iron deficiency even though they were taking daily prenatal supplements, Paul Seligman, M.D., and his colleagues at the University of Colorado Health Sciences Center became suspicious and decided to research the matter. They gave nonpregnant healthy women either iron supplements alone or iron in the form of prenatal multi–vitamin/mineral supplements. Of the four different brands of vitamin/mineral supplements tested, less than the needed 3.5 milligrams of iron were absorbed in each case. When 65 milligrams of supplemental iron alone were given, 8.1 milligrams were absorbed.

Further examination showed that the reason so little iron was absorbed in the multi–vitamin/mineral preparations was largely because the calcium carbonate and magnesium oxide in some of them interfered with iron absorption. When the researchers reformulated the supplements to contain less calcium and magnesium, 4.5 milligrams of iron were absorbed.

But the calcium carbonate and magnesium oxide did not account for all of the decrease in iron absorption. The researchers believe that additional factors, such as fillers, other vitamins and minerals, or the coating and compressing of the nutrients might also have played a role.

Dr. Seligman and his colleagues also had their subjects take the supplements on empty stomachs, because iron absorption may be as much as 75 percent less when the supplements are taken with meals.

Nutrition during the Menstruating Years

It has been known since ancient times that in the days preceding menstruation each month, some women experience a variety of symptoms ranging in intensity from unpleasant to debilitating. But the medical community did not seriously begin to consider Premenstrual Syndrome (PMS) a clinical disorder until 1931, when a physician named Robert T. Frank called it a syndrome of "indescribable tension and irritability." The symptoms, said Dr. Frank, were relieved with the onset of menstruation.

Although the definition of PMS has grown more sophisticated since 1931, there is much that remains unknown about the syndrome. It is generally recognized as a set of physical and/or emotional symptoms that begin every month after ovulation and end abruptly with the start of the menstrual flow. For some women, the syndrome lasts for the entire two weeks or so from ovulation to menstruation. For others, it appears for only a few days, or even for just one day, before the period begins. But it is this cyclical pattern—the timing of the symptoms—that defines PMS, more than the nature of the symptoms themselves, which range considerably in nature and severity from woman to woman. More than 150 PMS symptoms have been described. The most common include tension, depression, irritability, inability to concentrate, crying spells, headaches, breast tenderness, bloating, weight gain, acne, clumsiness, and cravings for chocolate or other sweet or salty foods.

Unfortunately, some physicians still consider PMS a neurotic condition rather than a clinical syndrome caused by an altered endocrinologic state. It is hoped that, as more information becomes available on PMS, physicians will reach a consensus on its treatment as a medical condition.

The Misleading Nutrition–PMS Connection

At this time, there are no well-conducted clinical trials that establish a direct relationship between nutrition and PMS. An added difficulty is the fact that the symptoms of PMS cannot be objectively viewed on X rays or in lab tests. Only the woman herself can say whether she feels better.

Of special concern to physicians and nutritionists is the proliferation of expensive and potentially harmful supplements and other "remedies" that have flooded the marketplace. We know these remedies are not based on scientific studies. So how do the proponents reach their conclusions? Usually, an isolated nutritional factor is used as the basis for conclusions that, in a scientific setting, would not be acceptable. In other cases, the conclusions are simply quackery. There is no evidence to support them—only questionable anecdotal references and hefty marketing budgets.

It is important that consumers understand the truth behind these claims. Not only are some of the remedies expensive, but they can cause severe problems, ranging from stomach irritation to calcium deficiency to nerve damage. These are the most popular theories:

THEORY 1: VITAMIN B-6 DEFICIENCY

The vitamin B-6 deficiency theory is perhaps the most widely held theory and has been making the rounds since the 1940s. Proponents claim that a deficiency of B-6 is somehow related to hormonal imbalance, in particular an imbalance of estrogen, which leads to depression or dramatic mood swings. In spite of there being no evidence that women with PMS have estrogen imbalances or B-6 deficiencies, practioners prescribe megadoses of the vitamin. In some instances, the recommended levels have been as high as 2,000 milligrams a day, 100 times the RDA of 2 milligrams.

Since B-6 is a water-soluble vitamin, it is believed that any excess amounts in the system will simply be excreted in urine and therefore cause no harm to the body. But research has shown that even doses much lower than 2,000 milligrams a day can cause damage to the nervous system, resulting in numbness, tingling, difficulty walking, and spinal cord problems. These symptoms have developed in women who have taken as little as 500 milligrams a day. Indeed, one woman suffered symptoms after taking only 200 milligrams a day over the course of three years. From a scientific point of view, supplements of vitamin B-6 have never proven to be more effective than a placebo, in spite of their popularity.

THEORY 2: A NEED FOR
EVENING PRIMROSE OIL

Some people believe that victims of PMS do not have enough of the enzyme needed to produce a fatty acid called gamma linolenic acid, leading to a deficiency in a very active biochemical called prostaglandin E-1. This deficiency, they think, may be involved in PMS symptoms such as breast tenderness. Their solution is oral ingestion of evening primrose oil, sometimes sold as Efamol, which they say contains the missing fatty acid and allows the balance to be restored.

Besides the fact that evening primrose oil, widely sold in health food stores, is expensive, it has never been demonstrated that a prostaglandin deficiency is what causes PMS symptoms or that any oil given in supplement form will correct such a deficiency. And evening primrose oil has never been shown to relieve any of the discomfort, physical or emotional, of PMS. It can, however, cause gastric irritation if taken on an empty stomach.

THEORY 3: TOO MUCH CALCIUM,
TOO LITTLE MAGNESIUM

Some experts have observed that some women with Premenstrual Syndrome have lower levels of the mineral magnesium than women who do not suffer from PMS. Therefore, the possibility exists that the condition may have something to do with a magnesium deficiency. According to the theory, the deficiency develops in part because of too much calcium consumption in the form of dairy products. Calcium is transported through part of the gastrointestinal tract via the same carrier that transports magnesium. Thus, calcium competes with magnesium for absorption and leaves a

woman with a magnesium shortfall. The supposed solution is to take a magnesium supplement.

The hitch is that although some women with PMS were found to have lower levels of magnesium in their blood cells than symptom-free women, their levels were still within normal range. The fact is that other than in cases of alcoholism or a malabsorption disorder, women of childbearing age in the United States generally have no trouble getting enough magnesium from the animal foods, nuts, seeds, legumes, green vegetables, whole-grain products, and milk they consume.

The real problem in taking megadoses of magnesium is that a woman can, in fact, impair her absorption of calcium by consuming too much magnesium. Furthermore, in very high doses, magnesium can be toxic. And magnesium salts like those in Milk of Magnesia will act as laxatives —even if you're not looking for that effect.

THEORY 4: MULTINUTRIENT DEFICIENCIES

Some people subscribe to the notion that women with PMS may be deficient in a wide range of nutrients, including vitamins A, C, E, B-6, and other B vitamins, as well as magnesium, iron, and zinc. Based on this assumption, Dr. Guy Abraham has developed a nutritional supplement called Optivite, which, if taken six times a day, as advised, contains 15,000 percent of the RDA for vitamin B-6, 2,500 percent of the USRDA for vitamin C, 1,600 percent of the allowance for thiamin, almost 1,500 percent of the accepted figure for riboflavin, more than 1,000 percent of the recommendation for vitamin B-12, and 200 to 300 percent of the requirement for vitamins A and E and pantothenic acid. Niacin and zinc are also included in amounts exceeding 100 percent of the USRDA.

The increasing popularity of this supplement has given rise to some Optivite clones that are identical, or nearly identical, to the original. The six tablets can cost up to about a dollar a day, depending on the brand. Needless to say, the safety of taking megadoses of so many nutrients for any length of time is questionable at best and quite dangerous at worst. It should also be pointed out that in a study published in the *American Journal of Clinical Nutrition,* in which the levels or activity of zinc and vitamins A, E, B-6, and thiamin were compared in PMS sufferers and non-PMS sufferers, "no evidence was found to support the hypothesis that premenstrual symptoms are caused by absolute or relative nutritional deficiencies."

Some Sound Nutritional Advice

The bottom line is that the "miracle" remedies won't cure PMS and might lead to serious problems. But a well-balanced, healthy diet will at least insure that PMS sufferers are getting all the nutrients they need.

Dr. Annette Rossignol, an epidemiologist now at Oregon State University, reported while at Tufts that there was evidence of a connection between PMS and caffeine. While a statistically significant association still does not prove a causal relationship, it might be prudent for PMS sufferers to cut back on products containing caffeine.

17

Growing Old with Grace

From the moment of birth, every human being starts on the process of growing older. We don't just wake up one day to find that our bones are brittle, our skin has wrinkled, and our bodies don't function as well as they once did. There is no cut-off point when we stop being "young" and start being "old." Yet that is exactly the way most of us have learned to view growing older—as a point in time when the good days are gone forever. Gerontophobia, or fear of aging, has infected our society for so long that it comes as no surprise that we have avoided investigating so many issues involving the elderly.

The study of nutrition and its relationship to the aging process is a new field, but as the life expectancy of Americans grows it is taking on great significance. Today, people are living some 30 years longer than they were at the turn of the century, and the number of elderly people is increasing at a rapid pace: By the year 2030, it is estimated that the number of Americans over the age of 65 will be double what it is today and twice the number of teenagers. And since people are living longer, they want to live those years more fully. Today the average, healthy 50-year-old woman has a life expectancy of 80 years; it's absurd to think that she should spend those 30 years "winding down."

Since 1982, Tufts has been involved in the study of aging at its federally sponsored USDA Human Nutrition Research Center on Aging. Research at the center focuses on how nutrition during the entire life cycle influences the way people age. The center has a staff of more than 200, including 50 research scientists with Ph.D. or M.D. degrees. During the years since its inception, the center's researchers have already uncovered a number of critical connections between nutrition and aging, including:

▶ Protein requirements for physically active older men are higher than the current RDA.

▶ Physical exercise markedly increases muscle size and strength in men and women, even at 90 years of age.

▶ Certain identifiable genetic factors might predict the risk of early heart disease and may be used to recommend diet therapy for high-risk individuals.

▶ A hormonal form of vitamin D might be related to skin aging and conditions such as psoriasis.

▶ The ability of the skin to synthesize vitamin D from sunlight decreases markedly with age, supporting the need for the elderly to be more dependent on dietary vitamin D than younger people.

▶ A decreased ability to produce stomach acid occurs in 20 percent of the elderly population and interferes with the absorption of several vitamins and minerals.

▶ Elderly women who ingest low levels of calcium lose that mineral from the spine at a significantly greater rate than those whose intakes exceed the RDA.

▶ Calcium supplements, when taken with a meal, impair the absorption of iron from that meal.

▶ Under experimental conditions, vitamin E has been shown to play an important role in the immune system and may act to partially reverse some age-related declines in immune response.

▶ There seems to be a dietary relationship between the delay of cataract or cataract-like changes in the eye lens and nutrients that act as antioxidants, such as vitamins C and E.

▶ Vitamins A and D may be involved in important skin protection functions.

▶ There is evidence that vitamin B-6 requirements are increased in the elderly and that vitamin A requirements may be reduced.

These and many other studies at Tufts provide new information that may have important effects on the health and vitality of the elderly. Unfortunately, nutrition research on the elderly shows that, for the most part, diet cannot miraculously reverse the health status of the current generation of elderly. Rather, it suggests that the sooner healthful patterns of nutritional behavior are practiced, the greater will be the effects of good nutrition on the vitality level and longevity of the older population.

For today's seniors, the health and nutrition picture is complex. Although life expectancy con-

tinues to increase, 80 percent of today's elderly have at least one chronic condition; among the most prevalent are osteoporosis , arthritis, hypertension, hearing and visual impairments, and cardiac conditions. On the average, individuals over the age of 75 make eight visits to their doctors every year; in 1985, approximately 5 million elderly in the United States required long-term care. In spite of this somewhat troubling picture, nutrition remains one of the controllable factors that can influence the overall health of the elderly, even those who already have one or more chronic conditions. For example, as discussed in chapters 18 and 20, cardiac conditions, hypertension, and osteoporosis can all be controlled, at least in part, with diet. In addition, an understanding of the physiological changes that occur with aging can help to prevent many diet-related health problems that commonly plague the elderly population.

Physiological Changes that Affect Nutrition

Many of the natural physiological changes that occur with age alter food preferences and nutritional requirements. They affect the way our bodies metabolize food, as well as the types of foods we are comfortably able to eat. Lean body mass decreases as our bodies lose muscle and our systems slow down. It is estimated that a 70-year-old man requires about 30 percent fewer calories than a 30-year-old man of the same size. With a decline in metabolism and physical exercise, calorie needs are less, and diets must become more nutrient-dense to assure that the proper intakes of nutrients are being maintained on the lower calorie diets.

Aging is also associated with alterations in smell, taste, and texture preferences in foods. Diets designed for young people are not as appetizing to people as they grow older, in part because many elderly people have teeth missing or dentures that fit poorly and cover taste receptors. Such people can find it hard to chew foods like crunchy vegetables and fruits, or meat.

As we grow older, the small intestine loses some of its ability to make lactase, the enzyme that digests milk sugar (lactose). Since the undigested lactose sits in the intestines and ferments, a number of elderly people are troubled by gas, bloating, and sometimes diarrhea after eating certain dairy products.

The intestines are affected in another way. Basically, with age everything slows down, so there is a tendency toward constipation, especially on diets low in fiber. Another change in the gastrointestinal tract is that the stomach produces less acid, which is needed to absorb some vitamins and minerals. A decrease in acid alters the normal bacterial flora found in the intestines, with a variety of nutritional ramifications.

There are also hormonal changes, such as a decrease in estrogen production in women, which causes calcium to be withdrawn from the bones and makes postmenopausal women more susceptible to osteoporosis (see chapter 20).

Getting Enough Fluids

Under normal conditions, the average adult loses roughly 2½ quarts of water a day, mostly in urine, but also in sweat, feces, and through breathing. This loss must be replaced or we become dehydrated and die. One way our bodies protect us is through the signal that we're thirsty. We are also protected by a mechanism that causes the kidneys to begin conserving water—reabsorbing it back into the blood instead of excreting it—when there is deprivation.

It has been found that, as people age, thirst signals become less strong. Studies conducted at Oxford and Johns Hopkins universities suggest that many elderly people fail to drink enough fluids, even when their bodies need it. To make matters worse, the kidneys do not act as efficiently to conserve water when it is needed. As a result,

elderly people are more prone than others to dehydration.

Since it is impossible to rely on thirst as a sole indicator of need, the elderly should create a regular regimen of fluid intake. Although approximately half the body's water stock is supplied by food, the remaining requirement should be consumed by drinking six to eight cups of fluid each day. For hydration, the best choice is water, but milk and juices can supply valuable nutrients as well. It is especially important to increase water intake during hot weather, since, in addition to replacing fluids lost through sweat, it acts as a body coolant, reducing the effects of body heat production and loss.

Socioeconomic Factors that Affect Nutrition

In the United States, aging is normally accompanied by a variety of psychologic, economic, and social changes that may affect the nutritional status of individuals. It is impossible to separate the socioeconomic and psychological issues from the biological realities when we evaluate the risk factors for the elderly in our society.

As a group, older Americans have a lower economic status than other adults in the United States. According to recent U.S. Senate studies, the decline in income most often results from retirement from the work force, the effects of inflation on fixed income, death of a wage-earning spouse, or failing health. Low income is clearly a major risk factor for inadequate nutrition in the elderly.

The process of evaluating nutrition and health factors for older people is complicated, and there are currently no firm guidelines for their nutritional requirements. The RDAs, for example, were developed largely from research on the nutrient needs of young, healthy people. The present standards for adults over 50 are almost identical to those for other adults because they were extrapolated from this research.

Studies of aging are also complicated by the many life-style changes that occur as people age. For example, the Ten State Nutrition Survey conducted in the 1970s found that two-thirds of the older population had changed their diets during the four years preceding the study, making it hard to evaluate long-term patterns.

In studying the elderly population, researchers have been stymied by the lack of correlation between certain nutrition-related findings. For example, over the past 20 years, several comprehensive nutritional surveys have been conducted that identified a substantial proportion of older men and women who fell below the RDA for calories, protein, vitamins, calcium, and iron. At the same time, studies have found that obesity is a real problem in the aged, especially in women. The two conflicting points are not hard to reconcile. It is clear that many elderly do not engage in work or exercise that uses many calories. Several credible studies have established the decline in physical activity as people age. One study of male executives in the Baltimore Longitudinal Study of Aging found a steady decline in average energy expenditure; other studies have supported this evidence. This decline is particularly unfortunate since recent studies at Tufts clearly demonstrate that even the very old may respond positively to exercise (see chapter 24).

Practical Vulnerabilities

Even when detrimental socioeconomic factors do not exist, many older people are vulnerable nutritionally simply because they lack the capacity to buy or prepare nutritional meals. Or they may be unable to shop for food, particularly if the weather is bad or they live far from the supermarket.

An elderly man or woman is far more susceptible to food poisoning than the average person, for two reasons. First, a declining power in the senses of taste, smell, and vision weakens the ability of elderly persons to easily recognize when a food has gone bad, when fresh foods are damaged, moldy, or off-color, when packaging is broken, or when dishes and utensils are not clean. They are less facile in identifying flavors and odors. A test conducted by Duke University demonstrated this. When asked to identify common odors such as chocolate, cinnamon, coffee, grape, onion, pepper, root beer, soy sauce, and tea, college students named the odors correctly 86 percent of the time. When the same test was administered to elderly subjects, they identified the odors correctly only 34 percent of the time.

Second, Tufts researchers have found that in at least 20 percent of the elderly, less stomach acid is being produced. Since stomach acid helps to digest food and kill microbes, an elderly person might become ill after eating food that would not cause a problem for a younger person.

Further, since the immune system appears to weaken with age, even a mild case of food poisoning can be a severe health problem for an older person. Add to that the fact that many older people suffer additional health complications, such as heart disease or diabetes, and it becomes easy to see why their bodies are less able to fight off infections.

Physical handling and ease of food preparation are other factors that influence health in seniors. Many rely heavily on canned or processed foods since they are easier to prepare. Or they may be limited in their ability to shop for a wide range of fresh fruits and vegetables. Additionally, package expiration dates may go unnoticed, or food may be saved beyond its safe consumption date out of frugality.

The Food and Drug Administration offers the following tips for people who want to help their older relatives and friends avoid trouble in the kitchen:

Be observant: Note any marked change in habits that might indicate an elderly person needs more help in the kitchen.

Watch nutrition: Check to see that older people are eating a variety of animal and dairy foods, cereals, grains, fruits, and vegetables.

Shop weekly: Either shop for elderly people or encourage them to shop every week and purchase perishable foods in small quantities. Sug-

---

AN EATING GUIDE FOR SENIORS

The elderly need to take special care to maintain a varied diet that is rich in all the nutrients they need. The following are some suggestions for nutrients that are sometimes a problem for the elderly.

Suggested Foods and Servings

Protein
2 scrambled or poached eggs
1 cup low-fat cottage cheese
3½ oz. tuna
3½ oz. broiled or baked chicken breast
1 cup low-fat milk
3½ oz. broiled lean ground beef or round steak
1 cup plain low-fat yogurt

Vitamin C
1 4-oz. glass orange juice
½ sliced tomato
1 cup sliced strawberries
½ cup cooked spinach
1 baked or mashed potato
½ honeydew melon
1 medium orange
1 4-oz. glass grapefruit juice

Vitamin A
1 cup low-fat fortified milk
1 cup cooked broccoli
½ cantaloupe
½ cup cooked carrots or 1 raw carrot
1 medium baked sweet potato

Vitamin E
1 slice whole-wheat or enriched bread with 1 tbsp. margarine
1 cup wheat flakes, bran cereal, or hot oatmeal, whole-grain or enriched
1 cup cooked whole-grain or enriched pasta
1 tbsp. vegetable oil-and-vinegar salad dressing on a green salad

Vitamin D
1 cup fortified low-fat milk

Calcium
1 cup low-fat milk
½ cup low-fat cottage cheese
3½ oz. canned salmon (with soft bones)
1 cup plain low-fat yogurt
½ cup ice milk

Niacin
1 slice whole-grain or enriched bread or 1 muffin or 4 wheat or rye crackers
½ cup (cooked) brown or enriched rice
3½ oz. lean ground beef
1 cup lima bean soup or ½ cup cooked lima beans
½ cup cooked peas

Folacin
3½ oz. broiled or baked beef liver
1 cup shredded cabbage coleslaw
1 cup cooked broccoli or cauliflower
1 cup cooked brussels sprouts
1 orange

Vitamin B-6
1 cup cooked corn or 1 piece of corn on the cob
½ cup low-fat cottage cheese
1 medium banana
1 3–4 oz. lamb chop
3½ oz. broiled halibut

Iron
3½–4 oz. shrimp or tuna
3½ oz. steamed clams
3½ oz. lean roast beef, broiled
3½ oz. broiled beef liver
3½ oz. broiled chicken breast
1 slice whole-grain or enriched bread or 1 medium enriched roll
1 cup lentil bean soup

gest that they look for single serving-sized prepared foods and not allow leftovers to linger in the refrigerator.

Help in cooking: Prepare batches of favorite foods and pack the portions in TV-dinner-size containers. Mark the containers clearly and store them in the freezer for easy preparation.

Ensure freezer safety: Date all packages to be stored in the freezer, using a dark magic marker. Suggest that older packages be moved forward as new items are added.

Provide easy snacking: Suggest that people with dentures keep a basket of soft fruit handy for snacks. Good fruits include bananas, grapes, and ripe pears.

Allow proper timing: Purchase a brightly colored, sufficiently loud timer for the elderly person who is getting forgetful but still likes to cook.

Use package aids: If hand strength and dexterity are a problem, there are special devices available to help. Your local Arthritis Foundation can supply information on locating gripper pads, can poppers, and other package-opening aids.

Check equipment: Make sure that your elderly relative or friend's refrigerator (safe at 40°F) and freezer (safe at 0°F) are running properly and that the freezer is defrosted when necessary.

Mixing Food and Medication

Since many elderly people take regular medication, it is important to know that some drugs may affect appetite and the metabolism of nutrients. When medication is prescribed, it is important to discuss with the doctor when it should be taken and whether it may affect nutritional needs.

The mere presence of food can change the chemical environment of the intestinal tract in such a way that the effects of certain drugs can be profoundly altered. Drugs and nutrients, when consumed together, may interact by binding tightly to each other and passing through the intestinal tract at the same time. The result is that the body is unable to properly utilize either the drug or the nutrient. Another possible undesirable reaction can occur with drugs that alter the metabolic environment of the body significantly enough for the nutrients or other substances in foods to behave quite differently in the blood and tissues than they would without drugs.

Those who are taking certain prescribed medications should be aware of the effects they may have on dietary needs and discuss these factors with their physician:

ANTIBIOTICS
In addition to killing harmful bacteria, antibiotics destroy beneficial bacteria in the intestines that synthesize nutrients such as vitamin K and folacin. Those taking antibiotics should be sure to include adequate amounts of these nutrients in the diet by eating green leafy vegetables. Also, certain foods may influence the effectiveness of antibiotics. For example, acidic beverages such as fruit juices destroy penicillin G and "uncoated" erythromycin, when consumed at the same time. And because calcium binds tightly with tetracycline, making it unabsorbable, dairy foods should not be consumed within several hours of taking this drug.

DIURETICS
Diuretics are often used to treat high blood pressure and water retention due to liver, kidney, or heart disease. They function by increasing the rate of urine formation. But in washing out excess fluid, some diuretics, such as Hydrodiuril and furosemide, may wash out potassium as well. People taking diuretics should take care to eat plenty of potassium-rich foods, such as fruit juices and bananas.

ANTICOAGULANTS
People with cardiovascular diseases are often treated with anticoagulants, which reduce the risk

of blood platelets sticking together and forming artery blockages. Certain foods can influence the effectiveness of these drugs. In large amounts, vitamin K, which helps blood clot, may reduce the effects of anticoagulants. And omega-3 fatty acids may increase their effectiveness.

CHOLESTEROL-LOWERING DRUGS

One strategy for lowering cholesterol levels is to remove bile acids from the intestinal tract, since the body must resort to its store of cholesterol to replace them. But because bile acids are necessary to absorb the fat-soluble vitamins (A, D, E, and K), these vitamins may be poorly assimilated when a drug known as cholestyramine is taken. In these cases, increased dietary intake may be advised.

Caution is needed, not only with prescription drugs, but with over-the-counter drugs as well. Many commonly used medicines can influence nutritional health:

ASPIRIN

Many arthritis sufferers tend to overuse aspirin. Although some doctors are now encouraging regular use of aspirin (based on the hypothesis that it helps slow blood-clot formation), consuming large amounts of aspirin over a long period of time can cause painless internal bleeding from the stomach that could ultimately lead to iron-deficiency anemia. Taking 12 to 15 aspirins a day —not an unusual dose for some arthritis sufferers —increases normal loss of blood from the stomach by five to thirteen times.

LAXATIVES

Persistent use of laxatives can result in the loss of vitamins and minerals because laxatives speed foods through the system before some of their nutrients can be adequately absorbed. Mineral oil, for example, can prevent the absorption of vitamins A, D, E, and K. Regular use of saline-type laxatives, such as Epsom salts and Milk of Magne-

sia, can deplete the body of fluid and mineral nutrients such as potassium.

ANTACIDS

Continued use of large quantities of antacids that contain the ingredient aluminum hydroxide, such as Rolaids or Maalox, may result in a phosphorus deficiency and thereby lead to osteomalacia, or "soft bones."

Elderly people must be sure to be honest with their doctors about their eating habits, alcohol consumption, and all of the medications they are taking. They should discuss potential side effects of drugs and never self-medicate or take more than the prescribed dosage.

Can We Slow Down the Aging Process?

Our search for the Fountain of Youth goes on. No doubt we humans will always be interested in finding ways to expand our lives and maintain a young look and vitality. We know that certain health and nutrition habits, carried over a lifetime, can dramatically improve health into the older years for many people. We also know that genetic factors play an important role in longevity. But the point of real controversy exists concerning the extent to which certain supplements might influence the aging process. Some manufacturers have aggressively promoted the idea that the aging process might be reversed or forestalled with supplement use.

Nutritional scientists have been vehement in their denial that many common ideas about supplements and aging are valid. According to Jeffrey Blumberg, Ph.D., and Robert Russell, M.D., of the Tufts School of Nutrition, in many cases the theories behind taking supplements of isolated nutrients are loosely based on intriguing hypotheses or rather remote studies on animals. But there is no sound evidence to support many of the claims that certain vitamins, minerals, or nonnutritive supplements can prolong life or effectively treat people who have common maladies of old age, such as arthritis, cancer, and heart disease.

There is interesting research taking place to see if nutrition is related to conditions such as Alzheimer's disease, cardiovascular disease, cancer, and cataracts—specifically, whether nutrition can protect against these and other degenerative diseases. But it can be dangerous for consumers to jump the gun on research and become involved with unproved nutrient and nonnutrient therapies. High doses of many minerals, such as selenium, and vitamins A, D, and B-6 can be harmful and may interfere with the metabolism of other nutrients. For example, high doses of vitamin E can interfere with the absorption of vitamin A.

And large amounts of some nutrients can interfere with the action of certain drugs.

Furthermore, despite claims to the contrary, there is no evidence that nutrients or special foods will help slow down the cosmetic changes that accompany aging, such as hair loss, graying hair, or wrinkles. Most of these changes are genetically programmed and you can't do anything about them. However, considering the fixation Americans have developed about aging skin, it's surprising that so many people continue to bake in the sun year after year. But then, think how many of us continue to smoke or develop chemical dependencies.

Our quest for health and long lives will not be satisfied by a magical antidote to aging. Rather, we must commit ourselves to a steady, commonsense approach to nutrition and health during every stage of our lives.

PART FOUR

Making the Diet–Health Connection

Diet management is a major factor in treating certain health problems. People with health problems must look for guidance to those who are treating them and who best understand their unique needs, but experts have reached some basic conclusions about diet and health, and this knowledge can work in tandem with medical and other therapies.

Unfortunately, those who are most physically needy often become the easiest victims of dietary misinformation. But the rules of common sense continue to apply. In fact, if common nutrition sense was used in this country, we could substantially cut down on incidences of our number one killer, heart disease. Most primary risk factors for heart disease—high blood cholesterol, high blood pressure, obesity, smoking—are controllable factors. Even those people who, because of family history, are naturally at greater risk can minimize their chances of suffering from this disease if they take the appropriate dietary measures.

The Tufts Low Cholesterol Diet may provide the first step in the process of improving cardiovascular health. Contrary to what many people fear, a heart-smart diet doesn't have to be dull and tasteless.

Other major health concerns, such as cancer, diabetes, and osteoporosis, also have nutritional connections. All of these are the subject of intense study in the Tufts laboratories and elsewhere. But it is important not to think of diet and disease as a simple cause-and-effect proposition. Nutrition is just one factor in the diagnosis and treatment of many diseases. Because we have a "quick fix" mentality, many people tend to exaggerate every small bit of dietary evidence. For example, after it was suggested that oats and oat bran might be positively related to lower blood cholesterol levels, oat bran became the new "miracle" food. Walk into a supermarket today and you'll be inundated with products that contain oat bran. While that's not necessarily bad, it is misleading. For one thing, oats are only one of many foods that might have this effect on cholesterol. For another thing, there's nothing magical about oats. People who consume large quantities of oat bran yet

205

continue to lead sedentary life-styles, smoke cigarettes, drink too much alcohol, or eat high-fat diets are not going to benefit.

We also want consumers to be aware that research into the nutrition-disease connection is in its infancy. There are many things that remain unknown about the specific dietary practices that might decrease the risk of certain cancers and other diseases. But doors have been opened and directions have been shown. For us, this knowledge represents an exciting new field of study. We believe that nutrition science will someday be able to uncover the links between nutrition and many diseases. But, for now, we suggest that people focus on those things that we do know and avoid participating in scientifically unproven practices.

18

Challenging Heart Disease

Coronary heart disease (CHD) is our nation's number one killer. Every year, almost 1 million Americans suffer heart attacks, and more than half of them die as a result. CHD has typically been a "silent" killer. There are few warning signals: The first "symptom" a victim might have is a massive heart attack.

A substantial amount of clinical and epidemiologic evidence has identified risk factors that are statistically associated with CHD. Many scientific studies have been conducted in a variety of circumstances and types of populations. While experts acknowledge that some contradictions exist and that they do not yet know all there is to know about CHD, there has been enough consistency in study results to establish certain risks, including blood pressure, diabetes, obesity, cigarette smoking, and a family history of CHD.

The leading cause of CHD is generally believed to be atherosclerosis, commonly known as hardening of the arteries, which involves the accumulation of fatty substances (primarily cholesterol) and fibrous tissues along the inner lining of medium and large arteries. Atherosclerosis starts with damage to the layer of cells lining an artery, caused by one or more of several irritants: The turbulent flow of blood, the impact of blood under excessive pressure (high blood pressure), possibly toxic chemicals, a high concentration of blood fats, or a bacterial or viral infection. If dam-

age to the artery wall occurs repeatedly because of untreated high blood pressure or other factors, it is believed that the body's normal repair processes are overwhelmed. Blood fats and platelets are attracted to the site of the injury, leading to an accumulation of cell debris and cholesterol. If the damage persists, smooth muscle cells migrate from adjacent areas and multiply, forming a mat of scarlike tissue. The resulting accumulation is called plaque. Plaque subsequently hardens with deposits of calcium. With continued insult to the artery, plaque grows larger, protruding into the interior of the artery and progressively narrowing the vessel.

Plaque is particularly dangerous when it forms in the coronary arteries, which deliver oxygen and nutrients to the heart muscle. If the narrowing becomes severe enough to impair the flow of oxygen, the result is a heart attack.

Heart attacks often occur without warning, but they are usually the result of the slow buildup of atherosclerotic plaques in the coronary arteries over a period of many years. A plaque rarely grows large enough to occlude a coronary artery completely by itself, but it can combine with a blood clot to abruptly shut off the flow of blood to the heart. When this happens, the result is a heart attack, or myocardial infarct. Blockage of an artery can also be caused by spasm of the vessels around the plaque, bleeding into a plaque, or dislodgment of a plaque from the artery wall, creating an obstruction downstream. Whatever the cause of the blockage, because of it the portion of the heart muscle that is nourished by the occluded artery becomes oxygen-starved and dies. If the damage occurs in a particularly vital spot, sudden death may result. Indeed, for about 25 percent of heart attack victims, sudden death is the first sign of the disease.

Less severe damage to the heart muscle may disrupt the electrical impulses emanating from the heart's internal pacemaker, causing abnormal heart rhythms. These "arrhythmias" are dangerous because they can lead to rapid, uncoordinated contractions (fibrillations) of the ventricles, the large chambers of the heart. Unless these ventricular fibrillations are corrected, they can lead to death within minutes.

The Cholesterol Connection

Scientists have been studying the implications of diet to CHD since the turn of the century, when researchers noticed that rabbits fed diets high in cholesterol developed arterial lesions resembling atherosclerosis in humans. But it wasn't until the 1950s, when CHD had already reached epidemic proportions, that saturated dietary fats were considered to be primary culprits in the development of the disease. In recent decades, many studies have deepened our understanding of the relationship between high blood cholesterol and CHD (see also chapter 5).

One of the most famous of these investigations is the long-running Framingham, Massachusetts, Heart Study, which has tracked incidents of CHD in men and later, entire families, since 1948. The study has found that men with average blood cholesterol levels of 260 have had three times the number of heart attacks as men with blood cholesterol levels that averaged 195. In 1988, the surgeon general's report concluded that high blood cholesterol is one of the major modifiable risk factors for CHD. Although there may be other factors that contribute to CHD, such as smoking and hypertension, the role of cholesterol is clearly a primary one.

Our bodies produce all the cholesterol they need, and we increase our blood cholesterol levels in two main ways: (1) by eating foods that contain cholesterol, and (2) by eating foods that are high in saturated fats, which result in a series of events causing a buildup of cholesterol in the blood.

Many studies back up our current understanding of the relationship between levels of cholesterol in the blood and risk for CHD. A landmark study published in 1984 showed convincingly for the first time that reducing cholesterol led to fewer heart attacks. The Lipid Research Clinics Coronary Primary Prevention Trial showed, in a study of 3,806 men, that a 9 percent reduction of blood cholesterol in the treatment group led to a 19 percent reduction in fatal and nonfatal heart attacks.

But, as discussed in chapter 5, it is not simply a matter of how much cholesterol is present in the blood; the method of transport must be considered. Cholesterol travels back and forth between the liver and the cells through the bloodstream, carried by lipoproteins. High-density lipoproteins (HDLs) are strong carriers that remove cholesterol from the cells and deliver it safely to the liver for processing. Low-density lipoproteins (LDLs) are more fragile, and they tend to leave deposits of cholesterol behind in the arteries, leading to plaque buildup. It is possible to reduce coronary risk either by lowering LDL levels or by increasing HDL levels. It is thought that polyunsaturated and monounsaturated fats might help lower LDL levels.

Testing Your Cholesterol Level

How do you know if your blood cholesterol level is too high? It is currently believed that the highest risk is present when blood cholesterol levels are greater than 240 milligrams per deciliter (mg/dl) of blood. Moderate risk exists when levels are between 200 and 239 mg/dl, and low risk exists when levels are below 200 mg/dl. It is estimated that 40 million Americans between the ages of 40 and 70 have blood cholesterol levels above 200 mg/dl.

Is there any value to have a cholesterol level that is lower than 200 mg/dl? Until a couple of years ago, the 200 milligram figure was considered to be a threshold, above which the risk for heart disease kept increasing with an increase in cholesterol concentration, but below which variations did not make a difference. However, the results of the largest cholesterol study conducted to date dispute the threshold concept. Called the Multiple Risk Factor Intervention Trial (MRFIT, or "Mr. Fit" for short), the study followed 356,000 men in 18 American cities for a period of six years. According to the study results, the relationship between cholesterol and heart disease is continuous. Even with very low levels to begin with, the risk for heart disease increases as the cholesterol concentrations rise. Indeed, "Mr. Fit" participants whose cholesterol ranged from 183 to 202 mg/dl were 31 percent more likely to die from coronary heart disease than those with an average of 164 mg/dl. And men whose cholesterol levels were 202 milligrams or below accounted for nearly one-fourth of all coronary-related deaths in the study.

Government guidelines suggest that all Americans over the age of 20 should have their blood cholesterol levels tested to determine their degree of risk. This test is conducted by having blood samples analyzed in a laboratory. In recent years, efforts have been made to standardize testing methods, according to guidelines issued by the National Cholesterol Education Program of the National Institutes of Health. The Centers for Disease Control (CDC) set up a network of standardized laboratories so that other labs can check the accuracy of their analyses. Today, major manufacturers of testing equipment are calibrating their equipment to CDC standards, vastly reducing the incidents of error in cholesterol testing.

There are a number of points you should bear in mind when you have a cholesterol test:

▶ Be sure to find out from your doctor if the laboratory that analyzes your blood sample is standardized in accordance with the CDC method. If it is not, the chances of an inaccurate reading may be increased.

▶ Sit down for at least five to ten minutes before you take the test. Standing can cause test results to be skewed by about 5 percent.

▶ Be aware that viral infections, certain medications, pregnancy, and recent surgical procedures may interfere with accurate test results. For example, it takes about two months after a heart attack, stroke, or cardiac surgery for the test to reflect an accurate picture of blood cholesterol level.

▶ Make sure the person who draws your blood is a medical technologist or someone who has had extensive training in correct testing methods. While most available equipment used to test cholesterol is capable of yielding accurate results, many machines are only as good as the technical background and training of the personnel who operate them. This is particularly true for desktop analyzers that test blood drawn from the prick of a finger (the fingerstick test) rather than from a vein.

▶ If you have a fingerstick test taken, don't let the test taker squeeze your finger. "Milking" the finger causes dilution of the blood sample, which produces inaccurately low test results.

▶ Make sure you've had at least two tests taken before beginning (or forgoing) dietary and/or medical treatment based on your blood cholesterol level. The tests should be spaced a month or two apart. If the results are within 30 points of each other, the average of the two is probably a safe estimate of your true blood cholesterol, because cholesterol totals vary somewhat from day to day and week to week. If the discrepancy between the two tests is more than 30 points, a third test is in order.

▶ If your cholesterol is over 200 mg/dl on two tests, make sure your doctor goes on to mea-

▶ NUTRITION QUIZ ◀

Have You Gotten the Cholesterol Message?

Test yourself to see how far you've come in your understanding of cholesterol and its relationship to diet and disease. Answer either True or False to these statements.

1. Saturated fat is found only in animal products.
   True _____   False _____

2. Cholesterol is found only in animal products.
   True _____   False _____

3. Hydrogenation makes fats more saturated.
   True _____   False _____

4. Losing excess weight will lower blood cholesterol.
   True _____   False _____

5. While lowering high blood cholesterol is important to decrease the risk for heart disease, other factors may be just as important.
   True _____   False _____

6. Exercise lowers the concentration of cholesterol in the blood.
   True _____   False _____

7. Saturated fats have more calories than unsaturated fats.
   True _____   False _____

8. The American Heart Association recommends that adults take in no more than 500 milligrams of cholesterol each day.
   True _____   False _____

9. The American Heart Association recommends that adults take in no more than 20 percent of their calories as fat.
   True _____   False _____

10. People whose blood cholesterol level is about 160 are at increased risk for developing cancer.
    True _____   False _____

ANSWERS

1. (False) Animal foods are the primary source of saturated fats, but they are not the only source. Saturated fat is also present in products made with coconut oil, palm kernel oil, and palm oil, all of which come from plants. What's more, the fat in coconut and palm kernel oil is actually more saturated than that found in animals.

These oils are most often found in snack products and other highly processed foods.

2. (True) Incidentally, the cholesterol is not only in the fat of the animal, where one might expect it to be, but also in the muscle tissue. So, while cutting away the visible fat on a piece of meat is a healthful practice, in that it reduces the amount of saturated fat to be eaten, it does not completely solve the problem of the food's cholesterol content.

3. (True) The process of hydrogenation, which food manufacturers often use in polyunsaturated liquid oils to solidify or partially solidify them, makes the oils more saturated. However, partially hydrogenated polyunsaturated oils and margarines may still be unsaturated, and are invariably less saturated than coconut and palm kernel oils.

4. (True) For some people, losing extra pounds is all it takes to completely correct an elevated concentration of cholesterol in the blood, since weight loss lowers the LDL levels.

5. (True) Three other important steps to take in order to reduce the chances of suffering a heart attack are to lower high blood pressure, quit smoking, and get rid of excess body fat.

6. (False) Exercise alone does not lower cholesterol levels. But if you couple it with a successful weight-reduction regime, it may indirectly contribute to lower blood cholesterol levels by bringing about a drop in weight. Furthermore, exercise helps raise HDL cholesterol, the kind that appears to protect against heart disease.

7. (False) Saturated fats in the diet, which are believed to be more likely than dietary cholesterol to raise the level of cholesterol in the blood, have the same number of calories (9 per gram) as unsaturated fat.

8. (False) The American Heart Association recommends that adults consume no more than 300 milligrams of cholesterol, and one egg yolk contains 213. (Egg yolks and organ meats are the foods highest in cholesterol.)

9. (False) While consuming only 20 percent of calories as fat is perfectly healthful (the Japanese do it and suffer less heart disease than Americans), it is a hard change to implement. For that reason, you are advised to aim for a diet that contains 30 percent calories as fat. Presently, the fat intake of the average American is closer to 40 percent of total calories.

10. (False) A few years ago the theory that low cholesterol levels may predispose the body to developing cancer gained momentum in a few scientific and lay circles. It now appears that the interpretation of the data was complicated by the fact that low blood cholesterol often results from, rather than predicts, cancer—probably due to weight loss and other outcomes of cancer.

sure cholesterol "fractions"—HDL cholesterol, LDL cholesterol, and triglyceride levels. Unlike total cholesterol levels, which can be measured with the fingerstick test, cholesterol fractions can only be determined with blood drawn from a vein following a 12-hour fast.

▶ When considering the results of any cholesterol test, remember that a number of factors, including diet, genetics, lack of exercise, and obesity, can influence cholesterol levels and the likelihood of heart disease.

What about High Triglycerides?

Triglycerides are your body's fat store. The bloodstream always contains some of them, and their levels are higher right after you've eaten. Elevated triglycerides, by themselves, are not thought to be a risk factor for CHD. However, several studies have shown that people who have high triglycerides also tend to have high cholesterol and low HDL levels and to be obese. This is in part due to the fact that many of the same factors that contribute to high serum cholesterol, such as diets high in calories and saturated fats, also cause high triglycerides.

The American Heart Association has set standards for triglycerides based on age and sex. The chart indicates the levels at which triglycerides are determined to be high.

Severe elevations of triglycerides—500 to 1,500 mg/dl—occur in only a very small number of people, and they're rarely caused by diet alone. But diets high in saturated fat, cholesterol, and alcohol, accompanied by lack of exercise and obesity, appear to be major contributors to less extreme elevations. Whether or not these less extreme levels present a health risk is open to debate, but certainly any of the factors mentioned would independently contribute to CHD.

The Dietary Connection

The leading factor in controlling cholesterol levels is diet. According to doctors at the Lipid

HIGH BLOOD TRIGLYCERIDE LEVELS

| Age | Blood Plasma Total Triglycerides (mg/dl) | |
	Male	Female
5–9	85	126
10–14	111	120
15–19	143	126
20–24	165	168
25–29	204	159
30–34	253	163
35–39	316	205
40–44	318	191
45–49	318	223
50–54	313	223
55–59	261	279
60–64	240	256
65–69	256	260
70 +	239	289

Metabolism Laboratory of the USDA Human Nutrition Research Center at Tufts University, diet can lower blood cholesterol by as much as 30 percent. The Tufts Low Cholesterol Diet, outlined in the next chapter, eliminates about one-fourth of the fat calories in the 38 to 40 percent fat diet that is typical for most Americans. Since, ounce for ounce, carbohydrates have less than half the calories of fat, a high-carbohydrate, low-fat diet also tends to cause weight loss, which can lower LDL levels. In fact, for some people, slimming down to a healthy body weight will completely correct elevated LDL concentrations.

The fat that needs to be restricted most is saturated fat, the kind that raises the LDLs and presently makes up about 15 percent of the calories in the American diet. If saturated fat were reduced from 15 percent of total calories to less than 10 percent, the goal of eating less than 30 percent fat calories would be achieved by most Americans. It's easy to see why. If a person who gets 38 percent of his or her calories as fat were to reduce the saturated fat intake from 15 percent to 8 percent of total calories (a drop of 7 percent), the net result would be 31 percent fat, close to the guideline of 30 percent.

Heavy sources of saturated fat include the marbleized fat you can see on beef, processed meats such as sausages and hot dogs, hard cheeses, butter, whole-milk dairy products, and snacks containing coconut, palm, and palm kernel oil, as well as cocoa butter. Healthful substitutions for these foods are lean cuts of meat in smaller portion sizes; beans (a low-fat source of protein); fruits and vegetables; margarine made with safflower, sunflower, or other polyunsaturated oils; skim milk; low-fat yogurt; and low-fat cottage cheese.

Since the soluble fiber in oats, fruits, and beans has been shown to reduce LDL levels, they are good foods to include in a low cholesterol diet. Similarly, many types of cold-water fish, which contain omega-3 fatty acids, may also bring down cholesterol levels. While the value of omega-3 fatty acids are questionable, fish certainly contain less fat, particularly less saturated fat, than meat, and are a good choice for a cholesterol-lowering diet.

The Hypertension Factor

One out of four Americans, or approximately 50 to 60 million people, are victims of hypertension, commonly referred to as high blood pressure. Sustained high blood pressure is a silent disease that can go unnoticed for years until it is picked up during a medical exam or suddenly results in a stroke, heart attack, or kidney failure.

In a small percentage of cases, the cause for the disease can be traced to some physiological malfunction, such as a kidney problem, a narrowing of the aorta (from which blood leaves the heart on its journey to the rest of the body), or a tumor in the adrenal glands. In these instances, the hypertension is called secondary hypertension and can often be cured by medical treatment. However, about 95 percent of the people who have high blood pressure have primary, or idiopathic, hypertension, which means that the cause of the disease cannot be determined and it is a lifetime ailment. This type of hypertension can be controlled with relative ease by medication and/or diet, and the chances for illness reduced. Although some high-risk groups have been identified—among them, blacks, the elderly, and people with a family history of hypertension—it is still not possible to predict with a degree of certainty who will end up with elevated blood pressure. That's why it is important for everyone to take precautions against the disease, particularly modifications in eating habits.

What the Readings Mean

Hypertension literally refers to a condition in which too much pressure is placed on the walls of the arteries. To understand how this happens, imagine that your arteries are so many garden hoses, and your blood is the water pumped through them. If you turn the water higher, more is pushed through in less time, increasing the pressure on the walls of the hoses. Or, if you pinch the hoses, the same amount of water is forced to circulate through narrower spaces, again increasing the pressure on the walls of the hoses. That's the basic mechanism of high blood pressure. It's a condition in which either the blood volume is increased or the arteries constrict. The extra pressure weakens the artery walls and thereby accelerates the wear and tear they undergo.

What does a blood pressure reading signify? Physicians consider approximately 120/80 (120 over 80) to 140/85 the normal range. The first, or upper, number represents the systolic pressure—that is, the pressure that is exerted when the heart contracts to pump out blood to all the arteries of the body. (A reading of 120 means that the heart is pumping hard enough to be able to drive a column of mercury up a tube to a height of 120 millimeters.) The second, or lower, number is the diastolic pressure—that is, the pressure exerted by the blood on the walls of the arteries between heart beats. While both numbers are important, physicians tend to be more concerned with diastolic pressure because, if the diastolic pressure is high, it means that the arteries are under great pressure even when the heart is relaxed and simply filling with blood in preparation for its next beat.

Obesity and Hypertension

It is believed that one of the best defenses against hypertension is to maintain a healthy weight. The incidence of hypertension among obese adults—that is, those people whose body weight is 30 percent or more above average—is estimated to be double that of nonobese people. And studies of large population groups have revealed that, in countries where weight does not increase with age, neither does blood pressure. In the United States, where people tend to gain weight as they grow older, about half the population has hypertension by age 74.

Overweight people who already have high blood pressure can often reduce it dramatically by getting rid of their excess pounds, even if they do not manage to lose them all. As little as a 5 percent reduction in weight has been associated with a reduction in blood pressure so significant that some patients are able to stop taking antihypertensive medication.

Furthermore, research results from Israel showed that some obese hypertensives were able to reduce their blood pressure to normal even when they lost only half of their excess weight. Why this happens is not fully understood, but it is known that the heart has to pump harder in overweight people, because of the amount of tissue the blood has to reach is greater than in thin individuals.

Obesity isn't always a factor in hypertension. Being overweight doesn't always lead to the disease. Nor does becoming or staying thin necessarily ward off high blood pressure. But in the absence of a clear understanding of how weight and blood pressure are related, it is wise to keep your weight close to the recommended level.

Dietary Risk Factors

It appears that only some people are what is called "salt sensitive." For these people, too much sodium in the diet can lead to a marked rise in blood pressure. Such individuals apparently have an altered ability to excrete excess sodium in their urine. The extra sodium remains in the blood, making it "thirsty"—not unlike the way in which salty foods bring on thirst—and thereby drawing water to the blood, increasing blood volume, which creates greater pressure as the blood is pumped through the arteries.

The trouble is that it is hard to pinpoint who is salt sensitive and who is not. Researchers at the Indiana University School of Medicine have gone so far as to discover a particular gene that predisposes people to sodium sensitivity under certain laboratory conditions. But there is still no way to say whether the carriers of that gene will benefit by restricting sodium in their day-to-day diets. So, how should you act, in light of these uncertainties? Perhaps the following figures will help answer that question.

Our bodies need only about 200 milligrams of sodium a day (equivalent to a tenth of a teaspoon of salt) to regulate the amount of fluid that passes in and out of the cells and to maintain the acid-alkali balance; these are fucntions necessary for life. The National Academy of Sciences reports that people can safely take in five to sixteen times that amount, or 1,100 to 3,300 milligrams. There are many sources of sodium in our diets, the most obvious being table salt. Sodium deficiency is not a concern in this country. Rather, it would seem that most Americans could stand to cut back on their sodium intake.

According to the Food and Drug Administration, even if only 10 to 15 percent of the population were potential candidates for hypertension because of salt sensitivity, a nationwide reduction in salt intake could still help protect as many as 23 to 35 million Americans against the risk of stroke, heart attack, and kidney failure.

Like salt, alcohol appears to increase the risk for high blood pressure. Statistically, between 5 and 11 percent of the cases of hypertension in men are attributed to alcohol consumption.

The evidence linking alcohol to increased blood pressure is strong. In one study, 20,000 people in Australia were observed and it was found that the more they drank, the higher their blood pressure became. The association between drinking and blood pressure grows even stronger after adjusting for age, obesity, and smoking.

In another study of patients entering a hospital, it was shown that over half of those who drank more than three ounces of alcohol a day were hypertensive. However, by the time their hospital stay was over and the drinking had stopped, fewer than 10 percent of the patients still had high blood pressure. When they were on their own again, just about all of those who remained abstinent continued to have normal blood pressure readings, while most of those who resumed drinking became hypertensive again.

Caffeine has been studied as to its possible contribution to hypertension. While caffeine consumption temporarily increases blood pressure, there does not appear to be an important relationship between reasonable caffeine consumption and hypertension.

Potentially Helpful Dietary Practices

The biomedical literature contains many studies that suggest that nutrients such as potassium, calcium, and some forms of fiber may help protect against hypertension. The data in these studies vary in quality and, in some cases, are almost anecdotal. For example, several years ago, it was noticed that the amount of salt eaten by the residents of two villages in Japan was very high, yet one village had a much lower incidence of hypertension than the other. Closer examination of the villagers' habits revealed that those with the lower are high in soluble fiber and a moderately good source of potassium.

It should not be too surprising that potassium might play a role in the regulation of high blood pressure, since it is a close relative of sodium. Like sodium, potassium is an electrolyte, a substance that helps regulate the water balance between the body cells and the blood. And, like sodium, it is essential for life. In fact, many people whose hypertension is so severe that they must take diuretics to rid their bodies of excess fluid must also take supplements to replace the potassium that is excreted along with the fluid. When the potassium level in the body falls too low, it can result in hypokalemia, a condition characterized by general weakness, an unexplained tingling sensation, cramps, an irregular heartbeat, and excessive thirst and urination.

Some scientists have suggested that it is not potassium per se that influences blood pressure, but the ratio between dietary sodium and potassium. It is an idea worth considering. Often, when people eat fewer of those highly processed, prepackaged foods that are high in sodium, they tend to increase their consumption of fresh items such as fruits and vegetables, which are low in sodium and high in potassium.

Recently, some researchers have been trying to link calcium intake and a lowered risk of hypertension. A number of studies, some quite controversial, point to a possible connection. Observation of participants in the Puerto Rico Heart Health Program found that individuals who drank no milk (which is high in calcium and potassium) had twice the incidences of hypertension compared to those who were heavy milk drinkers. In another study, more than 5,000 adults in southern California were surveyed for heart disease risk factors as part of a Lipid Research Clinics population study. Hypertensive men (but not women) had a significantly lower calcium intake from milk than those who did not have the disease. With an increase in milk consumption, diastolic blood pressure decreased significantly.

Calcium might even help control blood pressure when negative factors are present. In a study of hypertensive blacks conducted at Wayne State University in Detroit, it was found that those on high salt diets who were given supplemental calcium experienced reductions in blood pressure that were sometimes dramatic enough to produce normal blood pressure readings.

Despite all the promising clues concerning calcium's effect on blood pressure, the evidence is still much too sketchy to warrant increasing cal-

▶ NUTRITION QUIZ ◀

Evaluate Your CHD Risk

A variety of factors contribute to the risk of developing coronary heart disease. Your answers to the following points will help you become aware of the ways heredity and lifestyle might influence your CHD risk.

This test is not designed to replace physical examinations or clinical tests. Rather, our intention is to call attention, in a personal way, to the wide variety of factors that might increase or reduce your risk of CHD. If you have reason to be concerned about your risk, consult your doctor.

Add the points to the right of your answers, and compare your total to the scores at the bottom.

Age
_____ 20–40 (1)
_____ 40–55 (2)
_____ over 55 (3)

Sex
_____ male, over 45 (1)
_____ female, postmenopause (1)

Family History
_____ no family history of heart disease (0)
_____ 1 relative* who had a heart attack after age 60 (1)
_____ 2 relatives who had heart attacks after age 60 (2)
_____ 1 relative who had a heart attack before age 60 (3)
_____ more than 2 relatives who had heart attacks before age 50 (6)

Blood Pressure (systolic, or upper number)
_____ 101–120 (0)
_____ 121–140 (1)
_____ 141–160 (2)
_____ 161–180 (4)
_____ 181–208 (6)

Blood Cholesterol
_____ below 180 (0)
_____ 180–200 (1)
_____ 201–240 (2)
_____ 241–260 (3)
_____ over 260 (5)

Diet
_____ consume less than 30 percent calories as fat, 15–25 percent as protein, and 40–55 percent as complex carbohydrates, in a varied diet (0)
_____ consume 31–35 percent of daily calories as fat (1)
_____ consume 36–40 percent of daily calories as fat (2)
_____ consume 300 or fewer milligrams of cholesterol per day (0)
_____ consume 301–400 milligrams of cholesterol per day (1)
_____ consume 401–500 milligrams of cholesterol per day (2)
_____ consume 2,001–3,500 milligrams of sodium per day (1)
_____ consume more than 3,500 milligrams of sodium per day (2)

Smoking
_____ nonsmoker (0)
_____ ½ pack or less per day (1)
_____ ½ to 1 pack per day (2)
_____ more than one pack per day (3)
_____ 2 or more packs per day (5)

Weight
_____ within 10 percent of ideal weight (0)
_____ 10–20 percent overweight (1)
_____ 21–35 percent overweight (3)
_____ 36–50 percent overweight (5)
_____ more than 50 percent overweight (8)

Exercise
_____ 3–5 times a week for at least 20 minutes (0)
_____ 1–2 times a week for at least 20 minutes (1)
_____ occasionally (3)
_____ rarely or never (5)

Other factors
_____ history of diabetes (6)
_____ female taking oral contraceptives (1)
_____ alcohol consumption of more than 3 oz. per day (2)

Score
10 points or less = low risk
11–20 points = moderate risk
21–30 points = high risk
over 30 points = dangerously high risk

* Parent, grandparent, or sibling

cium for the purpose of controlling hypertension, especially if it's done in lieu of controlling dietary factors like sodium. While epidemiological evidence *suggests* that high calcium intake leads to lower blood pressure, it does not *prove* it. Lifestyle patterns or other nutrients that have not yet been accounted for may be the factors making the difference.

Several other dietary variables may be involved in controlling high blood pressure. One may be a higher ratio of polyunsaturated to saturated fat. In Finland, where the amount of fat consumed, particularly saturated fat, tends to be quite high, blood pressure fell when the total fat intake was decreased and the ratio of polyunsaturated to saturated fat was increased. This result was seen both in those with hypertension and in those with normal blood pressure. A single study such as this one does not prove that eating more polyunsaturates than saturates will keep your blood pressure down, but doing so won't hurt, and the practice would be consistent with dietary guidelines for reducing the risk of heart disease.

Dietary fiber has also been said to reduce blood pressure. A number of experiments have lent some support to the theory that the higher the fiber content of the diet, the lower the chance of developing hypertension. The evidence to support this conclusion is still incomplete.

Interestingly, all the measures mentioned—increasing polyunsaturated versus saturated fats; eating more fiber; keeping weight down; cutting back on alcohol; eating more fresh, low-sodium foods such as fruits and vegetables; eating low-fat, calcium-rich foods—are good ideas for a healthful diet in general. So, even though all the facts are not known about the relationship between diet and high blood pressure, following these guidelines will certainly help maintain overall health.

Exercise Aids Cardiovascular Fitness

According to the Centers for Disease Control, the sedentary life-style of many Americans may be as great a risk factor for CHD as high cholesterol or high blood pressure. The CDC made this claim after evaluating more than 40 studies that demonstrated the heart-beneficial effects of certain kinds of exercise programs.

One long-term study conducted by the Stanford University School of Medicine and Harvard's School of Public Health tested the relationship between health and exercise in 17,000 Harvard graduates. Researchers began the study in the mid-1960s, recruiting subjects from among alumni aged 37 to 74. The subjects were followed until 1978. By the conclusion of the study, 1,413 of the subjects had died, 45 percent of them from heart disease. In evaluating the risk factors, the researchers found that lack of exercise was of greater consequence than obesity, cigarette smoking, or a family history of heart disease. Exercise also appeared to lower the risk of high blood pressure and cut the risk of smoking by as much as one-third. It also seemed to reduce some of the risks from genetic predisposition to heart disease.

The type of exercise that appears to do the most good is aerobic—sustained exercise that increases the strength of the heart. Aerobic exercise appears to raise HDL cholesterol, increase muscle mass to alleviate stress on the heart, strengthen the heart, and stabilize the heart rate. See chapter 24 for advice on improving cardiovascular fitness with exercise.

The Tufts Low-Cholesterol Diet, outlined in the next chapter, is the first step to addressing the CHD danger in your own life. By reducing saturated fat, dietary cholesterol, and sodium, and increasing the percentage of high-carbohydrate, high-fiber foods, you can make a substantial dent in the risk factors for CHD. And you will no doubt be pleasantly surprised when you see how appealing and full of variety this diet is.

19

The Tufts Low-Cholesterol Diet

The Tufts Low-Cholesterol Diet is a 21-day meal plan designed to introduce you to low-cholesterol eating—the fun way. Each of the menus has been carefully planned to be consistent with the way people really eat and to incorporate the kinds of foods many people enjoy.

Each day's menu gets 50 to 60 percent of its calories from complex carbohydrates, with a minimum of 15 to 20 grams of fiber. Fewer than 30 percent of the calories come from fat, with only 10 percent of the total from saturated fat. In all, the daily menus fall well below the 300 milligrams of cholesterol that most experts consider the healthy limit.

The daily calorie total is approximately 1,800 calories. If you want to shave calories, it's easy to do so by eliminating the snacks (100 to 200 calories), having three ounces of meat instead of four, eliminating margarine, or having one slice of bread where two are called for. Men whose calorie needs are more than 1,800 should add calories to the complex carbohydrates—for example, having one to one and one-half cups of cereal instead of three-fourths cup, two muffins instead of one, or an extra baked potato or piece of corn on the cob.

We have tried to make the menus interesting by varying the types of breads, juices, and cereals.

But you should feel free to switch them around as you please.

Following the menus are a few delicious recipes that taste as rich as the fattiest foods you've ever eaten. The asterisk (*) next to a menu item indicates that a recipe for it is given.

21 Day Menus

Day 1

BREAKFAST
Apple juice, ½ cup
Crushed pineapple, ½ cup
*Cinnamon French Toast, 2 slices
Maple syrup, 2 tbsp.
1% milk, 1 cup
Freshly brewed coffee or tea

LUNCH
Cream of tomato soup (made with 1% milk)
Submarine sandwich:
    deli-sliced turkey, 1 oz.
    deli-sliced roast beef, 1 oz.
    deli-sliced mozzarella cheese, 1 oz.

219

lettuce, tomato, as desired

mayonnaise, 1 tsp.

mustard, as desired

Fresh, sliced nectarine, 1 medium

DINNER

Broiled center cut pork chop, sprinkled with rosemary, 4 oz.

Applesauce, ½ cup

Sauerkraut, ½ cup

Mashed potatoes:

1 medium potato mashed with 1% milk and 1 tsp. tub margarine

Steamed medley of zucchini and carrots, ⅔ cup, with 2 tsp. tub margarine

SNACK

Berries and yogurt:

low-fat French Vanilla yogurt, ½ cup

mixed fresh berries (raspberries, strawberries, blueberries), ½ cup

Day 2

BREAKFAST

Orange-pineapple juice, ½ cup

Bran flakes, ¾ cup, with 1 cup 1% milk and ½ sliced banana

Marbled rye-pumpernickel toast, 1 slice, with 1 tsp. tub margarine

Freshly brewed coffee or tea

LUNCH

Charbroiled hamburger:

lean ground beef, 3 oz.

tomato, onion, lettuce, as desired

ketchup, 1 tbsp.

mustard, as desired

sesame-seed bun

Fruit and cheese salad:

1%-fat cottage cheese, ¼ cup

fresh melon, ⅓ medium

pineapple, 1 slice (ring)

bed of leaf lettuce

DINNER

Chicken Oriental stir-fry:

boneless chicken breast (cut into thin strips), 4 oz.

Oriental vegetables (snow peas, bamboo shoots, mushrooms), ¾ cup

Green pepper and carrot strips, ½ cup

Vegetable oil (for stir-frying), 1½ tbsp.

Soy sauce, 2 tsp.

Steamed rice, 1 cup

Lemon-lime sorbet, ½ cup

Fortune cookie

SNACK

1% milk, 1 cup

Graham crackers, 4 squares

Day 3

BREAKFAST

Toasted English muffin, with 2 tsp tub margarine

Yogurt-Berry Swirl:

low-fat lemon yogurt, 1 cup

fresh blueberries, ¾ cup

Freshly brewed coffee or tea

LUNCH

*Curried chicken salad

Whole-wheat pita pocket, 1 medium, 6″ round

lettuce, tomato, as desired

Watermelon, 2″ x 4″ wedge

Grape Fizz:

grape juice, ½ cup

club soda, ½ cup

DINNER

Poached haddock with dill, 5 oz. (use ½ cup 1% milk as poaching liquid)

*Parmesan Noodles

Steamed zucchini and summer squash, ½ cup, with 1 tsp. tub margarine

White Zinfandel wine, 4 oz.

SNACK
Orange freeze:

orange sherbet, ½ cup, blended with 1 cup 1% milk

Day 4

BREAKFAST
Scrambled eggs:

1 egg plus 1 egg white, cooked in 1 tsp. tub margarine

Whole-wheat toast, 2 slices, with 1 tsp. strawberry jam, 2 tsp. tub margarine

Cantaloupe wedge, ⅓ medium

Freshly brewed coffee or tea

LUNCH
Roast beef sandwich:

lean roast beef, 3 oz.

lettuce, tomato, as desired

mustard, as desired

mayonnaise, 1½ tsp.

roll

Fresh peach, 1 medium

1% milk, 1 cup

DINNER
Roasted light-meat turkey, 5 oz., with 2 tbsp. meat juices (skim fat from drippings)

Stove-top stuffing, made with tub margarine, ⅓ cup

Cranberry sauce

Green beans, ½ cup, with 1 tsp. tub margarine.

Whole-grain dinner roll, with 1 tsp. tub margarine

SNACK
Fresh, sliced strawberries, 1 cup

Day 5

BREAKFAST
orange juice, ½ cup

Raisin Bran, ¾ cup, with 1 cup 1% milk

Cracked-wheat toast, 2 slices, with 2 tsp. tub margarine

Freshly brewed coffee or tea

LUNCH
*Cashew turkey salad, served on a bed of lettuce

Crusty pumpernickel roll

Celery sticks

Fresh pineapple, ¾ cup

Mandarin orange sparkling water

DINNER
*Mom's meat loaf, 1 serving

Corn on the cob, 1 medium, with 2 tsp. tub margarine

Steamed English peas, ⅔ cup, with 1 tsp. tub margarine

Italian-style broiled tomato:

½ tomato

1 tbsp. Parmesan cheese

sprinkling of basil

Fresh fruit salad (diner's choice), ½ cup

SNACK
Angel food cake, 1/12 medium cake

1% milk, 1 cup

Day 6

BREAKFAST
Pineapple-grapefruit juice, ½ cup

Italian vegetable omelette:

1 egg plus 2 egg whites

diced tomato, zucchini, mushrooms, ½ cup

1 tbsp. Parmesan cheese

2 tsp. tub margarine

Toasted Italian bread, 2 slices

Freshly brewed coffee or tea

LUNCH
Chicken with rice soup, 1 cup
French vegetable salad:
 leafy greens, 1 cup
 diced red and green pepper, ¼ cup
 sliced cucumber, ¼ cup
 garbanzo beans, ¼ cup
 French dressing, 1 tbsp.
Crusty French roll, with 1 tsp. tub margarine
Red Delicious apple, 1 medium
1% milk, 1 cup

DINNER
Parsley halibut bake:
 halibut steak, 5 oz.
 breadcrumbs, 2 tbsp.
 crumbled fresh parsley
 tub margarine, 2 tsp.
 lemon juice, 1 tbsp.
Butternut squash with nutmeg, ¾ cup
Fresh asparagus, 5 spears
Oven-crisped potatoes:
 sliced potato, ½ cup, with 2 tsp. hot margarine
Citrus sections, ½ cup

SNACK
Low-fat apple fruit yogurt, ½ cup
Ginger snaps, 3

Day 7

BREAKFAST
Cranberry juice cocktail, ½ cup
Low-fat peach or tropical fruit yogurt, 1 cup
Raisin toast, 2 slices, with 2 tsp. tub margarine
Freshly brewed coffee or tea

LUNCH
Tarragon chicken salad sandwich:
 diced chicken, ½ cup
 chopped celery, 1 large stalk

mix 1 tbsp. each mayonnaise and low-fat, plain yogurt; add tarragon
Small French roll
Marinated raw vegetables:
 carrots, broccoli florets, red pepper, with 1 tbsp. Italian dressing
Lemon spritzer

DINNER
Spicy taco salad:
 lean ground beef, browned and drained, 3 oz.
 shredded cheddar cheese, 1 tbsp.
 lettuce, diced tomato, as desired
 salsa, taco sauce, as desired
 Soft flour tortilla, 1
Steamed Mexican corn:
 corn, ¾ cup
 chopped red and green pepper, ¼ cup
Poached pear with cinnamon

SNACK
Blueberry cheese crumble:
 fresh blueberries, ¼ cup
 layered with 1%-fat cottage cheese, ½ cup
 sprinkled with 4 crumbled ginger snaps

Day 8

BREAKFAST
White grape juice, ½ cup
Bran flakes, ¾ cup, with 1 cup 1% milk
Toasted oatmeal bread, 1 slice, with 1 tsp. tub margarine
Freshly brewed coffee or tea

LUNCH
*Two-alarm chili
Saltines, 6
Side salad:
 red leaf lettuce
 tomato wedges

oil and vinegar, 1 tbsp.

basil to taste

Watermelon, 2″ × 4″ wedge

DINNER

Broiled salmon à l'orange:

   4 oz. salmon, cooked with 1 tsp. tub margarine, 2 tbsp. orange juice

Baked potato, 1 medium, with 2 tbsp. low-fat yogurt and 1 tbsp. chives

Steamed green beans, 1 cup, with 1 tsp. tub margarine

Red seedless grapes, 1 cup

Sparkling water with lemon slice

SNACK

Graham crackers, 4 squares, with 1 tbsp. peanut butter

1% milk, 1 cup

Day 9

BREAKFAST

Orange-grapefruit juice, ½ cup

Toasted poppy-seed bagel, with 2 tsp. tub margarine

1% cottage cheese, ½ cup, served in ½ cantaloupe

Freshly brewed coffee or tea

LUNCH

Ham sandwich on rye:

   deli-sliced ham, 3 oz.

   lettuce, tomato, as desired

   rye bread, 2 slices

   mayonnaise, 1 tsp.

   mustard, as desired

Marinated cucumbers, ½ cup, soaked in 1 tbsp. Italian dressing

Fresh bing cherries, ½ cup

1% milk, 1 cup

DINNER

Charbroiled porterhouse or sirloin steak (trimmed of fat), 4½ oz.

Baked potato, 1 medium, with 2 tsp. tub margarine

Fresh broccoli, 2 stalks, with 2 tsp. Parmesan cheese

Sourdough dinner roll, with 1 tsp. tub margarine

Boysenberry or pineapple sorbet, ½ cup

SNACK

1% milk, 1 cup

2 vanilla wafers

Day 10

BREAKFAST

Sparkling apple juice:

   ½ cup of apple juice

   ½ cup of club soda

Bran flakes, ¾ cup, with ½ sliced banana, 1 cup 1% milk

Toasted whole-grain bread, 1 slice, with 1 tsp. tub margarine

Freshly brewed coffee or tea

LUNCH

*Italian tuna pasta salad, served on a bed of leaf lettuce

Cherry tomatoes, 4

Crusty French roll, with 1 tsp. tub margarine

Red Delicious or Granny Smith apple, 1 medium

1% milk, 1 cup

DINNER

*Mexi-stuffed green pepper

Mixed green salad:

   leaf and red-leaf lettuce, 1 cup

   raw scallion, 1 tbsp.

   cucumber, ¼ cup

   French dressing, 1 tbsp.

Medley of sliced peach and pear, ½ cup each

SNACK
French vanilla ice milk, ½ cup
Ginger snaps, 2

Day 11

BREAKFAST
Pineapple juice, ½ cup
Wheat or corn flakes, ¾ cup, with 1 cup 1% milk
Whole-wheat toast, 1 slice, with 1 tsp. tub
    margarine
Fresh strawberries, ½ cup
Freshly brewed coffee or tea

LUNCH
*Chef Salad, with 1 tbsp. oil, 1 tbsp. balsamic
    vinegar
Pumpernickel roll
Fresh pineapple, ½ cup
Lemon spritzer

DINNER
Spaghetti and meat sauce:
    spaghetti, 2 cups, cooked
    tomato sauce, ⅔ cup
    lean ground beef, 3 oz., cooked
    Italian seasonings, as desired
    Parmesan cheese, 1 tbsp.
Italian bread, 1 slice
Romaine lettuce, with 1 tbsp. Italian dressing
Italian ice, ½ cup

SNACK
Mixed fresh fruit salad, ½ cup

Day 12

BREAKFAST
Fresh grapefruit, ½
Scrambled eggs:
    1 egg plus 1 egg white, cooked in 1 tsp. tub
    margarine

Whole-grain toast, 2 slices, with 1 tsp. tub
    margarine, 1 tsp. strawberry jam
Freshly brewed coffee of tea

LUNCH
Tuna salad sandwich:
    tuna, 3 oz., water-packed
    chopped celery, 1 tbsp.
    mayonnaise, 1½ tsp., mixed with 1½ tsp. plain
    yogurt
Sesame-seed bun, 1
Carrot sticks
Fresh plums, 2 small
1% milk, 1 cup

DINNER
*Chicken Parmesan, served over 1 cup of
    fettuccine
Spinach salad:
    fresh, chopped spinach, 1 cup
    grated carrots, ¼ cup
    chopped red pepper, ¼ cup
    oil and vinegar, 1 tbsp.
Toasted garlic bread:
    1 Italian roll, spread with 1 tsp. tub margarine,
    garlic powder

SNACK
Peach milkshake:
    1% milk, 1 cup, blended with ½ cup sliced
    peaches, 1 tbsp. sugar

Day 13

BREAKFAST
Grapefruit juice, ½ cup
Corn or bran flakes, ¾ cup, with ½ cup sliced
    peaches, 1 cup 1% milk
Freshly brewed coffee or tea

LUNCH
Cream of tomato soup, made with 1 cup 1% milk
Club sandwich:
   deli-sliced turkey and ham, 1 oz. each
   low-fat cheese, ½ oz.
   lettuce, tomato, as desired
   mayonnaise, 1 tsp.
   mustard, as desired
   whole-grain bread, 2 slices
Carrot and celery sticks

DINNER
Chicken in wine:
   skinless chicken breast, 5 oz., poached in ½ cup of red wine
Steamed wild rice, 1 cup, with 1 tsp. tub margarine
Fresh asparagus, 5 spears, with 1 tsp. tub margarine
Honeydew melon, ¼ medium

SNACK
Fig Newtons, 3
1% milk, 1 cup

Day 14

BREAKFAST
Orange juice, ½ cup
*Cinnamon french toast, with 2 tbsp. maple syrup
Blueberries, ¾ cup
Freshly brewed coffee or tea

LUNCH
Corned-beef sandwich:
   deli-sliced lean corned beef, 3 oz.
   rye bread, 2 slices
   spicy or regular mustard
Coleslaw:
   shredded cabbage, ½ cup
   shredded carrots, 2 tbsp.

mayonnaise, 1½ tsp., mixed with 1½ tsp. plain, low-fat yogurt
   sprinkling of caraway seeds
1% milk, 1 cup

DINNER
Broiled rainbow trout:
   5 oz. trout, broiled with 1 tbsp. lemon juice, 1 tsp. tub margarine
Spinach and orange salad:
   leaf spinach, 1 cup
   mandarin orange sections, ¼ cup
   toasted almond slivers, 1 tbsp.
   French dressing, 1 tbsp.
Steamed yellow and zucchini squash, ¼ cup each, with 1 tsp. tub margarine
Boiled red potatoes, 2 small, with 1 tsp. tub margarine, parsley
White-wine spritzer:
   ½ cup white wine
   ½ cup club soda

SNACK
Peach crumble:
   ½ cup fresh sliced peaches, sprinkled with 3 crushed graham cracker squares
1% milk, 1 cup

Day 15

BREAKFAST
Raisin bran cereal, ¾ cup, with 1 cup 1% milk
Whole-wheat toast, 2 slices, with 1 tsp. tub margarine, 1 tsp. orange marmalade
Banana and kiwi fruit salad:
   ½ medium banana
   1 sliced kiwi fruit
Freshly brewed coffee or tea

LUNCH
Ham sandwich:

    deli-sliced ham, 2 oz.

    lettuce, tomato, as desired

    mayonnaise, 1 tsp.

    mustard, as desired

    pumpernickel bread, 2 slices

Fresh orange or tangerine

1% milk, 1 cup

DINNER
*Spinach-chicken calzone

Broiled Italian tomatoes:

    2 tomato halves, broiled with 1 oz. shredded
    part-skim mozzarella cheese, dash of oregano

Raspberry sorbet

Ginger snaps, 3

SNACK
1% milk, 1 cup

Day 16

BREAKFAST
Grapefruit, ½ medium

Spanish omelette:

    1 egg plus 2 egg whites

    chopped red and green pepper, ¼ cup

    hot sauce, 1½ tbsp.

    sauté in 1 tsp. tub margarine

Toasted oatmeal bread, 2 slices, with 1 tsp. tub
    margarine, 1 tsp. grape jam

Freshly brewed coffee or tea

LUNCH
Stuffed pita bread sandwich:

    salad stuffing: 1 cup assorted vegetables
    (shredded carrots, chopped mushrooms,
    tomato, green pepper, shredded lettuce)

    shredded part-skim mozzarella cheese, 1 oz.

    pita pocket, 1, 6″ round

    drizzle with 1 tsp. Italian dressing, 1 tsp.
    flavored vinegar

Apple, 1 medium

1% milk, 1 cup

DINNER
Scallop scampi:

    sea scallops, 6 oz., broiled with 2 tbsp. tub
    margarine, garlic

Baked potato, 1 medium with low-fat yogurt,
    2 tbsp., chives

Steamed broccoli, ½ cup

Carrots with ginger, ½ cup, with 1 tsp. tub
    margarine

Lime sherbet, ½ cup, with ½ cup sliced
    strawberries

SNACK
Seedless green grapes, 12

Vanilla wafers, 3

1% milk, 1 cup

Day 17

BREAKFAST
Apple-cranberry juice, ½ cup

Fruit yogurt, 1 cup, low-fat

*Three-grain muffin, 1

Melon balls, made with ½ cup each cantaloupe,
    honeydew

Freshly brewed coffee or tea

LUNCH
Tuna Nicoise:

    tuna, 3½ oz., water-packed

    steamed green beans, ½ cup

    chopped pimento, 3 tbsp.

    chopped onion, 1 tbsp.

    celery sticks

    vinegar and olive oil with basil, 1 tbsp.

    served on a bed of lettuce

Crusty hard roll, 1

Red seedless grapes, 12

Fresh whole strawberries, 4   .

Lemon water

DINNER

Broiled tenderloin steak, 4 oz.

Corn on the cob, 1 ear, with 1 tsp. tub margarine

Steamed carrots with mushrooms, ½ cup

Linguini noodles, ½ cup, with 1 tsp. tub
    margarine, fresh parsley

Coffee ice-milk, ½ cup, with 1 tbsp. slivered
    almonds

SNACK

Angel food cake, ¹⁄₁₂ cake

1% milk, 1 cup

Day 18

BREAKFAST

Fresh-squeezed grapefruit juice, ½ cup

*Cinnamon French toast, with 2 tbsp. maple
    syrup

Berries and oranges:

    blueberries, ¼ cup

    mandarin orange sections, ¼ cup

Freshly brewed coffee or tea

LUNCH

Roast beef sandwich:

    deli-sliced roast beef, 2 oz.

    lettuce, tomato, as desired

    mayonnaise, 1½ tsp.

    bulky roll, 1

fresh plums, 2 small

1% milk, 1 cup

DINNER

Grilled chicken kabobs:

    cubed chicken breast, 4 oz.

    cherry tomatoes, 3

pearl onions, 2

green pepper, ½ medium

Steamed brown rice, ⅔ cup, with 1 tsp. tub
    margarine

Bibb lettuce, 1 cup, with ¼ cup herbed croutons,
    1 tbsp. vinegar and oil

SNACK

Lemon-berry parfait:

    ½ cup low-fat lemon yogurt, layered, with
    ¼ cup blueberries and 2 crushed graham
    cracker squares

Day 19

BREAKFAST

Pineapple-grapefruit juice, ½ cup

Oatmeal, ½ cup, with 2 tbsp. raisins and
    cinnamon, 1 cup 1% milk

Whole-wheat toast, 1 slice, with 1 tsp. strawberry
    jam

Freshly brewed coffee or tea

LUNCH

*Lentil-pasta soup, 1 cup

Spinach salad:

    chopped spinach, 1½ cups

    sliced mushrooms, ½ cup

    tomato wedges, ½ cup

    hard-boiled egg, 1

    low-calorie French dressing, 1 tbsp.

Fresh nectarine

DINNER

*Oriental beef stir-fry

Steamed rice, ⅔ cup

Fresh fruit salad:

    sliced strawberries, ½ cup

    pineapple chunks, ¼ cup

    chopped walnuts, 1 tbsp.

Fortune cookie

Sparkling water with lime

SNACK
Three-grain muffin, 1
1% milk, 1 cup

Day 20

BREAKFAST
Apple juice, ½ cup
Low-fat vanilla yogurt, 1 cup, with fresh peach
 slices, nutmeg
*Three-grain muffin, 1
Freshly brewed coffee or tea

LUNCH
*Curried Chicken and Rice Salad, served on a
 bed of lettuce
Crusty rye roll, 1 small
*Low-fat lemon cheesecake, 1 slice
Iced tea with lemon

DINNER
Broiled lemon cod:
 4 oz. cod, broiled with 1 tsp. tub margarine,
 2 tbsp. of lemon juice; sprinkle with basil
*Parmesan Noodles, ½ serving
Steamed broccoli, 3 stalks, with 1 tsp. tub
 margarine
Side salad:
 romaine lettuce, 1 cup
 sliced mushrooms, ¼ cup
 shredded park-skim mozzarella cheese, 1 oz.
 low-calorie Russian dressing, 1 tbsp.
1% milk, 1 cup

SNACK
Gingersnaps, 3
1% milk, 1 cup

Day 21

BREAKFAST
Fresh grapefruit, ½ medium
Bran flakes, ¾ cup, with 1 cup 1% milk

Cinnamon-raisin toast, 1 slice with 1 tsp. tub
 margarine, 1 tsp. apple jelly
Freshly brewed coffee or tea

LUNCH
*Lentil and pasta soup, 1 cup
Tuna salad sandwich:
 tuna, 3 oz., water-packed
 chopped celery, 2 tbsp.
 mayonnaise, 1½ tsp. plus 1½ tsp. plain yogurt
 lettuce, tomato
 marbled rye bread, 2 slices
Fresh pear
1% milk, 1 cup

DINNER
Glazed Cornish hen:
 ½ of a 1-lb. hen, skinned, roasted, and glazed
 with 1 tbsp. apricot jam during last few minutes
 of cooking; sprinkle with tarragon
Baked sweet potato, 1 medium, with 1 tsp. tub
 margarine
Steamed zucchini, 1 cup, sprinkled with lemon
 juice, dill
Pumpernickel dinner roll, 1 small with 1 tsp. tub
 margarine
Raspberry sorbet, ½ cup, with ½ cup of fresh
 blackberries

SNACK
Blueberry cheesecake crumble:
 ½ cup blueberries, topped with ½ cup low-fat
 vanilla yogurt, 4 crumbled vanilla wafers

Kitchen-Tested Recipes

Lentil and Pasta Soup

4 cups low-sodium chicken broth
4 cups water
1 cup dried lentils, rinsed
28-oz. can whole tomatoes, chopped with their
  juice
6 oz. tomato paste
1 tbsp. brown sugar
1 cup each sliced carrots and chopped celery
9-oz. package frozen Italian green beans
1 large onion
3 garlic cloves, minced
1 cup dry (uncooked) tubettini pasta
1 bay leaf
½ tsp. each basil, oregano, thyme, black pepper,
  marjoram
¼ cup wine vinegar

In large pot, combine broth, water, lentils, tomatoes, tomato paste, brown sugar, vegetables, and
garlic. Bring to a boil, lower heat, cover pot, and
simmer for 30 to 45 minutes. Add about 2 more
cups of water, pasta, spices, and vinegar and simmer for about 30 minutes more. Remove bay leaf
before serving.

Yield: 14 cups

Spinach-Chicken Calzone

10-oz. homemade or ready-to-bake pizza crust
¾ pound chicken, skinned, cooked, and shredded
10-oz. frozen chopped spinach, thawed and
  drained
1 cup fresh mushrooms, chopped
¼ cup grated Parmesan cheese
¼ cup 1%-fat cottage cheese
½ cup parsley flakes
½ tsp. oregano
1 tsp. garlic powder
1 tsp. onion powder
pepper to taste

Preheat oven to 375°F. On a lightly floured surface, roll dough to a 12″ × 14″ piece. Cut into six
equal squares and place on a cookie sheet coated
with vegetable oil spray. Combine remaining
ingredients to make filling. Divide filling equally
among the six squares by spooning it into the
middle of each. Fold squares in half diagonally.
Firmly press edges together and crimp with a fork
to make a tight seal. Lightly prick the top of each
calzone with the fork and bake for 20 to 25 minutes or until crust is golden brown.

Yield: 6 calzones

Three-Grain Muffins

1 cup bran flakes cereal
1 cup dry (uncooked) oatmeal
1 cup whole-wheat flour
1 tbsp. baking powder
1 tsp. cinnamon
½ tsp. nutmeg
1 cup skim milk
¼ cup egg substitute
3 tbsp. molasses
1 tbsp. corn or safflower oil
1½ medium apples, chopped

Preheat oven to 400°F. Combine bran flakes, oatmeal, flour, baking powder, and spices in a large bowl. In a separate bowl, mix the remaining ingredients and add to the dry cereal mixture. Stir contents until just moist. Coat 12 muffin tins with vegetable oil and divide batter equally among them. Bake 20 to 25 minutes until lightly browned.

Yield: 12 muffins

Low-Fat Lemon Cheesecake

Crust:
1 cup graham crackers, crushed
1 tbsp. margarine, melted
1 tsp. cinnamon

Filling:
4 cups low-fat lemon yogurt, drained
1 cup 1%-fat cottage cheese
¼ cup all-purpose flour
1 egg
½ cup egg substitute
¼ cup sugar
2 tsp. vanilla

Line a colander with cheesecloth and place in dish deep enough to collect liquid that drains from yogurt. Pour yogurt into lined colander to drain. Cover and refrigerate overnight.

Preheat oven to 300°F. Combine crust ingredients and press into bottom of a 9″ springform pan coated with nonstick vegetable oil spray. Combine filling ingredients and blend thoroughly with a hand mixer or food processor. Pour filling over prepared crust. Bake in preheated oven for approximately 1 hour (the edges will pull away from the pan when the filling is set). Set pan on rack and cool completely. Loosen edges with a knife before removing the pan sides. Chill and cut into 12 slices.

Yield: 12 slices

Cashew Turkey Salad

2 oz. turkey breast, cooked and chopped
7 cashews, broken into pieces
¼ cup green pepper, chopped
½ medium carrot, grated
1 tbsp. mayonnaise
1 tbsp. low-fat plain yogurt

Mix ingredients and chill.

Yield: 1 serving

Mom's Meat Loaf

1 lb. lean ground beef
2 eggs
8 tbsp. tomato sauce
2 tbsp. chopped onion
Italian seasoning

Mix meat, onion, Italian seasoning, and ½ of tomato sauce, and place mixture in a small loaf pan. Bake at 350°F for 30 to 40 minutes. Drain fat and top with remaining tomato sauce.

Yield: 4 servings

Parmesan Noodles

1 cup noodles, cooked
2 tsp. tub margarine
2 tbsp. Parmesan cheese
Fresh ground pepper

Mix thoroughly and serve hot.

Yield: 1 serving

Curried Chicken Salad

3 oz. chicken breast, cooked and diced
2 tsp. mayonnaise
2 tsp. low-fat plain yogurt
2 tbsp. raisins
2 tsp. chopped walnuts
curry powder to taste

Mix thoroughly and chill.

Yield: 1 serving

Curried Chicken and Rice Salad

2 oz. chicken, cooked and cubed
⅔ cup rice, steamed
½ cup grapes, sliced
1 tbsp. walnuts

Dressing:
2 tsp. mayonnaise mixed with 3 tsp. low-fat plain yogurt
Curry powder to taste

Mix chicken and rice in a bowl, cover and set in refrigerator to chill. Before serving, mix in thoroughly grapes, walnuts, dressing, and curry powder.

Two-Alarm Chili

3 oz. lean ground beef, cooked and drained
⅔ cup canned kidney beans
¼ cup chopped onion
2 tbsp. medium-hot salsa
3 tbsp. water

Mix together all ingredients and slowly cook over low to medium heat. Add more water, if necessary.

Yield: 1 serving

Chicken Parmesan

4 oz. boneless chicken breast
1 oz. part-skim mozzarella cheese
1 tsp. tub margarine
1 tbsp. Parmesan cheese
½ cup spaghetti sauce

Remove skin from chicken and sauté in margarine until cooked. Place chicken in oil-sprayed pan and cover with spaghetti sauce. Top with cheese. Bake at 350°F until cheese melts. Serve over linguine.

Yield: 1 serving

Cinnamon French Toast

2 slices wheat or raisin bread
1 egg plus 1 egg white
1 tbsp. 1% milk
cinnamon to taste
2 tsp. tub margarine

Mix egg, egg white, and milk. Add cinnamon and dip bread into egg mixture to coat. Sauté in oil-sprayed pan using tub margarine.

Chef Salad

2 cups assorted leafy greens (spinach, leaf
　　lettuce, iceberg lettuce)
1 oz. each of lean ham and turkey, cut in strips
1 oz. part-skim mozzarella cheese, cut in strips
¼ cup grated carrots
tomato, cut in wedges

Layer ingredients onto lettuce bed and top with 1 tbsp. vinegar and oil dressing.

Italian Tuna Pasta Salad

3 oz. water-packed tuna
1 cup cooked pasta, any kind
½ cup shredded raw carrots
½ cup shredded raw zucchini
2 tbsp. Italian dressing

Lightly mix all ingredients. Top with fresh ground pepper, if desired.

Oriental Beef Stir-Fry

4 oz. flank steak or other lean cut of beef
1 medium carrot
¼ cup snow peas
¼ cup water chestnuts
½ cup bean sprouts
2 tbsp. dry-roasted cashews
1 tbsp. sesame oil
1 tbsp. soy sauce

Cut beef into strips and carrots into thin slices. Sauté beef in wok or skillet until cooked. Add vegetables and stir-fry until tender crisp. Remove from heat and sprinkle with soy sauce.

Mexi-Stuffed Green Pepper

4 oz. lean ground round
⅓ cup boiled rice
¼ cup tomato sauce
1 tbsp. salsa
1 green pepper

Brown ground round in a skillet and drain off excess fat. Mix meat, cooked rice, tomato sauce, and salsa, and stuff into pepper. Bake at 350°F for 30 minutes.

20

Can Diet Cure What Ails You?

The link between diet and disease is not always as clearly defined as it is with coronary heart disease. And yet, we are reaching a point in our scientific research where certain conclusions can be formulated, based on the data that now exists, regarding the most pressing disease-related concerns of Americans today.

Our intention in this chapter is twofold. First, to offer a reliable perspective on the current state of scientific research; and second, to provide you with dietary guidelines where they exist. As you read, you may begin to appreciate why there is so much complexity involved in the process of finding specific connections between diet and disease. It is nearly impossible to isolate human beings from their environments and the wide range of factors that might increase or decrease their risks. Only after seeing consistent results in a number of different kinds of studies can any conclusions be drawn at all.

Nevertheless, scientists and health experts have reached preliminary conclusions about dietary factors that influence various types of cancers, diabetes, and osteoporosis.

New Data on the Cancer-Diet Connection

Cancer is the second leading cause of death in the United States. Not a single condition but rather a group of conditions, cancer results from the uncontrolled growth of cells originating from almost any tissue in the body. Many factors appear to influence the onset of these conditions, including the environment, heredity, and smoking. However, the most current data suggest that diet may play an important role, as well.

A great deal of research is going on worldwide about cancer and diet. And while there is gathering evidence that there are links between what we eat day-to-day and the long-term development of cancer (particularly of the breast and colon), there is also a growing body of conflicting evidence that these links may not be as specific as once believed. This disagreement is fueling a behind-the-scenes debate within the scientific community over whether the public is being misled with statements that may not be quite true. A host of practical questions are being raised: Will a high-fiber, low-fat diet prevent cancer? Are there such things as "protector nutrients" that can guard the body against cancer? Is supplement-taking ever warranted to fight cancer? What are the real cancer-causing dangers of carcinogens in our food supply? There are no final resolutions to most of these questions. However, an examination of what is currently being seen in research should help put the issues in perspective.

Lung Cancer

Lung cancer is the number one cause of cancer deaths for men, and it is approaching that status for women. The medical community is in agreement that cigarette smoking is the leading causal factor; smokers have a 20 to 30 times greater risk of contracting the disease than nonsmokers.

While no conclusive studies have linked diet to lung cancer, a growing body of evidence does suggest that beta-carotene, the vitamin A precursor, may help protect people against a common form of lung cancer, called squamous cell carcinoma. Other research indicates that vitamin E may help reduce the risk for developing any type of lung cancer. Research at Johns Hopkins University in Baltimore suggests that people with relatively low levels of beta-carotene in their blood may be at least four times as likely to fall victim to lung cancer as others; the risk for those who have low blood levels of vitamin E may be as much as two and a half times greater.

Scientists reporting in the *New England Journal of Medicine* found that the blood of 99 people who eventually developed lung cancer (most, but not all, were smokers) contained almost 14 percent less beta-carotene and 12 percent less vitamin E than the blood of 200 people who had similar smoking habits but remained free of lung disease. The mechanism by which beta-carotene and vitamin E may work to inhibit the development of lung cancer is not certain. It is known, however, that beta-carotene and vitamin E "trap" and "deactivate" free radicals, chemical components in the body that can harm cell structure and, in the process, presumably predispose tissues to cancerous growths.

Another study of 25,000 people over the course of a decade in Japan uncovered what appeared to

be a link between daily consumption of vegetables high in beta-carotene and a decreased risk of cancer of the lung, colon, stomach, prostate, and cervix.

To find out more about whether beta-carotene and vitamin E play a role in preventing cancer—and if they do, how so—scientists are conducting studies known as chemoprevention trials, in which large numbers of people are given supplemental doses of one or more substances and are then observed over a period of several years to see if they are less likely to contract cancer than others. Currently, some 25,000 male physicians throughout the United States are participating in a trial funded by the National Cancer Institute to determine if beta-carotene supplements will decrease the overall incidences of cancer. Other groups are being given vitamin E.

Even if the connection between these two nutrients and the avoidance of lung cancer proves to be valid, there is some concern that people might use the information to begin or continue practices that are harmful. For example, smokers should not take this information to mean that it's okay to smoke as long as they increase their intake of these two nutrients. According to Dr. Charles H. Hennekens of the Harvard Medical School, even if beta-carotene was effective in reducing lung cancer deaths by half, lifelong smokers would still have a 10 to 15 times greater risk than nonsmokers of contracting the disease. Cigarettes are associated with a much greater risk of lung cancer than low levels of beta-carotene and vitamin E. Furthermore these two nutrients may be only indirectly associated with a decreased risk of lung cancer. It may be that other, as yet undiscovered, substances in foods with beta-carotene and vitamin E are responsible for the protection against cancer that the researchers observed.

For this reason, it is not recommended that people take vitamin supplements of these nutrients, either in lieu of foods or in addition to foods. Rather, it is advised that people include in their diets the orange- and yellow-colored produce and the leafy green vegetables that contain beta-carotene, as well as the whole grains that contain vitamin E. Those who might take the early results of ongoing research to mean they should start taking large doses of certain nutrients in supplement form should be aware that this could be a dangerous practice. Although large doses of beta-carotene are relatively harmless, too much vitamin A can cause permanent liver damage. Selenium, a mineral that is currently being tested in anticancer studies, can be toxic in amounts easily obtainable from supplements. Even vitamin C, which, like vitamin E and beta-carotene, is being tested for its possible properties in warding off cancer, may cause problems when it is consumed in megadoses. Furthermore, nutrient tests being conducted are related to people's patterns of *food* intake, and there is currently no data that might justify self-treatment with nutrient supplements.

Colon Cancer

Colon cancer is second only to lung cancer as the leading cause of cancer deaths among men in the United States. Current speculation is that a high-fiber, low-fat diet can be a preventive factor. Many studies have been conducted in both humans and animals to assess the relationship between high-fat diets and colon cancer. To date, nineteen case-controlled human studies have been done. Of these, three found no effect, three found an increased risk, and thirteen observed a protective effect from fiber-containing foods, especially vegetables. Like other diet/cancer studies, the data are mixed—although scientific opinion leans in the direction of supporting a low-fat, high-fiber diet.

The theory stems, in part, from research demonstrating that a high intake of fat causes greater secretion of bile acids. And while bile acids are necessary to help the body digest fats, they or their breakdown products have also been shown to promote tumors in the colon (or large bowel) in laboratory animals. Dietary fiber may minimize the harmful affects of bile acids and thereby inhibit tumor development. But, even if it has a

positive effect, it has not yet been determined whether an increased fiber intake works independently of decreased fat intake or whether the two must operate in tandem for an optimal anticancer effect. In either case, fiber may help to decrease risk in one or more ways. It increases the bulk of the stool, which may dilute the concentration of cancer-causing agents. This increased bulk speeds the passage of stool through the colon and lessens the time carcinogens or carcinogenic substances in waste can do damage. It also may bind carcinogens that might otherwise remain free to work on producing a tumor.

One of the problems in assessing the precise relationship between fiber and colon cancer is that there are many different types of fiber and not all of them appear to be protective. While the insoluble fiber present in whole-wheat products has held up relatively consistently as a cancer inhibitor in research on rats, in some studies the soluble fiber found in oat bran and fruits have been shown to stimulate tumor production in laboratory experiments, possibly by increasing the concentration of bile acids. Of course, one problem with animal studies is that they often use potent carcinogens or unrealistically high levels of fiber.

To make matters even more confusing, Greenland Eskimos, who eat no fiber to speak of but whose diets are extremely high in fat, have a low rate of colon cancer.

These seeming inconsistencies might lead you to conclude that "you're damned if you do, and damned if you don't." But closer examination reveals that the type of fat Greenland Eskimos eat consists largely of the omega-3 fatty acids found in fish, which may not have the same effect on the secretion of bile acids as the typical saturated and polyunsaturated fats of the American diet.

Breast Cancer

Breast cancer is the leading cancer killer of women. In 1985, the latest year for which reliable figures are available, more than 40,000 women in the United States died of the disease. Against the backdrop of this distressing statistic, scientists are now debating whether women can reverse the trend by cutting back on the percentage of fat in their diets.

Several convincing studies back up the contention that there is a relationship. In fact, according to Leonard A. Cohen, Ph.D., of the American Health Foundation in Valhalla, New York, "The association between dietary fat and breast cancer comes closest to fulfilling the criteria epidemiologists look for when they make inferences about what causes disease."

One recent study, led by Dr. Paolo Toniolo of the New York University Medical Center, studied 750 Italian women. Those who ate the most fats, saturated fats, and animal protein had a three times greater chance of getting breast cancer than those who had the lowest intake of these foods. The study also showed that a high-calorie diet seemed to increase the risk of cancer; women who consumed more than 2,700 calories a day had almost twice the risk of breast cancer as those who ate fewer than 1,900 calories. (It is not certain whether the high calorie diets were culpable because they were also high in fat.)

Studies of Japanese women who eat a traditional diet that is only about 20 percent fat have shown that these women are less likely to contract breast cancer than women in countries, such as the United States, where the diet is higher in fat. In fact, breast cancer has been estimated to be four to five times as common in the United States as it is in Japan. Particularly telling is the evidence gathered on the granddaughters and great-granddaughters of Japanese families who migrated to Hawaii and the mainland of the United States and adopted diets higher in fat. The breast cancer rate among these Americanized women approaches that of other women in this country. The same has proved true for American-born women of Polish descent, who have a higher rate of breast cancer than their ancestors who ate a lower fat diet. Furthermore, in Japan today, where the diet has become more Westernized, the incidence of breast cancer is on the rise. These studies indicate that genetic factors are not the sole determinants in assessing breast cancer risk.

Despite this evidence, there are those who cautiously point out that none of these studies linking high-fat diets to breast cancer have proved a specific cause-and-effect relationship between the two. It is true that even the most carefully constructed epidemiological studies cannot rule out the possibility that other environmental influences or genetic variations account for some of the differences. Studies on laboratory animals cannot provide an absolute link either, since they cannot automatically be extrapolated to humans.

Skeptics of the dietary fat–breast cancer link also point to a recently completed Harvard study of almost 90,000 women, which revealed that those who took in 44 percent of their calories from fat were no more likely to develop breast cancer than those who consumed only 32 percent of their calories from fat. But is 32 percent fat low enough to draw the comparison? Not according to scientists whose research suggests that the risk of breast cancer does not decrease little by little as fat is cut out of the diet; instead, they believe there may be a cutoff point below which women are not at high risk for breast cancer and above which they are. In effect, there may be a "threshold point."

If that is true, where is the threshold? Not all scientists agree on the exact number, but most believe it is below 30 percent. Sherwood L. Gorbach, M.D., a professor of medicine at Tufts who has conducted numerous studies on the link between diet and breast cancer, recommends a diet consisting of 20 to 25 percent of fat calories. Dr. Gorbach is not convinced, however, that the threshold effect should rule women's thinking about lowering fat calories to the extent that they consider any effort to lower fat intake as irrelevant if it doesn't reach the recommended level. "To whatever extent you can lower your fat intake, you might be lowering your breast cancer risk," he says.

Prostate Cancer

The cause of prostate cancer, which affects 20 to 30 percent of all men in their lifetimes, is still a mystery. However, at least one study suggests that obesity and heavy consumption of meat and dairy products may play a role in the development of the disease. David A. Snowden, Ph.D., and his colleagues at the University of California, Loma Linda, examined the 1960 diet and weight records of more than 6,700 men over the age of 60, and focused their attention on those who died during the following twenty years because of prostate cancer.

Dr. Snowden's group found that heavy consumers of animal products were over three and a half times more likely to die of prostate cancer than light consumers of animal products. Heavy consumption was defined as eating cheese, eggs, meat, or poultry three or more times a week and drinking more than two glasses of milk each day. Light consumption entailed eating each of these foods on the average of one day a week and drinking less than a glass of milk every day. The researchers also found obesity to be a significant risk factor. Men who were one-third or more above their desirable weight in 1960 were two and a half times more likely to succumb to prostate cancer than men of normal weight.

It's worth noting that protate cancer is not usually fatal. Since this study examined only fatal victims of the disease and not survivors, it is uncertain whether diet is related to development of the disease or to survival once it occurs.

Although the evidence is not absolutely clear as it relates to prostate cancer, most experts would agree that obesity and a heavy consumption of high-fat and cholesterol-containing foods increase the risk factors for many illnesses.

Stomach Cancer

During the past 50 years, there has been a remarkable decline in stomach cancer in the United States and many other industrialized nations. It is believed that at least part of the reason for the decline is that people are eating less smoked and pickled foods. Salt-cured and salt-pickled foods have been linked to gastric cancer, possibly because the nitrates in these foods are converted to nitrosamines in the body. Nitrosamines have been shown to be carcinogenic.

Current Recommendations

While questions remain about which dietary components may protect against or contribute to the development of various kinds of cancer, most experts agree that by following a certain dietary pattern, health-conscious eaters can apply the best of what has been gleaned so far about reducing the chance of developing diet-related cancer. Even if it turns out that dietary measures do not reduce the risk as much as many scientists hope, this pattern will provide the balance of nutrients that is essential to the maintenance of general health, as well as assist in the fight against obesity and heart disease. Here are the suggested dietary guidelines:

▶ Eat fewer items that are high in fat, including heavily marbled meats, fried foods, cold cuts such as bologna and salami, bacon, whole milk and cream, creamed dishes, rich desserts, and meals prepared with lots of oil, butter, or margarine.

▶ Consume more low-fat dairy products, such as low-fat yogurt, cottage cheese, and skim milk; baked or broiled poultry without the skin, fish, and lean cuts of meat with all the fat trimmed away.

▶ Select fiber-rich whole-grain breads, cereals, and pastas (the ingredient list must contain the words "whole-grain" or "whole-wheat"), all types of fruits and vegetables, legumes, oat-based products, and, in moderation, nuts (which are relatively high in fat).

▶ Increase your daily intake of fruits and vegetables rich in beta-carotene, such as cantaloupe, apricots, sweet potatoes, spinach, and broccoli.

▶ Eat a variety of produce that contains appreciable amounts of vitamin C, which includes everything from citrus fruits to tomatoes to dark-green leafy vegetables.

▶ Get enough vitamin E by using small amounts of polyunsaturated oils when cooking and by eating a wide variety of vegetables and whole-grains.

Diabetes Can Be Controlled by Diet

Diabetes mellitus occurs when the pancreas either does not produce enough of the hormone insulin or when the cells of the body are not able to use it properly. In order to understand how diabetes causes problems, it helps to look at how the normal body functions.

When you eat food, your body must process the nutrients, carbohydrate, protein, and fat before the body cells can use them. Carbohydrate, for example, is converted in the process of digestion to a simple sugar, most often glucose. The glucose is then released from the intestines into the bloodstream, where it is transported to the body cells for use as an energy source or converted to fat and stored. Protein and fat are also broken into smaller components to be used by the cells.

When a person eats a meal, the pancreas releases insulin into the bloodstream to assist the cells in absorbing and utilizing the sources of energy glucose, fatty acids, and amino acids. Insulin is also involved in the synthesis of protein and the storage of glucose and fatty acids as glycogen and fat. Without insulin, or without the ability to properly utilize it, your body cannot adequately use the foods you eat. Hence, the glucose that comes from dietary sources accumulates in the blood and people are said to have "high blood sugar." Further, when blood glucose builds to a certain point, the kidneys, which filter all of the blood, are unable to handle the load, and some glucose

quite literally spills into the urine. The appearance of glucose in the urine is the major diagnostic test for diabetes.

Diet is known to be a critical factor in the management of diabetes. There are three different types of diabetes mellitus. One of them, gestational diabetes, is a temporary condition that sometimes afflicts pregnant women (see chapter 16 for more details). The other two forms are insulin-dependent diabetes (Type I) and noninsulin-dependent diabetes (Type II). Diabetes mellitus is the third leading cause of mortality in the United States and the second leading cause of blindness.

TYPE I: INSULIN-DEPENDENT DIABETES

Often called juvenile-onset diabetes, this form usually occurs in childhood and lasts throughout the diabetic's life. It is the most serious form of diabetes, accounting for about 10 percent of all cases. Those afflicted with Type I diabetes make little or no insulin, so they must rely on injected insulin to metabolize food. They also must make an effort to match their food intake to their insulin dose to minimize the fluctuations in their blood-sugar levels. Until recently, insulin was derived from animals. Modern molecular biology enables the production of an identical form from bacteria.

With the advent of home blood-glucose monitoring and the practice of taking two or more daily insulin injections, people with Type I diabetes are now able to more easily control their condition, and they have greater freedom in making food choices and timing their meals than they once did.

TYPE II: NONINSULIN-DEPENDENT DIABETES

Often called adult-onset diabetes, this is the most common form of diabetes. It can exist in varying degrees of mildness or severity. Type II diabetes is usually seen in adults over 30 years of age who have problems with obesity. Unlike those with Type I diabetes, who cannot produce enough insulin, Type II sufferers often produce enough, but are unable to use it properly, often because they are carrying too much weight. For these people, weight loss often makes it impossible for their bodies to begin using insulin in a normal way.

Although Type II diabetes is often hereditary, diet is considered to be the single most important factor in its control.

Dietary Guidelines for Diabetics

Even those diabetics who receive insulin treatments need to carefully monitor their diets. The American Dietetic Association and the American Diabetes Association have recommended an "exchange" program that is widely used in the United States. This system groups foods according to calories and carbohydrate, protein, and fat content. The Exchange Lists for Meal Planning (available from the American Diabetes Association National Service Center, 1660 Duke Street, Alexandria, VA 22314) includes six lists, each of which contains a group of foods that are similar in calorie and nutrient content. For example, the "bread" list includes foods that are equivalent to one slice of bread, such as a half cup of potatoes or half an English muffin.

Recently, the exchange system was updated to include "new" foods, such as kiwi fruit and tacos, along with commonly eaten items such as pizza. Along with the increased choices of foods in the six groups, a separate section called Foods for Occasional Use includes, for the first time, such sweet items as ice cream, cookies, and granola bars. The addition of these dessert foods reflects formal acceptance of what nutritionists have recognized for a long time: With caution, some sweets can be eaten by diabetics without causing a rapid rise in blood sugar.

Another change is that more emphasis is placed on starchy foods, such as whole-grain breads, cereals, and rice. The new recommendations suggest that 50 to 60 percent of the diet should come from complex carbohydrates and high-fiber foods.

However, scientists have learned that people with diabetes often have varying responses to car-

bohydrate sources, depending on the severity of their conditions. A diabetic's physician must prescribe a diet based on a careful evaluation of blood tests.

In general, the Committee on Food and Nutrition of the American Diabetes Association recommends the following guidelines for people with diabetes:

▶ Follow a diet high in complex carbohydrates, such as vegetables and whole grains, as well as fruits.

▶ Increase your intake of water-soluble fibers, such as oats, barley, lentils, and beans. In addition, increase your intake of fiber in general, with foods such as carrots, broccoli, dried fruits, pears, nuts, seeds, bran, and whole-grain foods. Studies show that high-fiber diets can help to lower blood-sugar levels, thereby reducing the need for insulin.

▶ Decrease your intake of high-fat foods, reducing your daily fat intake to no more than 30 percent of your total calories. Since both Type I and Type II diabetics run a higher risk of developing heart disease, this factor is particularly important.

▶ Decrease consumption of fatty meats, and use leaner cuts with the fat trimmed off before cooking. Eat chicken (preferably without the skin) and fish a few times each week.

▶ Cut down on high cholesterol foods in general to lower cholesterol intake to about 300 milligrams per day.

▶ Decrease consumption of candy and foods made with refined and processed sugars, to avoid overloading on highly absorbable sugars.

▶ Decrease intake of salt and foods with a high sodium content.

▶ Maintain regular meal and medication times. Eat the same amount of food at the same times each day, and take medication on a regular daily

► NUTRITION QUIZ ◄

Test Your Sugar Sense

Sugar has little to offer in the way of nutrient value. For all its calories (16 per level teaspoon), sugar provides no vitamins or minerals that are essential to good health.

But is sugar one of the culprits in disease? Does eating too much sugar lead to obesity? What is the role of sugar in the onset of diabetes?

Take this quiz to see how your answers match up with those given by experts.

1. People who eat a lot of sugar tend to be heavier than others.
   True _____   False _____

2. Excess sugar consumption can lead to diabetes.
   True _____   False _____

3. Sugar plays a role in the development of tooth cavities.
   True _____   False _____

4. Research has begun to implicate sugar as a risk factor for certain cancers, particularly cancer of the colon.
   True _____   False _____

5. Reactive hypoglycemia, a condition characterized by a sharp drop in blood sugar after meals, affects a larger percentage of the population than was once believed.
   True _____   False _____

6. Sugar interferes with the availability of certain vitamins and minerals to the body.
   True _____   False _____

ANSWERS

1. (False) Overweight people actually eat less sugar than thin people, according to epidemiological studies. Moreover, the amount of sugar someone eats is not necessarily a determinant of whether he will gain weight. Obesity results from a variety of factors, including life-style, genetics, and overall eating and activity patterns.

2. (False) Sugar in itself does not contribute to the development of diabetes. However, it does aggravate the condition once it exists. People who have diabetes have trouble keeping down their blood-sugar levels, so eating products that contain a lot of sugar makes the problem harder to control.

3. (True) It is not possible to say exactly how great sugar's role is in the development of cavities. The form in which it is consumed makes a difference. Sugar in sticky substances is more problematic than sugar in fruit or fruit juices. Other factors, such as the hardness of the tooth's surface, are also involved. But the amount of sugar

Americans eat does contribute to dental cavities. That's because the bacteria that cause tooth decay feed on sugar. Sugar also increases the chance that periodontal (gum) disease will occur. The more sugar a person eats, the more likely it is that his gums will recede, causing his teeth to loosen.

4. (False) No scientifically based data support the notion that high levels of sugar consumption increase an individual's risk of developing any type of cancer.

5. (False) Although many people believe they have reactive hypoglycemia, relatively few individuals suffer from this condition.

6. (False) Scientists have discovered no convincing evidence that people who eat large amounts of sugar have trouble metabolizing any nutrients.
Note: Taken as a whole, these answers indicate that sugar appears to cause no direct problems besides playing a role in the development of tooth decay. But that doesn't mean that a healthy diet is consistent with the consumption of a lot of sugar-filled snacks and beverages. Since sugar contributes no nutrients to the diet, its consumption should be limited to make room for foods with vitamins, minerals, and other essential nutrients.

schedule. It is advisable to spread out food consumption throughout the day.

▶ It has also been suggested that diabetics can substantially improve their condition by undertaking a regular program of exercise. Exercise lowers blood sugar and helps to control weight.

Preventing Osteoporosis in Later Life

Osteoporosis, or loss of bone mass, is universal in all people as they age. It is estimated that 15 to 20 million Americans currently suffer from the problem. Osteoporosis is a particularly severe condition that leaves the skeleton abnormally fragile. Each year the condition is responsible for about 1.3 million fractures of the vertebrae, hips, forearms, and other bones of people who are 45 years old or older. All people lose bone mass as they age. Bones reach their peak density about the age of 30, then begin to decline. At maturity,

men have more bone density than women, and blacks more than whites.

Postmenopausal women are at greatest risk for developing the disease because their protective levels of the hormone estrogen have declined. Following the onset of menopause, declining estrogen levels can lead to a rapid loss of bone mass.

The development of osteoporosis is hard to track because there are usually no symptoms of bone loss until the condition actually becomes a problem. Once it becomes detectable on X rays, as much as 50 percent of bone loss may have occurred already. And once bone is lost, it cannot be replenished. In that respect, osteoporosis cannot be "cured." The focus of action must be on prevention.

Intense public attention has been devoted to the calcium-osteoporosis connection in recent years. Few scientists believe that the disease is simply a case of calcium deficiency that can be halted by consuming large quantities of calcium-rich foods and/or suppplements. But osteoporosis is far more complex than that. Calcium deficiency is only one of several factors, including genetics, hormone levels, exercise, life-style, and general nutrition, that may lead to the condition. The casual assumption that calcium alone can eliminate the risk for osteoporosis has proved to be lucrative for many food manufacturers who have added the mineral to their products, and for the producers of nutrient supplements. (Sales of calcium supplements total more than $200 million a year.) But a serious review of the causes and preventions of osteoporosis must include a comprehensive analysis of all the factors. For example, certain other nutrients are needed to assure proper absorption of calcium; without these, even large quantities of calcium may be ineffective. Further, there is evidence that exercise may play an important role in osteoporosis prevention. There are also genetic factors that place certain individuals and populations at greater risk for developing the disease. For example, thin women and women with small bone structures seem to be at greater risk than larger, big-boned women. Also, white and Oriental women appear to be at greater risk than blacks. There's also a family connection. Women who have a history of osteoporosis in their families suffer a greater risk.

A Complex Nutritional Picture

Calcium is the key player in the formation and maintenance of the body's bones and teeth, which contain 99 percent of the body's calcium. It stands to reason that a sufficient supply of calcium is needed for building and maintaining the skeleton. But studies of the effects of dietary calcium on osteoporosis are relatively new and they are complicated by the need to evaluate not just the amount of calcium consumed but how much of that calcium is absorbed and retained by the body.

The factors that influence calcium absorption and utilization include the physical and chemical form of the calcium that is consumed, the way that calcium interacts with other nutrients, the

way that calcium is transported through and maintained in the body, and the way it is excreted by the kidneys.

Our body's ability to absorb calcium is influenced by the interaction of a variety of nutrients. The most important of these is vitamin D, which is converted to a hormone called calcitriol, which regulates the transport of calcium from the digestive tract to the bloodstream and its deposition into bone. However, this does not mean that large amounts of vitamin D will make a difference. Scientists have found that calcium absorption is enhanced by a "normal" intake of the vitamin. Patients who were given supplement doses of vitamin D in quantities of 50,000 to 150,000 IU per week showed no measurable improvement. Furthermore, vitamin D is potentially toxic in megadoses; it can lead to calcium deposits in the kidneys, blood vessels, heart, and lungs. Toxicity has been reported at dosages ranging from 10,000 IU per day taken for four months, to 200,000 IU per day taken over a period of two weeks.

Next to calcium, phosphorus is the most abundant mineral in our bodies. Bone consists of salts of calcium and phosphorus. Too much or too little dietary phosphorus may have a harmful effect on bone formation.

Another critical dietary factor is protein. Because much of the protein we consume is channeled into tissue (including bone) growth and maintenance, an adequate intake of protein is essential for prevention of bone loss. However, too much protein might be a contributing factor in the development of osteoporosis since it increases the amount of calcium excreted in the urine. High sodium intakes can also increase the amount of calcium lost in the urine, and massive fiber intakes can interfere with calcium absorption. Also, since bone is made up of many elements, they all contribute to the way calcium is utilized in the body. Among these, fluoride has attracted the most attention, since there are some data indicating that the bones of people raised on fluoridated water may be denser than those whose access to fluoride has been limited.

The Best Way to Meet Calcium Needs

The current RDA for calcium is 1,200 milligrams for persons 11–24 years old, who need larger amounts during the period of growth and bone development, and 800 milligrams for other adults. Heightened interest in the osteoporosis-calcium connection has led to heavy marketing of calcium supplements, as well as to the frequent fortification of foods that do not naturally contain the mineral. The supermarket shelves are filled with calcium-fortified foods, including orange juice, flour, bread, cereal, and even milk. Many people are convinced that it is a good idea to buy calcium-fortified products whenever they can, as well as to take calcium supplements, just to be sure they're getting what they need.

Calcium fortification is largely untested. Scientists are not certain to what extent it protects against osteoporosis or how effectively it is absorbed and used by the body. Nor are they certain how added calcium affects other nutrients.

There are also a number of problems with the calcium supplements on the market today. As discussed in chapter 6, many calcium supplements contain very little calcium. The best source, calcium carbonate, is only 40 percent calcium. Some people may need to take a calcium carbonate supplement if they are unable to reach the RDA level with diet alone. However, it also appears that consuming too much calcium carbonate can have the opposite-than-intended effect. Researchers at the Vitamin D and Bone Metabolism Laboratory at the Tufts USDA Center on Aging have found that, in high doses, calcium carbonate may actually lower the levels of calcitriol, leading to incomplete absorption of the calcium consumed.

To place the issue in context, it must be understood that the reason the medical and health communities have been talking up calcium is not because they have seen the need for people to consume it in larger quantities in supplement form. The emphasis is placed on encouraging people to regularly include high calcium sources in their diets. The average calcium consumption of women over age 50 in the United States is only about one-half the requirement. Calcium-rich foods are readily available in the American diet. For example, the following foods each contain between 300 and 350 milligrams, or slightly more than one-third the RDA:

8 oz. skim, low-fat, or whole milk

8 oz. buttermilk

1 cup low-fat or whole-milk yogurt

2 cups low-fat or whole-milk cottage cheese

½ cup part-skim ricotta cheese

1½ cups ice milk or ice cream

1½ oz. cheddar cheese

1½ slices American cheese

2½ oz. sardines with bones

4 oz. salmon with bones

Calcium is also found in a number of vegetables, but in much smaller amounts. It would be hard to meet the daily requirement for calcium with vegetables alone. For example, one-half cup of cooked mustard greens supplies only about 100 milligrams of calcium, and one-half cup of cooked broccoli supplies only 68 milligrams.

Further, there is some evidence that the calcium in certain foods may be poorly absorbed by the body. For example, studies now show that spinach, once thought to be an excellent source of the mineral (139 milligrams in one-half cup, cooked), may not be absorbed at a great enough level to be of much benefit. A group of scientists at Creighton University's Hard Tissue Research Center in Nebraska and at the Department of Foods and Nutrition at Purdue University in Indiana gave a group of men and women spinach and then traced the route its calcium took inside their bodies. They found that only about 5 percent of the mineral was absorbed. The rest was tied up by the oxalic acid contained in spinach and was excreted.

Preventing Osteoporosis: Start Young

Even though postmenopausal women are at greatest risk for developing the disease, it does not necessarily stand to reason that women should start taking larger amounts of calcium as they get older. For older women with osteoporosis, estrogen-replacement therapy might be of greater benefit than calcium supplements.

Estrogen is important to the normal utilization of calcium in women. Some researchers believe that adding estrogen, not calcium, is the best way to halt the disease.

In one study, reported in the *New England Journal of Medicine,* researchers in Denmark divided women into three groups. The first group was composed of women who received estrogen-replacement therapy for osteoporosis; the second group was composed of women who received 2,000 milligrams of supplemental calcium each day; and the third group was composed of women taking placebos. Researchers studied the changes in calcium metabolism among the three groups over a two-year period. They found that, while those on estrogen did not lose calcium, the high dosage supplements did not seem to slow the loss of calcium markedly.

To be effective, estrogen therapy must be started in the first few years after menopause, when the rate of bone loss is accelerated. It can't restore bone mass once it's lost. The necessity and implications of this treatment should also be discussed carefully with a physician, since estrogen therapy may increase the risk of other diseases for some women.

Most important, women need to pay attention to their calcium intake long before menopause occurs. Women who consume the recommended levels of calcium in the time between puberty and menopause are less likely to suffer from the disease.

The same holds true when describing the merits of exercise for reducing the risk of osteoporosis. Physical activity plays an important role in preserving bone. In particular, "weight bearing" activities such as walking, jogging, bicycling, and aerobics help maintain bone mass. But these activities may do little to halt bone loss in postmenopausal women. Researchers have found that premenopausal women who exercised regularly had a higher calcium content in their bones than those who did not. However, it is not clear whether exercise by postmenopausal women will protect against bone loss.

21

When You're Oversensitive to Food

Two out of five Americans believe they have adverse reactions or "allergies" to certain foods. Chronic headaches, arthritis, depression, skin rashes (such as hives), fatigue, weight fluctuations, and hyperactivity are just a few of the problems people attribute to food allergies. Some popular practitioners of "allergy cures" would have people believe that nearly everyone suffers them to some extent; they prescribe expensive supplements, injections, and complicated dietary regimens to combat these allergies. In fact, the number of people who suffer from food allergies is probably exaggerated. That's not to say that there's no such thing as a food *intolerance,* which is a food-related illness. But, unlike allergies, food intolerances have little or nothing to do with the immune system. Much of the mislabeling of problems as food allergies results from a lack of understanding about the difference between allergies and intolerances.

Identifying a True Food Allergy

A food allergy can best be described as an "overreaction" of the body's immune system, which includes the disease-fighting white blood cells, lymph tissues, thymus gland, and bone marrow. Substances, usually proteins, that are harmless for most people, trigger an allergic person's immune system to release antibodies that attack the proteins that are seen as unwelcome. Subsequently, the body releases chemicals, such as histamine, that irritate tissues. The most commonly affected tissues are those of the gastrointestinal tract, skin, and respiratory system. That's why the typical symptoms of food allergies are nausea, vomiting, diarrhea, skin rashes, or difficulty in breathing. In severe cases, fatal shock may occur.

About 90 percent of food allergies are caused by relatively few substances. The most common offenders are proteins in cow's milk, egg whites, peanuts, wheat, and soybeans. A number of foods commonly believed to be allergenic are not. Chocolate, for instance, rarely causes an immunologic reaction. And the notion that sugar is allergenic is simply false. Strawberries and tomatoes are often blamed for allergic reactions, but they too are rarely allergenic.

It's often difficult to pinpoint when a physical problem is actually the result of a food allergy, since the typical symptoms—diarrhea, vomiting, rashes—can be caused by any number of medical conditions. Even psychological factors, such as emotional stress, can bring on the same type of symptoms as those triggered by an allergic reaction to food. Indeed, just believing strongly

245

enough that a particular food will make you sick can cause you to become ill. Consider the case of a woman who complained of cramps and nausea after drinking as little as four drops of milk. When she was fed water through an opaque tube inserted into her stomach and was told it was milk, she experienced nausea and abdominal cramps within 10 minutes. When she was given milk and was told it was water, no symptoms occurred.

Because symptoms that can be attributed to food allergies are relatively common, laypeople and physicians alike often consider food allergies more prevalent than they are. In fact, it is not uncommon for physicians to label problems as food allergies when they can find no other explanation.

It is true that infants and toddlers have higher incidences of food allergies than adults. But studies of young children indicate that two-thirds of adverse reactions to foods reported by parents are not brought on when the children are given the suspect food disguised in a capsule.

Reputable Allergists and Reliable Tests

If you suspect you have a food allergy, the best way to insure that the problem is properly diagnosed is to consult a physician who has been certified by the American Board of Allergy and Immunology. Such a qualified allergist will take a detailed history of your family's medical problems, as well as a personal history, and follow it up with a thorough medical examination. Special attention will be paid to the details of your symptoms and when they occur in relation to eating food. You may be sent home with an assignment to keep a diary of everything you eat. You'll also be told to note when you eat it and to record any symptoms you develop. When "suspicious" foods are identified, the allergist will likely advise you to eliminate them for a period of time to see if the adverse symptoms disappear. Then you'll be told to add back the suspect foods one at a time to see whether the problems recur.

Sometimes it's hard to identify specific foods as the cause of the symptoms. If that's the case, the next step might be to follow a restrictive "elimination" diet in which all but very well tolerated foods are cut out. Gradually, items will be added back to see whether you develop a reaction in response to eating any of them. These "elimination" and "rechallenge" diets are also useful in identifying food intolerances.

Another method for determining food allergies is to use skin tests. Liquid extracts of single foods are placed either on your arm or back and pricked or scratched into the skin with a needle. If an itchy swelling appears within about 20 minutes, it means you had a "positive" response. One problem with skin tests, however, is that they are not completely reliable in showing a food that is causing a problem. In some cases, people develop skin reactions to foods that do not cause allergic reactions when eaten.

Still another test that is used to diagnose food allergies is called the RAST test, which involves mixing small samples of your blood with food extracts. If you are allergic to a particular food, measurable levels of allergy antibodies to that food will be detected. Because a RAST test is conducted outside the body, it has the advantage of being safer than a skin or challenge test for someone who might react severely to a specific food. But it has the disadvantage of being less accurate than a skin test.

If none of these tests reveals the source of your symptoms, the allergist may resort to a double-blind challenge. This test, usually performed under close supervision in the allergist's office or in a hospital, is one of the best ways of confirming both allergies and intolerances. The "challenge" involves giving the patient capsules of dried food suspected of causing reactions, as well as capsules containing a nonreactive substance. Neither the physician nor the patient knows which type of supplement is being administered at any given time. Thus, both are "blind." If symptoms occur after consumption of any of the food extracts but not after consumption of the nonreactive substance, the symptoms can truly be blamed on food. Double-blind challenges are especially valuable because they can detect, as well as rule out, allergies or intolerances to many foods and other substances, such as additives. They also eliminate nonfood factors that can cause symptoms, including psychological influences.

For all the legitimate ways to determine whether someone has a food allergy, there are at least as many tests and remedies that have never been proved accurate or effective. Nevertheless, quite a few of these approaches have popular followings and are employed by nontraditional physicians. The procedures have been promoted through such channels as best-selling books like *Dr. Berger's Immune Power Diet,* franchised clinics, and mail-order ads. Following is a review of some of the questionable theories and practices, many of which claim that foods are responsible for conditions ranging from anxiety to arthritis:

CLINICAL ECOLOGY

Clinical ecology sprang from a 1930s theory that food "allergies" cause a plethora of poorly defined problems, including headaches, itching, dizziness, insomnia, drowsiness, and epilepsy. Modern day "clinical ecologists" attribute similar ailments to hypersensitivities that certain people supposedly develop because their immune systems are damaged by chemically contaminated air, food and water. Consequently, clinical ecology patients are often placed on very strict "all natural" diets and may even be told to move to different locations.

An evaluation of clinical ecology methods shows that they do not meet the medically accepted requirements for treating illnesses. In one study, 50 patients who had been treated by clinical ecologists were found to have no food-induced immunologic abnormalities. Ironically, three out of five patients developed one or more new symptoms while undergoing clinical ecology treatment.

CYTOTOXIC TESTING

Also known as Bryan's test, leucocytotoxic testing and food sensitivity testing, cytotoxic testing involves taking small samples of blood, separating out the white blood cells, and mixing them with dried extracts of specific foods. If, upon examination with a microscope, the white cells change in shape or size in response to a particular food, the patient is said to have a "sensitivity" to that food.

The white blood cells are part of the immune system, and this gives the test its air of legitimacy. However, there is no evidence that the white blood cells of people with food allergies have defects that would cause them to take on a unique change in shape or size when they are exposed to foods outside the body. There *is* evidence that cytotoxic testing doesn't pick up food allergies when they really exist. In one study, the white blood cells of people with known food allergies reacted in the same way to allergenic as to non-allergenic foods. Further, test results appeared to be inconsistent, altering a person's cells on one day but not on the next. (Note: cytotoxic testing should not be confused with the RAST test, which involves a different type of reaction.)

PROVOCATION AND NEUTRALIZATION

Provocation and neutralization is a double-edged procedure. First, people are given doses of suspected allergenic foods—either as drops placed beneath the tongue or as injections—to provoke a reaction that corresponds to their complaints. Immediately following, weaker or stronger doses of the offending foods are introduced to neutralize the reaction. These tests are not effective and might be dangerous, since when someone has a real food allergy, the more of the offending food eaten, the more severe the reaction. Moreover, the patient's "reaction" in these cases is subjective, and the test is unable to reveal an immunologic cause.

Provocation and neutralization are not the same as the allergy shots or immunotherapy that patients sometimes receive from reputable allergists. These shots can be of value for individuals with allergies to such airborne substances as pollen. But they have not been shown to be effective in treating food allergies.

YEAST HYPERSENSITIVITY TREATMENT

Yeast hypersensitivity treatment is based on the theory that a host of ills, ranging from depression to headaches to schizophrenia to cancer, are caused by a sensitivity to yeast-like fungi called *Candida*. The belief is that the fungi multiply in the body and weaken the immune system. Treatment includes a diet in which all the yeast and mold-containing foods, as well as fruits and milk, are temporarily avoided. The patient is also told to stay away from refined carbohydrates and processed foods.

It is unreasonable to assume that *Candida* could cause the wide array of symptoms attributed to them, since they are ubiquitous organisms that inhabit the mouth, skin, and intestines of most healthy people without creating any problems. It's true that for a few people, *Candida* cause fungal infections on such areas as the skin and nails, but in no way do these individuals manifest the host of problems ascribed to "yeast sensitivity." Further, there is no evidence that the foods to be avoided stimulate yeast growth or weaken the immune system, as proponents of this theory claim.

In light of the proliferation of unscientific allergy theories that attribute all kinds of physical and psychological problems to food allergies or "sensitivities," it is easy to understand why so many individuals conclude that they suffer some sort of adverse reaction to food, even when they have never been tested and shown to have a problem. But there is no sound evidence that allergies and intolerances lead to many of the conditions they are said to bring about, including arthritis, anxiety, and muscle pains. Nor do they make people fat, a newly popular theory.

Many of the popular practitioners of food-allergy theories put the cart before the scientific horse, espousing untested dietary remedies based on little more than anecdotal case histories. A new medical treatment, such as a drug or diet, should not be recommended by physicians unless it has first been tested by researchers in what are known as clinical trials. In these experiments, the new treatment is tested under carefully controlled circumstances to make certain that no outside factors influence the results. To date, no clinical trial has conclusively demonstrated that food allergies or intolerances can bring on fatigue, depression, or other of the many problems ascribed to them. But it is easy to be swayed by the many "success stories" of people who reported dramatic health improvements when certain foods were avoided. Consider, for example, the dramatic turn for the better that is sometimes reported in hyperactive children when they are placed on additive-free diets. When the same children are placed on additive-free diets in a "blind" test, few, if any, show improvement.

Indeed, although many parents of hyperactive children will try just about any dietary technique to tame the unruly behavior, scientific studies have not shown that dietary intervention is of any value in most cases. (According to the American Academy of Allergy and Immunology, a small number of children do appear to become more hyperactive when they ingest some food dyes.) Perhaps the reason behavior sometimes improves with a special diet is that the new eating regimen requires the parents to devote more attention to their child.

What Are Food Intolerances?

Food intolerances are different from food allergies, either because they are unrelated to the immune system or because the immune system reacts in a different way than it does to allergenic proteins in foods. One such condition is lactose intolerance. People with this condition cannot adequately digest lactose, or milk sugar. Consuming products like milk and ice cream may lead to gas, diarrhea, and stomach cramps.

Another food intolerance is "gluten enteropathy," more commonly known as celiac disease. A person who suffers from it cannot eat gluten, a protein in wheat, rye, barley, and, to a lesser extent, oat products, without damaging the small intestine. The result is chronic diarrhea and abdominal pain.

Certain additives may cause intolerances, too. Tartrazine, or FD & C Yellow (Dye) # 5, for example, may induce asthma attacks in a very small minority of asthmatics. For that reason, manufacturers of foods containing this dye are now required to list it with the ingredients.

Sulfites can also bring on attacks in a few people who have asthma. They are used as preservatives in certain processed foods and dried fruits. Although previous estimates were higher, the number of sulfite-sensitive adult asthmatics now appears to be limited to fewer than 100,000 people in the United States.

Health problems that are not directly related to food do show some improvement in a minority of cases when the suspect food is eliminated. For example, while most headaches are not triggered by food, there is evidence that some migraine sufferers find relief by eliminating certain items. A cluster of other problems—asthma, for example—are thought to be specifically tied to milk and milk-based products in a very small number of children. Dairy products are also said to be the cause for persistent stuffy noses in some toddlers. Ear infections, too, have been linked to milk products in some preschoolers. But since ear infections usually disappear during the summer months, it is unlikely that milk is the cause.

A condition that may be aggravated by certain foods in afflicted children is eczema, a chronic itchy and scaly skin rash. Avoiding certain foods may partially alleviate the symptoms but will not make the condition go away.

Understanding Lactose Intolerance

For some people, eating milk products can cause severe abdominal cramps, bloating, and diarrhea. These people are "lactose-intolerant"—that is, they do not have enough lactase, the enzyme needed to digest lactose, the sugar found in milk and milk products. Lactose intolerance affects an estimated 50 million Americans. It can occur in one of three ways:

▶ After the age of two, some people gradually stop producing sufficient quantities of lactase, which breaks down lactose into the simple sugars glucose and galactose. The condition, which is usually inherited by non-Caucasians affects an estimated 70 percent of the world's population to some degree. People of African, Asian, and Mediterranean descent are more prone to lactose intolerance than others.

▶ A rare congenital disorder makes some people unable to produce lactase from the time they are born or to produce it only in limited amounts.

▶ Any illness that affects the lactase-producing cells of the small intestine, such as inflammatory bowel disease or even the flu, can induce a temporary lactase deficiency. However, in these cases, the condition is more likely to be temporary; once the damaged cells recover, they begin producing the enzyme again.

People who are milk-intolerant are usually lactose-intolerant and experience stomach upset and gas after drinking milk. In rare instances, however, the same symptoms are the result of a different problem, that is, an allergy to the protein in milk. For this reason, some physicians use a hydrogen breath test to diagnose lactose intolerance. When food containing lactose is not digested, hydrogen gas is produced, and its rate of expiration can be measured from the mouth. The more hydrogen gas produced, the more lactose-intolerant the patient is.

Lactose intolerance is not the same as milk intolerance. It is possible for most lactose-intolerant people to handle moderate amounts of milk or milk products over the course of a day without pain. If lactose-containing foods are eaten in conjunction with other foods, the chances of developing the symptoms are decreased. The intensity of symptoms increases as more lactose is consumed. When the concentration of undigested lactose becomes particularly high, the large intestine responds by drawing water from the surrounding tissues, causing watery diarrhea.

Milk is the food with the most lactose. Yogurt has the highest, although lactose-intolerant people don't appear to suffer from eating yogurt that has active cultures. That's because the bacteria in yogurt produces lactase that breaks down the milk sugar on its own. The same thing occurs in the production of cheese—generally, hard, aged cheeses, such as Swiss and cheddar, contain less lactose than softer cheeses.

Sweet acidophilus milk is sometimes said to be good for milk-intolerant people, but because it does not have reduced levels of milk sugar they do not tolerate it any better than regular milk. Cultured buttermilk is slightly lower in lactose content than regular milk, but it does not agree with most milk-intolerant people either.

Fortunately, there are a number of dairy products on the market designed for those who are milk-intolerant. These specially treated products make it possible for milk-intolerant people to benefit from the major nutrients found in milk foods, such as calcium, vitamins A and D, riboflavin, and protein. LactAid, a company that caters specifically to people with the problem, adds a lactase solution to milk, ice cream, and cottage cheese. As a result, much of the lactose in these foods is broken down to glucose and galactose before it reaches the body. This gives the products a sweeter taste since each of these sugars is sweeter on its own than in the combined form of lactose. For those who want to add lactase to their own milk, LactAid now supplies lactase in both liquid and tablet form. The liquid version has to be added to milk 24 hours before serving in order for the lactose to be sufficiently broken down. The tablets are swallowed before a meal and go to work almost immediately.

There are also many nondairy products that can be used as alternatives to dairy foods. Ice cream can be replaced by a number of desserts made with tofu or fruit instead of with milk. And soymilk, although not a perfect substitute for cow's milk since it lacks calcium and some vitamins, is widely available in health-food stores, including in fortified forms.

Diet-Induced Skin Reactions

A number of well-known vitamin deficiency states are associated with abnormalities of the skin. For example, severe vitamin C deficiency, leading to *scurvy*, is accompanied by bleeding of the skin and gums. Deficiency of niacin leads to *pellagra*, which is characterized by a severe skin rash on parts of the body exposed to the sun. Deficiencies of other B vitamins and vitamin A may be associated with *dermatitis* and mucous-membrane changes such as mouth ulcers and redness and cracking at the corners of the mouth. However, these symptoms appear only with very severe deficiencies.

There's no truth to the assumption that topical application of vitamins or ingesting special vitamin supplements will improve your skin. In some cases, they might even hurt skin. For example, too much vitamin A can make the skin rough and dry. High doses of niacin cause itching and flushing in some people. And despite vitamin E's wide use as a topical solution, there is no proof that it provides anything more effective than the soothing qualities of the oil in which it is contained. Vitamin E even causes acne and rashes in some people.

There is also no evidence to support the notion that vitamin treatments can slow down or reverse the effects of aging on the skin. One of the causes of wrinkling is exposure to the ultraviolet rays of the sun, and the only known way to prevent the sun's damaging effects is to wear sunscreeen and avoid sunbathing.

What about the relationship of the foods we eat to the tendency to get *acne?* In spite of the wide belief that certain foods, such as sugar, chocolate, and dairy products, cause acne, the relationship has never been proved. Today, most dermatologists minimize the effects of diet on acne, except when patients do not respond to other treatments and the specific food or food group can be identified as causing the problem.

The latest "wonder" treatment for acne and aging skin is Retin-A, made from a synthetic derivative of vitamin A. It has been effective in some severe cases of acne, but it appears to work as a drug, not a vitamin, and must be used only under close medical supervision because of the possible side effects. It must never be used by pregnant women (or shortly prior to pregnancy) because of the potential for birth defects.

One allergenic skin disease that is clearly associated with food is urticaria, or *hives,* which afflicts one in five Americans. The most common food offenders are eggs, nuts, beans, chocolate, strawberries, tomatoes, fish, pork, corn, citrus fruits, and certain condiments and spices. Some synthetic food additives, such as the dye tartrazine (FD & C yellow dye #5) and the preservative sodium benzoate, can also cause hives, as can the naturally occurring salicylates in almonds, apples, peaches, potatoes, and a number of other foods. In addition, the small amounts of salicylates and benzoates in blueberries, bananas, green peas, lingonberries, and licorice may cause problems for some people. Salicylates are also found in aspirin-containing compounds.

It is often difficult to isolate the cause of hives, which may be related to drugs and yeast infections as well as foods. However, if specific foods are identified by a dermatologist or allergist as causing the problem, it is important to be sure that major amounts of nutrients are not eliminated from your diet, and that you replace forbidden foods with other that offer the same nutrients.

Atopic eczema, or *dermatitis,* is an itchy, red, and scaly rash that tends to run in families. There is some debate about the extent to which diet contributes to this hereditary condition, but at least one study has shown that children with eczema improved when they eliminated certain foods. Another study reported that oral supplements of evening primrose seed oil had beneficial effects, but the research on its benefits remains in the experimental stages.

The cause of *psoriasis,* characterized by red, scaly patches that result from skin cells being produced at a greater-than normal rate, is still not known. Research in progress suggests that an abnormality in the production of certain metabolic products of a fatty acid, arachidonic acid, may play an important role. Since body levels of some of these metabolic products may be affected by certain foods, it is conceivable that diet may play a role in its cure. But the matter is still in research, and supposedly effective treatments, such as lecithin and other vitamins, are of no benefit.

Some people develop rashes simply from touching certain foods. For example, mangoes contain an allergen similar to poison ivy allergens and can cause a similar rash. Oils of cinnamon, oranges, and certain preservatives can produce hand dermatitis, especially for people who have repeated exposure, such as bakers and chefs. In certain instances, a chemical, drug, or food that causes a rash upon skin contact can produce a similar result when it's taken orally. Cashew nuts, for example, contain a chemical related to poison ivy allergens, and a generalized rash from eating cashews has been observed in a few exceptionally sensitive people.

Rosacea is a chronic facial eruption in which acne-like blemishes appear along with redness and flushing. A number of foods and drinks have long been recognized as factors that exacerbate the condition. For example, alcoholic beverages and spicy foods are thought to agitate rosacea by causing repeated flushing.

The relationship of diet to skin problems is hard to study since many of the conditions undergo spontaneous remission. Although scientists have not ruled out even some of the most outlandish claims, neither have they found evidence to substantiate them. Caution is in order until proper scientific research confirms courses of treatment.

PART FIVE

Keeping Fit and Trim

Obesity has become a crisis in the United States for young and old alike, increasing the risks for heart disease, hypertension, diabetes, and other health problems. There is evidence that obesity, as we know it today, is a relatively new condition, related to both the increased availability of food and the technology that has made the process of procuring and preparing food less strenuous. In fact, anthropologists and other scientists speculate that the efficiency with which our bodies store calories might have an ancestral basis: The storage mechanism helped prevent starvation during prehistoric times when food was scarce. For this reason, plumpness was often considered a sign of affluence and good health. In women, it was often equated with fertility and maternity, since adequate fat stores are essential for the successful bearing and nurturing of infants. Today, in industrial societies, the emphasis has changed to the point where being lean is associated with health and affluence, and excess weight is considered unhealthy and undesirable.

But the question of ideal weight and body fat is far more complicated than a simple fat versus lean evaluation. For, at the same time that we express concern with the growing problem of obesity in the United States, we also observe with concern the intensification of a lean-body bias that has spawned a $30 billion weight-loss industry. All too often, the emphasis of this industry is placed on arbitrary cosmetic standards rather than true health concerns. While sidestepping the legitimate questions of nutrient sufficiency, many weight-loss programs stress the social advantages of being thin. The thin-body bias of our society has created new issues for nutritionists, including the damaging effects of chronic dieting and how to address a new population of people who engage in forced starvation. Nevertheless, health-damaging obesity grows as a problem in a society where diet and weight-loss are obsessional concerns.

253

It is our intention in this section to examine the fundamental issues regarding nutrition and obesity, and to reframe the dialogue about weight and fat. Specifically, we will focus on:

▶ The distinction between cosmetic and health concerns regarding body fat and weight

▶ The different criteria for determining healthy weight

▶ The genetic factors that influence body shape and size

▶ The research about the health-related dangers of obesity

▶ The ways that our cultural thin-body bias often interferes with achieving healthy weight

▶ The new health crisis presented by the large number of people with eating disorders

▶ The criteria for legitimate approaches to weight loss and nutritional well-being

▶ A weight-loss approach that emphasizes nutrition and self-sufficiency

▶ The role of physical exercise in fitness and health, and practical guidelines for exercise programs

We believe that it is time for health professionals in this country to take a stand against the weight-loss-diet charlatans whose scientifically unproven, gimmicky, and often unhealthful approaches to diet have distracted the public from focusing on the true issues of health and fitness. It is our conviction that if people would stop following false promises and, instead, listen to the evidence that scientists now have about how to maintain a healthful body size and weight, the problem of obesity could be successfully addressed in our society.

22

Fight Fat Nutritionally

According to the 1985 National Health Interview Survey, nearly 50 percent of all American women and 30 percent of all American men report that they are engaged in the process of losing weight, either by reducing calorie intake, increasing physical exercise, or both. While this involvement indicates a positive trend of increased interest in health and fitness, it also raises new questions for health and nutrition professionals about how to define healthy versus unhealthy weight, and what are the most appropriate and nutritionally responsible methods for treating obesity.

Defining Ideal Weight

The most commonly used measure of healthy weight has been the Metropolitan Life Insurance Company's height and weight tables, first developed in the 1940s and revised in 1959 and again in 1983. The tables were established based on the evaluation of the weight-for-height ratios of insured persons with the greatest longevity. The tables give a range of weight-for-height, with the midpoint being considered the "ideal" for most people (see table).

In recent years, the validity of using these tables as a basis for evaluating healthy weight has been seriously questioned by a number of health researchers and nutrition experts. Not only do the tables fail to consider the percentage of body fat and fat distribution, the methodologies used might not have been accurate determinants for judging the overall population. In particular, critics cite the self-selection aspects of the study; although data was collected on nearly 5 million people, they were all purchasers of life insurance and may not be indicative of the general population since, statistically, insured people tend to be generally healthier and have longer life spans than the overall population. The insured population also tends to be predominantly white, middle-class males who are not necessarily representative of other groups. Furthermore, the data were not scientifically gathered or always consistent. Some study subjects answered questions about weight on insurance forms but were not independently weighed; others, who were weighed, sometimes wore shoes and clothing and sometimes did not.

The largest issue, however, relates to the overall criteria for determining ideal healthy weight. Height-to-weight tables are certainly valuable measures that help people determine safe weight ranges. But it is clear that it's not appropriate to think of them as rigid standards; rather, they offer general guidelines. Since the Metropolitan tables

Metropolitan Life Insurance Company
Desirable Weights in Pounds for Ages 25–29

| Height | 1959 table | | 1983 table | |
	Men	Women	Men	Women
4′10″		91-119		100-131
4′11″		93-122		101-134
5′0″		96-125		103-137
5′1″	107-136	99-128	123-145	105-140
5′2″	110-139	102-131	125-148	108-144
5′3″	113-143	105-135	127-151	111-148
5′4″	116-147	108-139	129-155	114-152
5′5″	119-151	111-143	131-159	117-156
5′6″	123-156	115-147	133-163	120-160
5′7″	127-161	119-151	135-167	123-164
5′8″	131-165	123-155	137-171	126-167
5′9″	135-169	127-160	139-175	129-170
5′10″	139-174	131-165	141-179	132-173
5′11″	143-179	135-170	144-183	135-176
6′0″	147-184		147-187	
6′1″	151-189		150-192	
6′2″	155-194		153-197	
6′3″	159-199		157-202	

The Metropolitan Life Insurance Company tables of desirable weights (copyright, 1983, Metropolitan Life Insurance Company) were most recently revised in 1983. Here is shown a comparison with the earlier 1959 table. The low number refers to a person with a "small" frame size; the high number refers to a person with a "large" frame size; and "medium" frame size. The Metropolitan Life Insurance Company offers these guidelines for measuring your frame size: Extend one arm and bend the forearm upward at a 90 degree angle.

Keep fingers straight and turn the inside of your wrist toward your body. Place the thumb and index finger of your other hand on the two prominent bones on either side of your bent elbow. Pull your fingers away, maintaining the space between them. Measure the space between your fingers and compare it with the numbers on the table below. If your measurement is lower than these, you have a small frame; if it is higher, you have a large frame; if it falls within the range, you have a medium frame.

MEN		WOMEN	
5′2″ - 5′3″	2½″ - 2 ⅞″	4′10″ - 4′11″	2¼″ - 2½″
5′4″ - 5′7″	2⅝″ - 2⅞″	5′0″ - 5′3″	2¼″ - 2½″
5′8″ - 5′11″	2¾″ - 3⅛″	5′4″ - 5′7″	2 ⅜″ - 3⅝″
6′0″ - 6′3″	2 ⅞″ - 3¼″	5′8″ - 5′11″	2⅜″ - 2 ⅝″
6′4″	2⅞″ - 3¼″	6′0″	2½″ - 2¾″

Gerontology Research Center
Recommended Weights in Pounds for Both Sexes

Height	20-29yr	30-39yr	40-49yr	50-59yr	60-69yr
4'10"	84-111	92-119	99-127	107-135	115-142
4'11"	87-115	95-123	103-131	111-139	119-147
5'0"	90-119	98-127	106-135	114-143	123-152
5'1"	93-123	101-131	110-140	118-148	127-157
5'2"	96-127	105-136	113-144	122-153	131-163
5'3"	99-131	108-140	117-149	126-158	135-168
5'4"	102-135	112-145	121-154	130-163	140-173
5'5"	106-140	115-149	125-159	134-168	144-179
5'6"	109-144	119-154	129-164	138-174	148-184
5'7"	112-148	122-159	133-169	143-179	153-190
5'8"	116-153	126-163	137-174	147-184	158-196
5'9"	119-157	130-168	141-179	151-190	162-201
5'10"	122-162	134-173	145-184	156-195	167-207
5'11"	126-167	137-178	149-190	160-201	172-213
6'0"	129-171	141-183	153-195	165-207	177-219
6'1"	133-176	145-188	157-200	169-213	182-225
6'2"	137-181	149-194	162-206	174-219	187-232
6'3"	141-186	153-199	166-212	179-225	192-238
6'4"	144-191	157-205	171-218	184-231	197-244

were first published, investigators in the field have discovered important new evidence that age, body composition, and body fat distribution are as important, and sometimes more important, than overall weight.

Taking Age into Account

There are a number of conflicting views regarding the accuracy of weight-to-height measures. Surveys of health and longevity and average height-to-weight ratios have been hampered by a number of shifting factors, in particular, the changes in weight patterns that occur as people age. Many scientists now believe that height-

weight charts must take age into account in order to be accurate.

In 1984, the Gerontology Research Center published a table adapted from earlier work of Reubin Andres, Edwin L. Bierman, and William R. Hazzard. The table provides recommended weight-to-height ratios for men and women in five age groups: 20 to 29 years, 30 to 39 years, 40 to 49 years, 50 to 59 years, and 60 to 69 years (see table). The age-adapted tables indicate changing weight patterns with age. For example, a 5'4" woman between the ages of 30 and 39 might have a healthy weight range of 112 to 145 pounds; between the ages of 40 and 49, the healthy range becomes 121 to 154 pounds. By contrast the Metropolitan tables give only one range for all women who are 5′4″, which is 124 to 138 pounds.

Evaluating Body Composition

It was traditionally assumed that excess weight was mostly the result of excess fat. While this is generally true, it is not always the case. To use one clear example, a boxer might have a weight that is substantially greater than that given for his height, but it is still possible that he has a "healthy" weight, since a high percentage of his weight is accounted for by muscle, not fat. Also, some people have larger body frames than those given in traditional height-weight charts; in their cases, weight and height alone would not be a valid measure for determining excess fat.

An accurate measurement of body composition (overall percentage of fat-to-lean tissue) can only be conducted in a clinical setting. The test most commonly used measures the skin-fold thickness in the shoulder and triceps areas. The amount of adipose (fat) tissue determined by the test is then subtracted from the total body weight to find the percent of fat to total weight.

There are a variety of more accurate (and more complex) ways of measuring body fat, but skin-fold measures are adequate for most people. In fact, the average person doesn't need a scientific method to determine the presence of excess fat. A good home method involves grasping the skin beneath the upper arm between both thumbs. If more than an inch of skin sticks out, there is probably excess fat in the body.

Body-Fat Distribution

New evidence suggests that excess body fat in some locations is more dangerous than in others. Studies show that people (usually men) who have excess fat in their abdominal areas suffer many health risks while people (usually women) who carry extra fat in their buttocks, hips, and thighs suffer few health risks associated with this fat. This theory, often referred to as "belly versus butt,"

proposes that, except in cases of overall obesity, having extra padding on the lower part of the body is not necessarily a health risk, while carrying fat in the stomach and upper body may be very risky.

The female hormone estrogen actually encourages fat in the hips, thighs, and buttocks, since the reserve is needed in late pregnancy and during breast-feeding. The often-voiced complaint of many women that "My hips are too fat," seems to be irrelevant from a health standpoint; in fact, anorexics and women who engage in semistarvation diets often stop menstruating, the body's signal that they're not carrying enough fat stores to support the reproductive process.

On the other hand, excess fat cells in the abdominal area are more likely to be associated with increased health hazards, including interference with the metabolism of insulin (leading to diabetes) and an increase in the liver's production of triglycerides and cholesterol (leading to heart disease and strokes).

To some extent, fat distribution is observable —you can see that you have broad hips or a potbelly. But clinical tests are available that measure fat distribution with some accuracy. The most common method measures the ratio of the abdominal area to the widest portion of the hips. The waist-to-hip ratio is then measured against criteria, different for men and women, that are used to determine a healthy ratio. Waist-to-hip ratio can be determined with a tape measure: Measure the circumference of the waist, then the widest part of the hip, and divide the first number by the second. The average healthy ratio is below 0.8 for women and 1.0 for men.

Genetics Makes a Difference

We do not completely understand all the factors that lead to obesity, but we know that it is much more complicated than what you eat and how much you exercise. In addition to overeating and underexercising, there is evidence that heredity and altered metabolic functions also contribute to obesity.

Some of the most significant studies relating obesity to heredity versus environment have been conducted by Canadian researcher Dr. Claude Bouchard and his colleagues. In one study, Bouchard fed an additional 1,000 calories a day to six sets of identical twins. When the results were evaluated, it was found that weight gain within the sets of twins was almost identical, while weight gain among the different groups differed greatly. The same pattern was observed when exercise was increased by several hours a day. So, although the weight gain varied notably among unrelated individuals who consumed the same number of calories, it tended to be fairly consistent between twins, suggesting that genetics plays a role in the determination of body weight.

Another study, conducted by Albert Stunkard and his colleagues at the University of Pennsylvania, examined the adult heights and weights of more than 4,000 people who were adopted as children, and compared them with both their adoptive and biological parents. Results indicated that the heights and weights of the adoptees were similar to their biological parents and not to their adoptive parents, suggesting that environmental factors may have less control over certain aspects of body size than heredity.

New studies are also being conducted that suggest hereditary implications for both metabolic rate (the efficiency with which people use calories) and fat-cell size and number. All of these studies are designed to identify whether some people might have hereditary tendencies toward obesity.

But there is a separate issue related to weight and heredity that applies to our cultural stereotypes. Scientists know that physical characteristics, such as eye and hair color, are genetically determined. So too are height and body shape. Those people who ignore the hereditary realities of their body size and shape are bound to be frustrated when ceaseless dieting and exercise does

not produce a body that is identical to that of their favorite movie star. In our society, we tend to be intolerant of people who don't fit an idealized norm, and this prejudice causes needless pain for people who have inherited stockier physiques.

The Fallacies of Chronic Dieting

All of the factors described above must be taken into account when deciding whether to embark upon a weight-loss regimen. And new evidence shows that chronic dieting, sometimes called the "yo-yo syndrome," can be ineffective. Current studies indicate that chronic dieters might actually find it harder and harder to lose weight over time, even if they follow the same diet practices. According to Kelly Brownell, Ph.D., a professor of psychiatry at the University of Pennsylvania School of Medicine, the more often you diet, the more your body might actually resist shedding pounds.

In a study with laboratory rats, Dr. Brownell observed that after the animals regained weight they had lost on a weight-reducing regimen, it took them more than twice as long to lose weight the second time, even though the number of calories they were fed on the weight-loss diet did not change. The difference is thought to be the result of a slowdown in the metabolic rate. The body may respond to repeated efforts at weight loss by automatically lowering its metabolic rate to protect against what it interprets as too much starvation. In studies conducted with high school and college wrestlers, Dr. Brownell found that those who lose and gain pounds frequently have significantly lower metabolic rates than wrestlers who maintain steady weights.

C. Wayne Callaway, M.D., an endocrinologist who has studied the effects of chronic dieting on patients at the Mayo Clinic and at George Washington University Medical Center in Washington, D.C., reported patients whose metabolic rates were so low that they were unable to lose weight

▶ NUTRITION QUIZ ◀

Are You Caught in the Thin Obsession?

For many Americans, the "thin obsession" is a way of life: being thin is equivalent to being desirable, successful, and worthwhile. It is more important than talent, intellectual ability, personality, or any of the other factors that make humans attractive to one another. Take this test to find out whether you're a victim of the thin obsession.

1. The first thing you notice about other people is their weight.
   True _____   False _____

2. You believe people who are overweight are lazy, lack discipline, or don't care about themselves.
   True _____   False _____

3. You believe that thin people are more attractive to the opposite sex.
   True _____   False _____

4. Staying thin is a way of proving to yourself that you have discipline, stamina, and control.
   True _____   False _____

5. At times, you have put off socializing, taking a vacation, interviewing for a job, or otherwise putting yourself in a public situation until you have lost a few pounds.
   True _____   False _____

6. Even though you know that extreme dieting can compromise you nutritionally, you feel that it is sometimes worth it to lose weight fast.
   True _____   False _____

7. If you gain any weight at all, you feel disgusted with yourself.
   True _____   False _____

8. You don't think you'll ever be "too thin."
   True _____   False _____

Examine your responses. The more times you answered "True," the more you are obsessed with body shape and weight.

on diets containing as few as 800 calories a day. Noted Dr. Callaway, "The patients assumed that they needed to consume fewer and fewer calories in order to lose when, in fact, they needed to consume more calories to restore their metabolic balance."

Dr. Callaway further pointed out that most extreme low-calorie diets have a diuretic effect in the early stages that causes a large initial weight loss, which is mostly water. But in what is also believed to be a protective impulse, the kidneys, being depleted of too much water and essential minerals, begin to cause the body to retain water. The weight loss stops, and large water-weight gains may occur, leading the dieter to believe that he or she has failed.

Diets that are very low in calories and that promote dietary practices that cause deficiencies in essential nutrients are in abundant supply in America. The consensus among health professionals is that these diets are not healthy and usually not successful. The failure rate of low-calorie diets is estimated to be as high as 90 percent. Although statistics are not available regarding the percentage of dieters who have unhealthy weights, it is obvious that many people are consuming nutritionally deficient diets to match the lean-body standards of our culture. The intense social pressure to be thin has led to an entire population of weight- and food-obsessed individuals for whom losing five, ten, or twenty pounds is a primary focus. Even if some of these people do have unhealthy weights, chronic dieting patterns are likely to cause greater health risks in the long run.

Overcoming the 10-Pound Obsession

People who diet as a way of life do more than just limit their daily calorie intake. They spend an inordinate amount of psychological energy worrying about what they will, will not, or did eat. They develop a type of "diet head" that prompts them to set strict rules for how many calories they allow themselves per meal or per day and for which foods are "forbidden." The "diet head" may lead to daily weigh-ins and to extreme anxiety if the scale registers even the slightest upward fluctuation. It may also lead to a cycle of starving followed by overeating, and then guilt and self-disgust at their lack of control.

University of Toronto psychologists Janet Polivy, Ph.D., and C. Peter Herman, Ph.D., have coined the term "restrained eaters" to describe this population of people who are obsessively concerned about eating and overeating and who, as a result, are almost always dieting. They contend that the very rigidity of the restraint these people impose upon themselves causes them to end up losing control and overeating. In other words, once the dieter breaks the self-imposed "rules" by eating a forbidden food or consuming more than the allowed calories, what Polivy and Herman call the "what-the-hell" effect occurs, and they overeat.

The diet-obsessed segment of the population is not helped by the many conflicting messages they receive every day from the media. For example, one magazine ran an article entitled "Are You a Fitaholic?" as a way of helping people cope with an "addiction" to exercise, only to follow it several months later with a positive story about a woman who maintained her weight loss by combining five different exercise programs which took more than an hour and a half each day. Another magazine published, in the same issue, a feature about the dangers of anorexia and a diet plan that restricted calories to 800 per day.

Readers of popular magazines can also be confused by articles with titles like "It's No Longer 'In' to Be Pencil-Thin," that share pages with advertisements that use tall, thin models. And, while some of our favorite movie and television stars are showing more curves these days, not many average people can hope to look as curvaceously glamorous as they do.

These mixed messages contribute to a central problem that weight-obsessed people have: They lose touch with the normal body mechanisms that prompt people to eat when they are hungry and to stop eating when they become full. Of course, everyone overeats once in a while or, conversely, does not eat for one reason or another. But for chronic dieters, ignoring hunger pains, as well as feelings of satiety, is a way of life. They often pass up food they really want in order to keep their weight down and then eat beyond the point of feeling full when they do start eating.

Chronic dieters often feel deprived, not only because they so often avoid eating when they're hungry, but also because they define foods as being either "good" or "bad." The "bad" foods are often those they find most pleasurable and therefore have to seek control over. They are incapable of participating in special occasions in a relaxed manner; a party or dinner out becomes an occasion to dread because the "bad" food temptations will be so great. While others around them are enjoying the pleasures of food, the chronic dieters are feeling deprived and depressed. If they do give in and allow themselves a forbidden food, they are ridden with guilt and even depression.

If you are a chronic dieter, the best way to control your diet is to drop some of the controls. Establish a normal eating pattern so that your hunger cues will return. Eat regular meals so you won't be thinking about food all the time. Stop applying "good" and "bad" labels to food. If a beloved food is not low in calories, don't deprive yourself completely. Rather, allow an occasional treat and limit the portion size.

You can also avoid feelings of depression and failure if you stop relying on arbitrary external measures of diet success or failure. For example, daily weight fluctuations are meaningless. Everyone's weight shifts slightly from day to day, but it is the balance of water that is shifting, not fat. Many women retain five or more pounds of water prior to their menstrual periods, but this weight gain is not related to the success or failure of a diet program. Besides, factors such as fat distribution and total body mass can't be recorded on the scale. People who are exercising and building muscle may even find that they weigh more, since muscle is heavier than fat. If you are trying to lose weight, you'll get a more accurate reading by weighing yourself once a week or even once every two weeks.

Eating Disorders—A Growing Crisis

Anorexia nervosa, the syndrome of self-induced starvation, is estimated to be two to four times as common today as it was 30 years ago. Bulimia nervosa, a related syndrome characterized by recurrent episodes of binge eating and subsequent vomiting, laxative abuse, or fasting, also appears to be growing more common. Some researchers believe that the two eating disorders together may afflict as many as 1 to 5 percent of high school and college women.

According to Marilyn Crim, M.D., Ph.D., assistant professor at the Tufts School of Nutrition, part of the problem lies in the way that self-esteem is tied to body image for many women. "Thinness has become synonymous with excellence in our society," says Dr. Crim. "And in the last few decades, the message has become 'the thinner, the better.' The Miss Americas and the *Playboy* centerfolds have become thinner and thinner since the early 1960s, while the average woman has become heavier. So the goal to be thin has moved further out of reach, and that contributes to people being obsessive about it."

Anorexia nervosa, which is most common in young girls, is often related to the quest for perfection, which includes meeting the standards for the thin-body ideal. Sometimes the message is passed on from thin-obsessed mothers to their daughters, but, even when it's not, there are plenty of places for young girls to pick up the message. The pattern of anorexia may begin as early as nine or ten years old, but it often intensifies during puberty. Then, as the girl's breasts begin to develop and her body becomes rounder, she seeks to remain lean by furiously dieting and exercising. In some cases, anorexia is brought on by feelings of shame over her emerging sexuality, and the young girl seeks to control her development and remain a nonsexual little girl.

Unfortunately, anorexia often remains undiagnosed until its victims are already extremely wasted. In part, that's because losing weight and controlling food intake is seen as such a positive

Do You Have the "Diet Head"?

Chronic dieters do more than just diet. They have a "diet head"—a set of self-punishing habits they use to control their food intake and their weight. Sometimes these habits are so ingrained that the dieters don't even realize they're obsessed about food. Might that be true for you? Take this quiz and find out.

1. How often do you diet in a conscious effort to control your weight?
   (a) rarely or never   (b) sometimes   (c) usually   (d) always

2. Would a five-pound fluctuation in your weight affect the way you feel about yourself?
   (a) not at all   (b) slightly   (c) moderately   (d) greatly

3. Do you feel guilty if you overeat or skip an exercise session?
   (a) rarely   (b) sometimes   (c) usually   (d) always

4. How likely are you to eat less than you really want?
   (a) unlikely   (b) somewhat likely   (c) often likely   (d) very likely

5. To what extent do you diet all day and then overeat at night, pledging that you'll start your diet again tomorrow?
   (a) never   (b) occasionally   (c) often   (d) constantly

6. If you are on a diet and you eat a food that is not "allowed," do you then go on a splurge and eat other high-calorie foods?
   (a) never   (b) occasionally   (c) often   (d) always

7. How frequently do you avoid bringing "forbidden" foods into the house?
   (a) never   (b) sometimes   (c) often   (d) very often.

8. How much food do you typically eat when you attend social events, such as parties or picnics?
   (a) just enough to feel satisfied   (b) a little too much   (c) enough to feel uncomfortable   (d) enough to feel sick

9. How often do you weigh yourself?
   (a) hardly ever   (b) once a week   (c) once a day   (d) more than once a day

10. How many times have you lost, and then regained, more than five pounds in the past ten years?
    (a) never   (b) rarely   (c)more than five times   (d) more than ten times

This quiz was adapted from the "Three Factor Eating Questionnaire" developed by Dr. Albert J. Stunkard and Dr. Samuel Messick, published in the *Journal of Psychosomatic Research*. The more you circled "c" or "d," the more likely it is that you have self-punishing diet habits and excessive concern about your weight.

thing in our society. It's also due to the fact that the anorexic girl is usually compulsive about perfection in all arenas, not just with her body. She'll get perfect grades in school, be exceptionally neat, and not behave in rebellious ways. Parents are often delighted that their child is not a "problem," and they praise this behavior, thereby reinforcing it.

Anorexia nervosa can be a life-threatening disease, with symptoms that are common in malnourished populations suffering famine conditions. If not treated, victims will continue until they literally starve themselves to death. It is not uncommon for hospitals to admit patients who are as much as 40 percent below normal body weight. Treatment is never easy. Those with anorexia nervosa resist it because they fear weight gain.

Bulimia is a form of anorexia, but its characteristics differ. Dr. Crim says, "The feeling I get from bulimic patients is that they see themselves as failed anorexics. Anorexia is the gold standard for them." Indeed bulimics often have a great deal in common with anorexics. They also tend to be young women, although the onset of bulimia usually occurs in somewhat older individuals. Bulimics are also obsessed with the idea of being thin and usually begin with a period of dieting.

Bulimics will binge, most often in secret, on rich foods like cookies, cake, and candy. Bingeing episodes are usually terminated only with abdominal pain, self-induced vomiting (purging), sleep, or the arrival of another person.

Bulimia is harder to diagnose than anorexia nervosa since many bulimics are of normal weight. Also, since bulimia usually starts when girls are in their late teens or early twenties, they're more easily able to hide their condition than are younger teenagers who are more closely supervised.

While bulimia may not lead to the type of severe malnutrition seen in anorexics, over time, serious complications can arise. Constant vomiting can lead to acid erosion of the esophagus, the gums, and the teeth. Those who use vomit-inducing chemicals run the risk of ripping the esophagus, a rare but potentially fatal complication. Constant vomiting can also lead to dehydration, loss of potassium, and kidney damage.

DIAGNOSTIC CRITERIA FOR ANOREXIA AND BULIMIA

Anorexia Nervosa

A. Refusal to maintain body weight over a minimal normal weight for age and height, e.g., weight loss leading to maintenance of body weight 15 percent below that expected; or failure to make expected weight gain during period of growth, leading to body weight 15 percent below that expected

B. Intense fear of gaining weight or becoming fat, even though underweight

C. Disturbance in the way in which one's body weight, size, or shape is experienced, e.g., the person claims to "feel fat" even when emaciated, or believes that one area of the body is "too fat" even when obviously underweight

D. In females, absence of at least three consecutive menstrual cycles when these would otherwise be expected to occur (primary or secondary amenorrhea). A woman is considered to have amenorrhea if her periods occur only following administration of a hormone, such as estrogen

Bulimia

A. Recurrent episodes of binge eating (rapid consumption of a large amount of food in a discrete period of time)

B. A feeling of lack of control over eating behavior during the eating binges

C. Regular occurrence of self-induced vomiting, use of laxatives or diuretics, strict dieting or fasting, or vigorous exercise to prevent weight gain

D. A minimum average of two binge eating episodes a week for at least 3 months

E. Persistent overconcern with body shape and weight

Source: *Diagnostic and Statistical Manual of Mental Disorders,* 3rd edition, revised. American Psychiatric Association, 1987.

Treatment for anorexia nervosa and bulimia requires medical, nutritional, and psychological intervention and, according to Dr. Crim, usually takes a minimum of one to two years. People who have reason to be concerned might want to contact one of the organizations listed in The Nutrition Hotline at the back of this book.

Options for Weight Loss

For those segments of the population who are above their healthy weight and need to lose, there are hundreds of diet options available. For some people, group support or structured programs are helpful. The best ones will include behavior modification and psychological support for those who need it. They emphasize sensible eating patterns and nutritious foods, and avoid gimmickry or the promotion of special foods and supplements. They allow sufficient calories and encourage dieters to participate in exercise programs in conjunction with the diet.

Occasionally, more extreme dietary procedures are needed. But, according to Tufts weight control experts Robin Kanarek, Ph.D., and Nilla Orthen-Gambill, Ph.D., these extreme measures, such as gastric balloons or liquid formula diets, are usually warranted only if the excess weight poses a greater health hazard than the reduction method itself.

In light of that advice, how are people to evaluate the increasing popularity of liquid diets? These formula diets returned to vogue in the late 1980s, spurred on by celebrity dieters such as television talk-show host Oprah Winfrey, who proudly modeled her "size 10 body" for millions of TV viewers. Oprah's regimen of choice was Optifast, one of several liquid diet programs currently being marketed. Unlike the liquid protein diets of the 1970s whose incomplete nutritional content led to a number of deaths, these new liquid formulas contain high-quality protein, as well as necessary amounts of vitamins and minerals.

More than 300,000 people have gone through Optifast since its inception in 1976, paying the heavy price of $2,500 for the 26-week regimen. Other companies currently marketing liquid formula diets include Medifast, Ultra Slim-Fast, and a fasting program called HMR.

Optifast, which is offered only through clinics and hospitals on an outpatient basis, was designed for severely overweight people, and the company says that only people who are at least 50 pounds overweight or 30 percent above their "reference" weight (as shown on the Metropolitan height-to-weight charts) are allowed to participate. The program involves patients taking the formula—powder dissolved in water—about five times a day for twelve weeks. They are then gradually reintroduced to solid foods that are consistent with a healthy diet; they also undertake a behavior modification program.

For people whose obesity puts them at high risk for disease, Optifast and other very low calorie liquid diets might be an appropriate medically supervised treatment. Four out of five patients who stick with it (up to half drop out) lose an average of 40 pounds. Whether the weight stays off is another matter. According to George Blackburn, M.D., Ph.D., chief of the Nutrition/Metabolism Laboratory at the New England Deaconess Hospital in Boston, the propensity to regain weight you lose that fast is three times as great as when it is lost more slowly. "People who lose 25 pounds and keep it off and then go on to lose another 25 pounds have a much better chance of keeping off 40 to 50 pounds of excess weight," he says. Dr. Blackburn also suggests that the message Oprah communicated to her millions of viewers should have stressed the health issue rather than putting so much emphasis on "the glorification of size 10." If the concern is health, many Americans can substantially lower their risks of disease by losing 20 or 30 out of a desired 50 pounds, even if they don't measure up to the current standards of (thin) beauty.

Another consideration when evaluating liquid formula diets is the fact that not every person's body responds in the same way. Some people lose more lean muscle tissue than others during a fast, even if their goal is to lose fat and spare muscle. For this reason, a "one formula fits all" approach is questionable. Further, even when programs are set up as "medically supervised," the extent of the supervision must be examined. For some people, a heavily restricted liquid diet could lead to serious problems—such as thyroid imbalances or heart stress—and they should be monitored frequently, even daily.

Choosing a Safe and Successful Diet Program

Liquid diets and other extreme regimens are not appropriate for the average American. But it's easy to become confused by the plethora of weight-loss programs, all of which claim to have the method that "really works." In the next chapter, we introduce an approach that can help you achieve self-sufficiency while you learn how to structure a healthy, low-calorie, low-fat diet. However, if you are the type of person who normally responds better in group or structured environments, there are many different programs available. How to choose? We propose a checklist that includes three sets of questions: one set for your own personal evaluation of your goals and expectations, one set to use in a consultation with your doctor, and one for the directors of any program you might consider joining.

QUESTIONS TO ASK YOURSELF

What are your reasons for wanting to lose weight—are they health-related or mostly cosmetic? Your motivations are an important factor.

If you equate a certain body style with specific benefits, such as a more successful career, a better love life, or just happier feelings in general, you are setting yourself up for potential problems. While a diet and fitness program can be a positive motivating factor in getting other areas in your life moving, losing weight, in itself, will not guarantee that your life will change.

Have you dieted before? If you are a "chronic dieter" who goes on diets once or twice a year, you may be setting yourself up for yet another defeat unless you address the issue of why other diets have failed. Chronic dieters cling to the belief that past failures are caused either by their own lack of discipline (which they're determined to overcome "this time") or by the programs they have tried, which have never been the "right" programs. The simple truth is that diet specialists have not yet discovered the one "miracle" diet that helps everyone to lose weight overnight. What you might have perceived as lack of discipline on your part was probably yet another diet hoax failing. One exercise you might try before pursuing a new weight loss program is to chart your weight-loss history, noting the type of diet you went on, how long it lasted, how much weight you lost, why you stopped dieting, how long it took you to regain the weight, and what were the factors that contributed to your regaining. Use this chart as a basis for evaluating future programs. You're likely to find some trends in your experience—such as repeated failure with very low-calorie diets or greater success in group programs—that will give you a firmer grasp of what seems to work best.

What do your parents, grandparents, siblings, and other relatives look like? Scientists know that genetic factors play a role in body shape, and there are some things that can't be changed. Many people who are not overweight by commonly used standards continue to diet in order to be thinner overall or to slim down thighs, legs, or hips. But you cannot simply point to a picture in a magazine and say, "I want to look like her." No matter how much you diet, you cannot change your genetically given shape, any more than you can change the color of your eyes.

Do you have special health considerations that must be discussed with your physician? Evaluate your personal medical history, as well as that of your family, to determine if you are at risk for heart disease, high blood pressure, or diabetes. Also note food allergies, gastrointestinal complaints, and medications you might be taking. Your ability to completely evaluate health risk factors will enable your physician to advise you better.

QUESTIONS TO ASK YOUR DOCTOR

Does your current weight, medical history, and evaluation of risk factors make it necessary for you to lose weight for health reasons? There's nothing wrong with wanting to lose a few pounds for cosmetic reasons, but it should be viewed as an issue separate from health.

Do laboratory tests indicate that you have special medical concerns, such as high cholesterol, high blood pressure, or high blood sugar?

Are there any factors that would make certain diet approaches either good or bad for your health? Along with that, does your doctor have any recommendations of his or her own, or any literature available about effective programs?

QUESTIONS TO ASK THE PROGRAM DIRECTORS

Does the program provide a comprehensive approach that includes diet, exercise, and behavior modification? The most effective programs seem to be more well-rounded than simply helping you shed a few pounds fast.

Is the program individualized? No single program works in the same way for everyone. Standardized diets that use the same format for everyone inevitably fail for those who don't fit the norm.

Does the program make fantastic claims? There's no such thing as a diet that allows you to lose a huge amount of weight overnight while eating anything you want. Most diets that offer rapid initial weight loss are low-carbohydrate diets that have a diuretic effect. But losing water is not the same as losing fat, and such diets have no staying power.

Is the program medically supervised? Don't hesitate to find out about the credentials of those who direct and monitor the program. Sometimes counselors are merely successful graduates of the program and have no medical or nutritional training. The presence of trained medical personal (with expertise in weight control), nutritionists, dieticians, exercise physiologists, and behavior modification specialists will tell you a lot about a program's viability.

Does the program relate realistically to your life-style? If you are not dangerously obese, your best course is to plan a gradual, steady weight loss. This process will include developing new, healthier eating habits. Many people fail on diets that require too much special shopping and preparation, or eating foods at times that don't fit their normal schedules. Some programs require that you weigh yourself daily, a practice that is both inconvenient and probably pointless. (Most metabolism and weight control specialists believe that daily weighing tells you little about real fat loss.)

Does the program recommend a nutritious diet? Never trust a program that emphasizes one or two "magic" foods, depends heavily on only one type of food (such as a high-protein diet), or otherwise deprive you of the nutrients you need.

Does the program offer help with maintenance? Once you've lost the weight, the key is to keep it off. You will need maintenance support— not just behavior modification but practical guidelines as well, such as shopping and cooking advice.

Can you afford it? There are many different kinds of programs in different price ranges. Some are quite expensive. Be sure to find out all the details in advance, such as what the program's guarantee is, whether you have to pay the entire amount up front, whether you'll get part or all of your money back if you drop out, and whether there are hidden costs for items like prepackaged foods or support materials.

23

Take Charge of Your Weight Control

As a first step in your weight-loss program, you might want to try the Tufts Low-Cholesterol Diet in chapter 19. Since, by its nature, a low-cholesterol diet is going to be high in complex carbohydrates and fiber and low in saturated fat and cholesterol, most people will lose some weight on such a diet. It will also give you an appreciation of just how appetizing "healthy" food can be. The menus are fun to follow and the recipes are delicious originals.

But even if you participate in a structured weight control program in the beginning, your goal should be to eventually achieve self-sufficiency in managing a healthy diet. If you are a chronic dieter, this might be a foreign concept because you've grown so accustomed to others telling you what you can and cannot eat. You may feel comfortable with the familiarity of that approach, even if the diets themselves have never worked for you. Maybe you're afraid that, left to fend for yourself, you'll lose control and fail.

On the other hand, it's likely that the more comfortable you become with selecting your own foods and managing your own diet and fitness plan, the less obsessed you'll become with food and the less likely you'll be to binge.

The following guidelines and food lists will help you begin to figure out how to construct a nutritious weight-loss diet on your own.

How Many Calories Do You Need?

Obsessive calorie-counting is not the way to achieve normal, healthy dietary habits. And if you follow the guidelines for healthy eating, you'll probably find that your calorie intake automatically declines. Both human and animal studies have shown that when fatty foods are replaced by those high in complex carbohydrates, subjects do not consume the same number of calories.

However, if you want to get a general idea of how many calories you should eat each day to encourage weight loss, there is a method for calculating this number individually. Many weight-loss programs place everyone on the same number of calories per day, but this practice is not very effective. People are different, and two people will have different results with the same number of calories.

As you calculate your calorie needs, don't forget that reducing calories too much will only create a slowdown in your metabolic rate and a tendency to retain water. Keep your calories at a reasonable level to encourage a slow, steady weight loss.

To find out how many calories you should consume to lose weight, you must first determine how many calories you need to maintain your

269

current weight. To calculate this number, first you must estimate how many calories you require to maintain your normal bodily functions at rest, in other words, your Basal Metabolic Rate (BMR). Add to that the number of additional calories you use for your daily activities. The total becomes the number of calories you use to maintain your weight. You can estimate this number by using the following equation:

1. BMR = current weight × 10

2. multiply result × 0.30 (for daily activities)

3. add BMR number and activity number together

It is estimated that the average sedentary American uses only an additional 30 percent of his or her calories on activity. If you are very active, you might want to raise your activity calorie level to 40 percent for a more accurate reading.

Once you know the daily calorie intake that keeps you at your present weight, you can lose weight by creating a negative energy balance, that is, taking in fewer calories than you use up. Specifically, to lose one pound of fat, you need to consume about 3,500 calories less than you use (by either eating less or engaging in more physical activity). We suggest that you do not cut your calorie intake below 1,200 calories per day. A better method might be to cut your calorie intake to your BMR, which means consuming 30 percent fewer calories per day. If you add exercise on top of this, you will increase the rate of weight loss.

At first glance, a weight loss of only one or two pounds a week may seem like very little, especially if you're familiar with the many diets that promise weight losses of five to ten pounds per week. But remember: On those diets you were losing mostly water, not fat. And you probably didn't achieve or maintain long-term weight loss. If you want to successfully achieve permanent weight loss, the slow, steady approach is your best and most nutritionally sound course. When you add a sensible exercise program, you can lose an additional pound or two a month.

Plan Your Weekly Menus

Construct your eating plans, using the food lists below as a general guideline. These lists are provided to give you a start. They are not intended to be rigid lists of "allowable" foods. To achieve your goal of becoming knowledgeable about foods and comfortable with the idea of managing your own diet, you need to avoid making "good" and "bad" food rules for yourself.

You might also want to use suggestions from other parts of the book. For example, the frozen dinners listed in chapter 12 all contain fewer than 300 calories.

As you construct your weekly menu plan, follow these guidelines to insure that you meet your nutrient requirements and are attentive to the recommendations for lowering fat and cholesterol:

▶ Consume approximately 50 to 60 percent of your daily calories in the form of complex carbohydrates. Sources of complex carbohydrates include fruit, vegetables, breads, cereals, and legumes.

▶ Consume 15 to 20 percent of your daily calories in the form of protein. The best protein sources are animal foods: meat, poultry, fish, and dairy products. These are "complete" proteins that supply all of the amino acids your body needs. (See chapter 1 for details on how to combine "incomplete" vegetable protein sources to make a complete protein meal.)

Example: How Many Calories Do You Use?

Adult women: 140 pounds

140 × 10 = 1,400
1,400 × 0.30 = 420
1,400 + 420 = 1,820 calories

Example: Daily Calories for Weight Loss

Adult woman—Weight: 140 pounds
               BMR: 1,400 calories per day
               Activity: 420 calories per day
               Total: 1,820 calories per day
               (− 0.30):   1,400 calories per day
               Deficit: 420 calories per day *
               Weight Loss: Roughly 1 pound per week

* Does not account for increased physical exercise. To lose more, increase exercise rather than cutting calories further (see chapter 24).

Consume 30 percent or fewer of your daily calories in the form of fats. No more than 10 percent of total daily calories should be saturated fats. Saturated fats include all animal foods as well as coconut and palm oils. Unsaturated fats include vegetable oils and margarine.

▶ Consume no more than 300 milligrams of cholesterol each day. Cholesterol is found only in animal foods. (See chapter 5 for cholesterol content of common foods.)

▶ Limit your sodium intake to between 1,000 and 3,000 milligrams each day. In addition to common table salt, sodium is found in many processed foods and some seasonings.

▶ While you're trying to lose weight, avoid alcohol. Its calories are "empty" in the sense that they supply no nutrients. On a controlled-calorie diet, you could end up wasting 20 to 30 percent of your daily calories with just a couple of beers or glasses of wine.

▶ Assume a balance of essential vitamins and minerals by eating a variety of foods every day. Consume at least 2 servings of dairy foods per day; 2 servings of meat, poultry, or fish; 4 servings of vegetables and fruits; and 4 servings of whole-grain bread, cereal, and pasta.

▶ Refer frequently to the sections in this book on shopping for and preparing food. They contain easy-to-execute guidelines for making your meals interesting, healthy, and low in calories and fat.

Change Your "Diet Head"

Here are a few suggestions to help you avoid being obsessed by food and weight loss while you're dieting:

Become active: Use the suggestions in chapter 24 to find a regular program of exercise, preferably aerobic. Exercise will not only contribute your fat loss but also increase your cardiovascular fitness and decrease your risk for osteoporosis. There's another benefit to exercise. It will cut down on your cravings for food.

Stop weighing yourself: People with weight obsessions usually weigh themselves every day. Some even weigh themselves several times a day or after every meal. When you do this, you're just tracking the amount of water you lose and gain over the course of a day. Limit your weighing sessions to once a week. And don't forget that there might be times you retain a little water—women often do so before their menstrual periods, for example. You can even test to see if you're retaining water: Push your finger against your shinbone and hold it for a few seconds. When you take your finger away, the skin will bounce back if there's no water retention. A dimple will remain if you're retaining water.

Don't make yourself miserable: If you're planning to attend a party or other special occasion, acknowledge in advance that you're going to splurge a little on a small dessert or other favorite food. If you go in with the attitude that you're not going to deprive yourself, you won't be as likely to binge.

Drop the idea of "good food, bad food:" Of course, if you're trying to lose weight, there are some foods that won't be a regular part of your diet. But your most successful route to life-time weight control is to avoid labeling any foods as bad. It won't harm you to have a treat once or twice a week. Calorie counting isn't, after all, a precise science. Eating 200 or 300 extra calories once a week isn't going to throw your diet off course. If it really bothers you, add some exercise —a better idea than cutting back on other nutrient-rich foods.

Avoid unrealistic goals: It's good to have weight-loss goals, but try to keep them general and avoid linking them to important factors in your life. If you say, "I'm going to lose ten pounds before my vacation in Hawaii this October," you are essentially saying that having a good time in Hawaii is dependent on your having lost ten pounds. Losing weight and getting fit is one way to improve yourself, but don't make it the requirement for your enjoyment in every other arena of your life. If you're a chronic dieter, this tendency has likely been a part of your problem in the past.

Focus on health, not weight: Except for those few people with medical complications, eating a healthy, well-balanced diet that is high in complex carbohydrates and low in fat and exercising several times a week will lead to weight loss and healthy weight maintenance. If you focus on improving your overall health and fitness instead of "going on a diet," you will most certainly benefit. And you may find, for the first time in your life, that you're enjoying yourself instead of suffering.

SAMPLE FOODS AND SERVINGS FOR A WEIGHT-LOSS DIET

Servings 100 Calories or Lower

Serving	Calories
1 medium apple	80
½ cantaloupe	80
10 seedless grapes	35
1 medium orange	90
1 peach	40
1 cup sliced pineapple	80
1 plum	30
1 cup strawberries	55
1 cup blueberries	82
½ grapefruit	50
3 small apricots	55
½ cup unsweetened applesauce	53
1 cup cooked carrots	50
1 cup cooked collard greens	65
1 cup cooked spinach	40
1 cup cooked summer squash	30
1 medium steamed artichoke	53
1 cup cooked asparagus	30
1 cup cooked green beans	30
1 cup cooked broccoli	40
1 cup cooked cauliflower	30
1 cup boiled eggplant	38
½ cup cooked green peas	67
1 slice cracked-wheat bread	65
1 slice whole-wheat bread	60
1 slice rye bread	65
1 slice French bread	72
2 bread sticks	86
3 rye crackers	72
4 saltines (low sodium)	52
4 wheat crackers	64
1 oz. bran flakes	90
1 oz. shredded wheat	100
1 corn tortilla	32
4 oz. tofu	82
4 oz. low-fat (1%) cottage cheese	82
1 oz. part-skim mozzarella cheese	80
1 poached egg	80
1 cup skim milk	85
½ cup vanilla ice milk	90

Servings 200 Calories or Lower

Serving	Calories
1 cup orange juice	110
1 pear	100
6 dried prunes	120
1 medium baked potato	145
1 cup cooked winter squash	130
1 medium baked sweet potato	160
1 medium bran muffin	110
1 English muffin	130
1 medium nut muffin	165
1 cup cooked farina	135
1 oz. corn flakes	110
1 cup cooked oatmeal	145
1 cup cooked long-grain brown rice	173
1 cup cooked macaroni	192
1 cup cooked egg noodles	200
1 cup cooked plain spaghetti	192
½ cup cooked lima beans	130
½ cup cooked navy beans	112
1 oz. sunflower seeds	162
½ cup part-skim ricotta cheese	171
1 cup low-fat (1%) milk	105
1 cup non-fat plain yogurt	125
3 oz. roasted chicken, skinless, white meat	165
1 roasted chicken drumstick, skinless	172
3½ oz. water-packed tuna, no salt	127
3 oz. steamed shrimp	102
3 oz. broiled or baked oysters	133
3 oz. poached salmon	126
3 oz. broiled or baked salmon	149
3 oz. broiled or baked perch fillet	113
3 oz. broiled or baked sea bass	117
3 oz. broiled or baked flounder	101
3 oz. broiled or baked scallops	106
3 oz. broiled, lean, top loin	172
3 oz. roasted, lean, round eye	155
3 oz. broiled liver	137
3 oz. broiled, lean, veal steak	123

Servings 300 Calories or Lower

Serving	Calories
1 cup cooked spaghetti with tomato sauce	260
1 cup cooked lentil beans	210
1 cup low-fat fruit yogurt	230
3 oz. lean ground beef	217

24

Build a Better Body

We include a chapter on exercise in a book about nutrition because exercise is such a vital part of keeping fit and healthy. Many studies have demonstrated that not only is exercise a good way to lose weight, it also is a key to basic health. Some of these benefits include cardiovascular fitness (with physical activities that increase the heart rate), a possible increase in bone mass that may diminish the risk of osteoporosis, and even a lessening of anxiety and stress.

So, whether your goal is to lose weight, improve health, or both, exercise is the ideal companion to a nutritious diet.

Exercise: Separating Fact from Fiction

There are as many false ideas about exercise as there are about nutrition. One reason might be that, like diet, exercise has grown into a major industry, dedicated to selling fitness-conscious Americans on the idea that they "must" have special supplements, drinks, foods, lotions, equipment, and so on. Americans are gullible about buying into this promotion, not only because we're always on the lookout for a quick answer, but also because we aren't very well educated

about exercise. Most of us learned about exercise in inadequate school programs, where the focus was on sports performance, not health. It's easy to see why we would be so filled with misconceptions. Let's look at some of the most common.

Fiction: No pain, no gain.

Fact: If belief in this maxim stands between you and the decision to improve your physical fitness, you'll be relieved to learn that you don't have to push yourself until it hurts to enjoy the benefits of exercise. In fact, excessive exercise increases the chances of bone, joint, and muscle injury, not to mention making your workout seem more like punishment than pleasure.

For most people, simply exercising for 15 to 60 minutes, three to five times a week, will improve cardiovascular fitness and contribute to weight loss. Cardiovascular fitness can be achieved if your heart is working at 70 to 80 percent of its maximum. Below is a list of the average 70 percent-capacity heart rate of people of various ages. Check yourself against the average this way: When you have completed your exercise, apply your fingertips to the artery on the inside of your wrist, just below the bone. Count the number of heart beats in a 10-second period and multiply it by six. That's the number of times your heart is beating per minute. Check yourself against these averages:

AGE	HEART RATE AT 70 PERCENT CAPACITY (AVERAGE)
20	140
25	137
30	133
35	130
40	126
45	123
50	119
55	116
60	112
65	109
70	105

If you think the weight-loss benefits won't be there unless you push yourself to the limit, consider this: if a 150-pound person spent one hour per day, three days a week, on a brisk walk, that would account for 900 calories a week, enough to lose about 13 pounds a year without even making one change in diet. What's more, most of those pounds come from stored body fat, not the lean body tissue that sometimes is lost with diet alone.

Fiction: Excess weight can be sweated off.

Fact: If this were true, we could all lose our excess weight by lounging around in saunas or steam rooms. Although it's not uncommon for exercisers who hop on a scale after a workout to find that they've lost weight, it's a result of perspiration. Once fluids are taken back in, that weight will return.

Fiction: Exercise will just make you hungrier.

Fact: Many skeptical dieters think they'll grow so famished from exercising that they will eat back all they've lost. Ordinary exercise does not decrease appetite, but neither does it increase it. In one study, obese women at St. Luke's-Roosevelt Hospital Center in New York City, followed a rigorous daily routine of walking a treadmill for a period of two months. Not only did they not in-

crease the amount of food they ate, but they walked off enough calories to lose an average of 15 pounds each.

It should be noted that already-slim women who were also put on a treadmill routine did increase their calorie intake to compensate for the extra calories they were burning. But they did not raise their "input" over their "output" and gained no weight.

Fiction: Spot-exercising causes more fat to be lost from a particular part of the body.

Fact: If only that were true! While the idea that fat-free thighs can be achieved by concentrating on leg-lifts or that a flat stomach can be had through sit-ups alone is an enticing thought, it seems to be fallacious. Researchers at the University of Massachusetts helped dispel the notion about spot-reducing several years ago when they put a small group of college men on a four-week sit-up program. When they evaluated the results they found that the amount of fat in the men's abdomens was not reduced to any greater extent than the fat in their buttocks or bases of their shoulder blades. In other words, fat lost through spot-reducing is not selectively drawn from fat surrounding the area being exercised. Rather, it is pulled from deposits throughout the body. Happily, exercising a group of muscles at a sepcific spot on the body can tone and firm them, but if there is excess fat in that spot it won't be lost by concentrating on that area.

Fiction: Special techniques other than exercise are needed to get rid of cellulite.

Fact: Cellulite, that lumpy, dimply flesh that collects on the hips, thighs, and buttocks and is supposed to be particularly hard to "break up," does not even exist. It's nothing more than a name that clever marketers have given to fat that collects directly under the skin. Thus, the claims that special exercises or products will "get rid" of it are completely spurious. The only way to smooth out those fat deposits is to follow the same kind of

Fitness Level Scorecard

Dr. James Rippe, director of exercise physiology at the University of Massachusetts Medical School, developed this test to help people determine their level of fitness. Clock out a mile using the odometer in your car, then walk it as fast as you can, and calculate your fitness score according to these guidelines:

	Time (Minutes: Seconds)	
	Male	**Female**
excellent	less than 10:12	less than 11:40
good	10:13–11:42	11:41–13:08
high average	11:43–13:13	13:09–14:36
low average	13:14–14:44	14:37–16:04
fair	14:45–16:23	16:05–17:31
poor	more than 16:24	more than 17:32

diet and exercise regimen that will get rid of fat all over the body.

Fiction: If women participate in strength training, they'll grow big muscles.

Fact: This is rarely true. Most women who routinely engage in weight-lifting programs are able to increase their muscle strength without surrendering their feminine physiques to man-size muscles. It's thought that the presence of hormones, particularly the male hormone testosterone, is responsible for the fact that men are much more prone to muscle enlargement through exercise than women.

Fiction: After a certain age, people shouldn't exercise.

Fact: Tufts School of Nutrition physiologist William Evans, Ph.D., found just the opposite to be true when he conducted tests at the Tufts-USDA Human Nutrition Research Center on Aging. When he put men aged 60 to 72 years on a weight-lifting program, they markedly increased both the size and strength of their thigh muscles after just 12 weeks. Even a group of men and women averaging 90 years of age increased the muscle area of their thighs by about 10 percent. And the amount of weight they were able to lift went from an average of 17.6 pounds to 44 pounds.

Many of the participants—a number of whom relied on canes and walkers to move about—were able to walk a little faster, take longer strides, and get in and out of their chairs more easily. One 90-year-old woman reported that before "pumping iron" she was always tired and rarely lifted anything heavier than a quart of milk. But after getting involved in the program she found that she had more strength in her arms and legs, and was capable of greater endurance during exertion, and had more overall energy. A man three years her junior who also participated in the weight-training program commented that "psychologically, it's a good feeling to see that you're not deteriorating."

Incidentally, Dr. Evans pointed out that elderly people who successfully strengthened their muscles at Tufts were eating well before they began. Had they not been, he believed the outcome would not have been so dramatic.

Getting Started on Fitness

If you're new to exercising, the first thing to do is see your doctor for a complete physical checkup. Such an exam is particularly important if you have any medical complications, are over the age of 60, or have any muscle or bone impairments.

If you want to maximize both the fat-burning and cardiovascular effects of an exercise regimen, your best choice is an aerobic exercise program. Aerobic exercise keeps the heart rate up to the 70

Exercise	Pros	Cons
walking	—not as stressful as jogging on bones and joints —good for obese or elderly people —convenient—no special arrrangements needed	—results take longer to show than more high-intensity methods —must be done briskly or all benefits won't be realized
jogging	—one of the best methods for losing weight fast —can be done alone, with few expenses or special arrangements	—impact stress is too high for many people, especially the obese and elderly —injuries to the bones and joints are common
aerobics class	—low-impact aerobics are a good workout —some people find the group setting more fun than exercising alone —trained teachers make sure you're performing the exercises properly for maximum benefit	—can lead to injuries, especially in high-impact aerobics —doesn't allow for a personal pace, and the group pace can be too strenuous for some people
bicycling	—many people find biking fun, and it lends itself to group and family rides —at a leisurely speed, it uses as many calories in an hour as 45 minutes of an aerobics class; faster, the rate nearly doubles	—won't be beneficial if you stop and start, so you need an open road or bike path —can be relatively expensive —injuries are common
swimming	—easy to incorporate into leisure activities alone or with a group —places little stress on the joints and doesn't cause overheating, making it good for the elderly and obese.	—for maximum aerobic benefits, you must do relatively fast laps; some people find this boring —not everyone has easy accessibility to a pool

or 80 percent level mentioned above, in a sustained effort. Calisthenics, for example, is not aerobic since it involves stopping and starting. To gain the full benefit of aerobic exercise, it should be done a minimum of three times a week. In the accompanying box, examine the pros and cons of these favorite aerobic activities.

Tips to Make Your Workout Work

To get the most benefit from your exercise program and to avoid injuries, remember these points:

Always warm up and cool down: Before you start exercising, make sure your muscle tendons are stretched to give you more flexibility and

---

HOW MANY CALORIES DO YOU SPEND EXERCISING?

This list gives the average calories spent per hour by a 150-pound person

Bicycling, 6 MPH	240 calories
Bicycling, 12 MPH	410 calories
Running, 10 MPH	1,280 calories
Cross-country skiing	700 calories
Jogging, 5½ MPH	740 calories
Jogging, 7 MPH	920 calories
Jumping rope	750 calories
Running in place	650 calories
Swimming, 25 yds./min.	275 calories
Swimming, 50 yds./min.	500 calories
Tennis, singles	400 calories
Walking, 2 MPH	240 calories
Walking, 3 MPH	320 calories
Walking, 4½ MPH	440 calories

The calories spent in a particular activity vary in proportion to your body weight. For example, a 100-pound person would decrease these numbers by ⅓; a 200-pound person would increase them by 1½.

Source: American Heart Association

---

avoid injury. After exercising, reinforce the flexibility of your muscles by stretching again. During this period of reduced activity, your heartbeat will gradually return to normal. Here are two sample stretches:

Knee bend: Place feet and knees together and squat down with your arms along the sides of your knees and fingers on the floor.
　　　　　　Straighten legs, leaving fingers on the floor and directing buttocks in the air. Repeat 8 times.

Calf stretch: Stand 3 to 4 feet from a vertical surface (like a fence, wall, or tree). Lean forward against the surface, bending your arms and keeping your right heel firmly planted. As you lean forward, drop your right hip, stretching the right calf and bending the left leg slightly. Hold for 10 seconds, then reverse and stretch the left leg. Repeat 8 times for each leg.

While you're exercising, be sure to breathe fully: Breathing is an important part of the workout, and holding your breath will hold you back. Inhale from the abdomen, expanding your chest with air, and then exhale, also from the abdomen, pushing the air out with a "whoosh." The rhythm of your breathing should coincide with the movement of your body. For example, if you are doing leg lifts, exhale as you lift your leg and inhale as you lower it.

If you are doing even mild weight-bearing exercises, be sure you wear the proper shoes, which will provide the necessary cushioning and support: There are many kinds of shoes to choose from. The personnel at a sporting-goods store should be able to explain the benefits of different brands and styles.

Don't push yourself: Start slowly and work up your speed and endurance over a period of weeks. If you try to do too much too soon, you'll suffer an injury or have so many muscle pains you won't be able to crawl to your next exercise session. Try to develop a slow but consistent three-day-a-week pattern.

Nutrition Notes for Athletes

The serious athlete has specific nutritional and health considerations that might not exist for the more casual exerciser. Of primary interest to the athlete are maintaining top physical condition and gaining a competitive edge. To achieve the former, there is no need for the athlete to eat more than the balanced, healthy diet recommended for the average American—in spite of the fact that an entire industry of health supplements and dietary products exists. The sports industry has long promoted the viewpoint that the dietary needs of athletes are vastly different from those of normal people.

Certainly it is true that athletes must pay special attention to their diets, since nutrition is linked in a very direct way with physical stamina and performance. But it is important that athletes learn to understand their true needs to avoid sabotaging their health as well as to save money they might otherwise spend on expensive and useless supplements.

Carbohydrate Loading

One dietary practice, carbohydrate loading, may be beneficial if it is done properly. Carbohydrate loading means eating a diet that is very high in complex carbohydrates—about 65 to 70 percent of total calories—for four to five days prior to a sustained event that lasts more than two hours. This practice is common for marathon runners and long-distance swimmers, for example, who will be competing for several hours at a stretch.

Carbohydrate loading allows the muscles to store extra carbohydrate in the form of glycogen, a rapidly available fuel source that they and the rest of the body use to work. Normally, we have enough glycogen in our bodies to last an hour and a half to two hours of continuous exercise. So only athletes who go without a break for two hours or more really benefit from the practice.

One of the most important studies demonstrating the effects of carbohydrate loading was performed by Dr. Per-Olof Astrand, a noted exercise physiologist from Stockholm. In the study, nine men were fed different diets during a period of three days; they then worked to exhaustion on stationary bicycles. Those who ate a diet of only fats and protein lasted less than an hour on the bicycles. Those who ate a balanced diet of carbohydrates, proteins, and fats lasted just under two hours. Those who ate a high carbohydrate diet lasted an average of two hours and forty-seven minutes on the bicycles.

To be really effective, carbohydrate loading must be done properly. As the day of the event approaches, the athlete should gradually taper off the amount of exercise, and do no exercise the day before. This time off will allow the body to hang onto the glycogen that has been formed from the carbohydrate so it will be available during the event.

Carbohydrate loading is a practice that should not take place more than three or four times a year, and some experts recommend that it be done only under medical guidance because, taken to an extreme, it presents risks. In any case, it is a practice that has real value only in continuous endurance sports. It does not apply to stop-and-start games like basketball and football. If the event lasts an hour or less, the body has no need for the extra fuel supply.

Packing Protein

Since we know that protein is needed to build muscle and tissues, many athletes assume that large quantities of protein will make them more muscular. Some eat diets that are full of high-protein, high-fat, and high-cholesterol foods as a result of this misconception. Others take supplements of amino acids, the building blocks from which proteins are constructed.

Although research suggests that the protein requirements of some athletes, particularly marathon runners, may be higher than those of the average person, this finding should be considered in light of the fact that the average American diet already includes much more than the requirement for protein. For example, a single whole chicken breast provides 52 grams of protein, almost the entire RDA for the average adult male. The average diet can easily surpass this allowance. So athletes who need to consume more than the RDA for protein could do so very easily without consuming massive amounts.

Protein overloading comes with a number of risks, in addition to the well-known disadvantages of a diet high in fat and cholesterol. The body uses only so much protein at a time, and the excess is either burned for energy or converted to fat for storage. In either case, the nitrogen component must be stripped away and excreted through the kidneys. Overloading on protein can put the kidneys under stress.

The supplement industry lures athletes with a variety of products, including protein powder, protein drink, and protein tablets, designed to increase protein consumption without adding fat and cholesterol. It's easy to see how athletes might be attracted to this idea. But, in fact, taking supplementary protein is a complete waste of money.

Fluids Are Essential

Vigorous exercise can mask the normal signals that tell us we're thirsty, and athletes lose a lot of water through perspiration. For this reason, they must take care to consume plenty of fluids, both before exertion and every 20 minutes or so during endurance exercise. Warm weather depletes body fluids further, so fluids should be consumed every 10 to 15 minutes. The best source of fluid is water.

Sports Supplements Should Be Avoided

Supposed "high energy" supplements containing vitamin E and certain B vitamins are a waste of money for those who meet their RDA through diet. There is no scientific evidence that an extra supply of these vitamins increases endurance or prevents fatigue. The nutrients athletes need are in abundant supply in mixed diets.

Some people believe that athletes need to take salt tablets to replace the salt lost from the body through sweat. But consuming too much salt in the form of tablets will further dehydrate the body by lowering the level of water in the blood. Too much salt will also cause potassium loss, undermining the operation of muscle cells.

There is rarely enough salt lost in sweat to require additional salt intake. The best way to replace fluids lost through sweat is by drinking water. Only in very unusual cases (such as when five to ten pounds of weight are lost during the event) might salt replacement need to occur, and then it should not be in a concentrated dose but in lightly salted drink or a small amount of salt sprinkled on food.

Potassium and magnesium, which are important for maintaining energy, body temperature, and the proper functioning of muscle cells, are also lost in high-intensity exercise, but again it is of no value to take supplements. Both are available in many foods. Potassium is found in dried fruits and nuts, bananas, and oranges. Magnesium can be found in nuts, meat, fish, milk, whole grains, and dark-green leafy vegetables.

Iron for Women Athletes

A condition known as sports anemia sometimes afflicts women athletes. The reasons for this low blood-hemoglobin level are not known for certain, but the condition tends to appear during the early stages of training. It is suspected that the culprits may include menstrual blood loss, poor iron intake, decreased absorption and increased loss of iron, expanded blood volume, decreased production or greater destruction of red blood cells, and inadequate dietary protein.

The best way to avoid iron deficiency leading to sports anemia is to consume plenty of iron in the diet. The best sources are animal products such as liver, meat, fish, and poultry.

Eating Disorders and Athletes

The popular image of an athlete is that of a vigorous, healthy person. But in recent years, specialists in sports medicine and collegiate athletic trainers have found an alarming incidence of young athletes who suffer from eating disorders, such as anorexia nervosa and bulimia.

What would cause a perfectly healthy young athlete at the peak of performance to reject food? The primary factor appears to be the extreme emphasis on leanness, both self-imposed and encouraged by coaches, in such weight-regulated activities as wrestling, lightweight crew, running, basketball, soccer, and figure skating.

Of all athletic-type performers, ballerinas have received the most attention from the sports medicine community regarding their restricted diets. Several years ago, *The Physician and Sports Medicine* published a study of 34 high-level classical ballet dancers made by L. H. Calabrese and his colleagues, showing that their average nutrient consumption was only 71.4 percent of the RDA. In another study, Paul E. Garfunkel and David M. Garner, researchers from the University of Toronto, estimated that among 112 Canadian dance students, the incidence of anorexia nervosa was 5 percent.

Another study found that some of the most bizarre and dangerous eating habits occur among wrestlers striving to qualify for lower weight classes. Investigators Sarah H. Short, Ph.D., Ed.D., R.D., and William Short, Sc.D., reported in the *Journal of the American Dietetic Association* that wrestlers tried to control their weight by using diuretics and laxatives, inducing vomiting, wearing plastic suits to force perspiration, and taking contrast (hot-and-cold) showers to make them-

selves urinate. Moreover, it was not uncommon for wrestlers to lose weight using these methods on numerous occasions during the season, since successful wrestlers compete in up to 30 matches per year.

The Shorts made their point in a case report of a 19-year-old collegiate wrestler who, before competition, lost 21 percent of his preseason body weight by crash dieting, forced vomiting, and heavy use of laxatives and diuretics. A typical "meal" for this athlete the day before a match consisted of root beer, a peppermint patty, and a piece of butterscotch candy. After the match, he would usually gorge at a pancake house, consuming almost 5,000 calories at one sitting. The Shorts reported that, although the wrestler took a daily multivitamin supplement, he showed symptoms consistent with vitamin A and riboflavin deficiencies, in addition to the strain his eating behavior placed on his heart, digestive system, liver, and kidneys.

Obsessive runners also seem to share some of the traits of individuals with anorexia nervosa. According to one study in the *New England Journal of Medicine*, these traits include extraordinarily high self-expectations, tolerance of physical discomfort, denial of the potential for serious disability, and a tendency toward depression as they struggle for a sense of identity and control.

Besides extreme emaciation, other symptoms of eating disorders include absence of menstruation in women, extreme hyperactivity and denial of fatigue, a bizarre preoccupation with food, trouble sleeping, and extreme paleness (a sign of anemia).

Poor dietary patterns are often found among bodybuilders who are judged for their physiques rather than for their athletic prowess. Research indicates that muscle builders develop their physiques through exercise and lifting weights (and sometimes by taking steroids), and not because of healthy diet practices. To make their muscles bigger, bodybuilders often consume large quantities of protein, packing away huge amounts of meat and eggs and consuming protein drinks. But eating large amounts of protein does not build muscle; it's exercise, not diet, that achieves that. As laboratory tests have shown, even animals on restricted diets will build muscle if they exercise.

The body is not able to store protein it does not use, and the excess is used either for energy or to build fat. The waste products of excess protein metabolism are lost in the urine, placing a load on the kidneys. Furthermore, the cholesterol and fat in many protein foods add problems for bodybuilders who have a predisposition toward heart disease.

In the month before competition, many bodybuilders subsist on diets that are almost entirely protein. According to Tufts sports nutrition expert William Evans, this is a dangerous and ultimately self-defeating practice. Carbohydrate is needed to provide energy for the grueling daily regimen of exercise bodybuilders put themselves through. If muscle carbohydrate stores become depleted, which will occur on a low-carbohydrate diet, bodybuilders will experience chronic fatigue.

Because eating disorders can have lethal consequences, it is important that athletes and their trainers recognize the dangers of pushing the goal of achieving leanness beyond the point where it will ultimately harm performance.

PART SIX

Ask the Experts: Tufts Answers Your Most Important Questions

Making Nutritious Choices

Q. Are there any nutritional differences between extra-virgin, virgin, fine, and ungraded olive oil?

A. None to speak of. The designations are related to variations in fragrance and flavor resulting from differences in the way oil is extracted from the olive. Extra-virgin olive oil, with its pleasant aroma and strong flavor, comes from the first "pressing" of an olive and is minimally pressed. If the olives are "cold pressed," a method that involves little processing and yields less oil, the finished product is even finer. The lower the grade of olive oil, the more pressings the olives have gone through to extract the oil and the more processing it has undergone.

Q. Does the oil in a can of sardines contain omega-3 fatty acids?

A. The oil in which sardines are packed varies according to brand. It may be olive, cottonseed, soybean, or sardine oil. Of these oils, only sardine oil (which appears on ingredient lists as sild sardine oil) contains omega-3 fatty acids, which some people believe lower cholesterol. Sild sar-

dines, incidentally, are young herring fish imported from Norway and only one of five types of sardines.

Q. Are kosher meats too salty for people on low-sodium diets?

A. The koshering process, which involves treating raw meat and poultry with salt to leach out the blood, can give them twice as much sodium as nonkosher meat. However, you can remove some of the excess salt in kosher beef or veal without compromising the nutrients by soaking it in water for one hour before cooking, a process that does not seem to be particularly effective with chicken.

Q. Are the salt substitutes sold in supermarkets more nutritious than regular table salt? What about taste?

A. Salt substitutes consist primarily of potassium chloride, which differs from ordinary sodium chloride (table salt) in that potassium takes the place of sodium in the molecule. Although potassium is harmless for most people, individuals with kidney damage may have trouble getting rid of excess potassium, which can accumulate to toxic levels. Also, be aware that the taste of potas-

283

sium chloride is distinctive and may take some getting used to. As an alternative to salt substitutes, you could consider making greater use of herbs and other seasonings that contain no sodium.

Q. Many recipes, especially for desserts, call for salt. Will the elimination of salt interfere with the success of the desserts?

A. Because salt is added to enhance flavor, if it's left out it will not interfere with the texture and quality of pie crusts, cakes, custards, puddings, and the like. It is even doubtful that you would perceive a difference in the taste. On the other hand, in the case of desserts made with yeast, it is necessary to add salt to control the rate of yeast fermentation and to help in the structure and texture of the finished product. And, when it comes to taste, you might notice the absence of salt in these recipes. The amount of salt used in most desserts and breads is not significant compared with the quantities we sprinkle on foods or consume when eating highly processed or salty snack foods.

Q. Is the salt content of foods the same as sodium?

A. No. Salt is about 40 percent sodium and 60 percent chloride—hence its technical name, sodium chloride. Only about one-third of the sodium in the typical American diet comes from table salt. You get the rest from sodium naturally present in foods and from the small amounts that are present in drinking water, as well as from salt and sodium added during food processing.

Q. What are egg substitutes made from?

A. Egg substitutes, which usually come in liquid form, are made primarily from egg whites, which means they do not contain fat and cholesterol, which eggs contain only in the yolks. In supermarkets, egg substitutes are stored in the frozen-food section. Look for small cartons with names like Eggbeaters or Scramblers.

One quarter cup of egg substitute will generally replace a whole egg, both in egg dishes like omelettes and in baked goods and casseroles.

Q. Why is veal much higher in cholesterol than other cuts of beef?

A. Cholesterol is a fat-like substance that concentrates in the muscle (meaty portion) of an animal, rather than in the fat. Since young animals have more muscle fibers because they are in a rapid growth stage, they are greater sources of cholesterol than older animals. Veal is the flesh of one- to four-month-old calves.

Q. Is honey more nutritious than sugar?

A. Unlike refined sugar, honey does contain small quantities of essential minerals (mainly potassium, calcium, and phosphorus), but they're present in such minute amounts that they have little value for human nutrition. Honey and sugar have roughly the same number of calories per serving. The only major difference is that, while table sugar consists of pure sucrose, honey contains a mixture of fructose, glucose, and smaller amounts of other sugars.

Q. Since raisins, which are dehydrated grapes, are a good source of iron, does that mean that grapes are also a good source of iron?

A. No. Since grapes have much more water than raisins, the nutrients are not as concentrated. In fact, ounce for ounce, raisins have almost nine times the iron of grapes. Three and a half ounces of raisins provide close to 20 percent of the USRDA for iron.

Knowing What's in the Package

Q. Is it true that some diet foods contain at least 20 percent more calories than is stated on the label? If so, why are food manufacturers allowed to do this?

A. By law, foods that come under the Food and Drug Administration's jurisdiction—which includes just about everything except meat and poultry products—can contain up to 20 percent more calories, carbohydrate, fat, and sodium than the label lists. This variance is allowed partly because the nutritional content of natural foods varies. For example, two oranges of the same size may not have the same carbohydrate content; two similar pieces of cheese may have different sodium or fat levels. Therefore, a product that lists 100 calories on the label may actually have as many as 120 calories. But according to FDA sources, the agency's ongoing surveillance rarely reveals calorie discrepancies that great.

Q. What is an organic food?

A. "Organic" has come to have two meanings. To scientists, it signifies that a substance contains carbon. Since carbohydrates, fats, proteins, and vitamins contain molecules of carbon, they are technically organic. The word has also been used to describe a food grown without the use of chemical fertilizers and pesticides. But the federal government has never turned that popular definition into law. Some states, however, including California and New Hampshire, have passed their own laws regarding the use of this term in order to protect consumers from unethical marketers who might label a product "organic" in order to charge higher prices. The wording of the laws varies, but they generally restrict the use of the terms "organic" and "organically grown" to products that are grown without factory-produced chemicals.

Q. What do such terms as "sell by" or "best if used by" on food containers mean?

A. The "sell by" or "pull" date indicates the last day a product should be offered for sale on the supermarket shelf. Most foods are still good to eat up to a week beyond this date because manufacturers factor in time to allow for home storage.

The "best if used by" date marks the end of the period during which a food will be at peak freshness. It can still be used after this date, but it may be a little stale or lacking in some other quality that affects taste or texture.

The "expiration" date is the last day on which a food should be eaten. After that time, safety and quality are not guaranteed.

The "pack" date is the day a food is packaged or processed for retail sale. Its purpose is primarily to help companies and retailers rotate food.

All of these terms are used by food companies on a voluntary basis. The Food and Drug Administration has no regulations or guidelines on dating food for freshness.

Q. Is it true that significant amounts of nutrients are lost from milk stored in see-through containers? Is milk in an opaque carton a better nutritional buy than milk packaged in a plastic container?

A. Packaging food in containers that allow the light to pass through can promote a slow destruction of nutrients. In the case of milk, exposure to supermarket fluorescent lights can exert a dramatic effect on its vitamin A content. Studies of milk stored in see-through containers, either glass or plastic, have demonstrated that milk can lose as much as half its vitamin A content (and small amounts of its riboflavin content) in just a couple of days. Milk in paperboard cartons loses little of its vitamin A. But vitamin A is so widely available in other foods—fruits, vegetables, meats, cheeses, and eggs—that it is not likely that the nutrient loss from milk stored in see-through containers will be injurious to anyone's health.

Keeping Food Safe

Q. Why must crustaceans like lobster and crab be cooked alive?

A. Cruel as it may seem, throwing a still-moving lobster into boiling water reduces the risk of food poisoning. Meat from crustaceans, because of its unique texture, acts as a sponge for bacteria that tend to grow extremely rapidly once these sea creatures die. Because there is no way to tell if bacteria are present, it is wise to avoid eating crustaceans that have died before being cooked. That should not be difficult, since public health policy forbids the sale of prekilled crustaceans (other than shrimp) in fish markets and restaurants.

Shrimp, incidentally, does not have the same rampant bacteria problem as lobsters and crab. You can safely cook and eat dead shrimp as long as it has been handled under sanitary conditions and refrigerated.

Q. Will bay leaves cause harm if they are left in foods?

A. Bay leaves, often used to season soups and stews, are not nutritionally harmful. But their sharp edges make them a potential hazard. People have suffered perforations of the intestines by swallowing bay leaves. Be sure to remove them before serving or eating food.

Q. Why are certain types of ceramic cooking ware considered to be unsafe?

A. Lead is used in glazes that are applied to ceramic ware to create a smooth surface. When glazes are not applied correctly, or when the ceramic ware is not fired at a high enough temperature, the lead in glazes can leach into food. An accumulation of too much lead in the body over a period of years can lead to severe toxicity. At its most devastating, lead poisoning can lead to chronic illnesses of the nervous system, reproductive system, cardiovascular system, and kidneys. It is especially dangerous for very young children, who are affected by much smaller quantities of lead in their systems.

To avoid danger: Store food in plastic or glass containers; line ceramic bowls with plastic or foil to protect food; don't use untested ceramics (especially products from Mexico, China, Italy, or Spain) to serve food.

Q. Are oranges that have a greenish color ripe? Are they safe to eat?

A. Such oranges have undergone a natural process called "regreening," which happens when a ripe orange fruit pulls some of the green chlorophyll pigment from the leaves and stem of the tree back into the peel. Regreened oranges are actually riper than others and often sweeter. And they're perfectly safe to eat.

Q. Will any harm come from eating peanut shells along with the nut?

A. Peanut shells are not meant to be eaten, and two physicians from Oregon Health Sciences University presented some pretty convincing evidence of the potential danger that exists for people who do eat them. The doctors described the case of a young man who had a nightly snack of 15 to 30 peanuts with the shells. He came to them with complaints of long-standing abdominal pain, loose and frequent bowel movements, and painful defecation. Needless to say, he was advised to kick the peanut shell habit, and the intestinal symptoms gradually subsided. It's not surprising that shells can wreak havoc with your intestines when you consider that they're an abrasive used in grinding and polishing.

Q. Is barbecuing a safe way to cook meat?

A. The greatest hazard of barbecuing is that the cook will not use enough caution and get burned. Some people suggest that the barbecuing itself is dangerous, because the smoke, which is absorbed by the meat, contains benzopyrene, which, in its pure form, has been known to cause cancer in laboratory animals. However, in order to experience the same results, people would have to consume unrealistically large quantities of barbecued meat at a time.

Q. If the refrigerator door is accidentally left open a crack for several hours, will the food be harmed?

A. With the door open, your refrigerator runs constantly to keep its temperature setting. If it's set at 40°F or lower and running properly, your perishable food is probably still cold enough to be safe. If food is cold to the touch, it should be fine. The items you have to be most careful to check are raw meats and casseroles, especially if they are stored at the front of the refrigerator near the door.

Q. Is it true that salmonella illness can be caused by eating raw eggs?

A. Although cracked, unwashed eggs and eggs that have not been refrigerated, probably present the most danger, there is some evidence that raw eggs, like raw meat and poultry, may breed the bacteria that leads to salmonella poisoning. Researchers at the Centers for Disease Control discovered that a number of cases of salmonella poisoning that occured in the northeastern part of the country could be traced to raw eggs or uncooked products made with raw eggs. If you want 100 percent certainty that you will not have problems, avoid eating foods like Caesar salad and hollandaise sauce that contain raw eggs. Cook your eggs well-done: 7 minutes when boiling, 5 minutes when poaching, and 3 minutes on each side when frying. Cooking eggs longer might make them tougher, but it will eliminate any potential dangers.

Q. Do antibiotics used in raising animals contribute to food-borne illnesses?

A. Many cattle ranchers routinely add antibiotics to cattle feed to help animals grow faster and stay infection-free. However, because the doses they use are very low, it's possible for bacteria that normally reside in animal meat to develop a resistance to the drugs over time. If the drug-resistant bacteria then infect a person, treatment with the same strain of antibiotic may not work. According to experts at the Centers for Disease Control, this is not because the bacteria are more vicious, but only because doctors are limited in the drugs they

can use to treat them. For this reason, the National Cattlemen's Association, an industry trade group, has urged its members to stop using antibiotics. Still, the number of ranchers and farmers raising "drug-free" cattle is small.

The future may bring changes. For one thing, the FDA is working to ban the use of antibiotics in cattle feed. And some health organizations are encouraging ranchers to limit, and perhaps eventually to exclude, the use of antibiotics and other potentially harmful drugs.

Concerns of the Ages

Q. Is sugar one of the causes of hyperactivity in children?

A. Many theories have held that limiting sugar and sugar-containing foods will "calm" a child who suffers from hyperactivity. Some parents, in the fear that their children will become more excitable after they eat table sugar or sucrose, try to cut out sugar-containing foods altogether. But there is no reliable evidence of a direct link between sugar consumption and hyperactivity.

In one study, researchers measured the effects of sugar on 50 hyperactive boys and girls whose mothers claimed that their behavior worsened after they ate foods that contained sugar. On three different occasions, the mothers were asked to compare their children's behavior after they drank a glass of lemonade that contained about two and a half ounces of sugar, with their behavior after they drank lemonade sweetened with saccharin. The mothers reported no differences in behavior.

Q. What is the safest way for working mothers to store breast milk until they get home?

A. More and more new mothers are opting to breast-feed, even if they work outside the home. It is easy enough to use a breast pump to extract milk during the day, but how can the milk be most safely stored until the end of the day?

Refrigeration is best, if you have access to a refrigerator where you work. However, breast milk can be safely left at room temperature for about an hour, depending on the temperature. Unlike cow's milk, nonrefrigerated mother's milk is a poor breeding ground for organisms that can cause illness. The reason is that human milk contains appreciable amounts of protective substances, such as lactoferrin, that inhibit the growth of bacteria. To be on the safe side, mothers should store their milk in a cool place, out of direct sunlight.

Q. Is fruit juice a good way to supply added nutrients to a baby's diet?

A. Occasional fruit juice is fine. It does contain some vitamin C, although it is not the only source. But juice should not be used as a substitute for the breast milk or formula the baby would otherwise consume. Milk provides protein and other nutrients essential to a baby's development.

One concern relates to tooth decay. Babies sometimes suck on a juice bottle for long periods of time, using it as a pacifier. This constant exposure to the sugar in juices can lead to cavities in tiny teeth.

Another concern is that too much apple juice might lead to chronic diarrhea in some children. In one study, investigators found that some children who consumed 8 to 12 ounces of apple juice per day had chronic watery stools. When parents were told to discontinue giving these children apple juice, the bowel movement consistency and frequency normalized.

Q. Can certain nutrients improve childrens' performance in school by giving them more "brain power"?

A. While extravagant claims to this effect are considered utter nonsense by health professionals, some studies do occasionally reflect positive results with nutritional supplements under certain circumstances. One such study, reported in the British journal *The Lancet,* found that 30 Welsh school children who were given a daily vitamin/mineral supplement showed improvement in their ability to reason out the answers to questions that did not require verbal skills. (One of the accepted ways to prove so-called nonverbal intelligence is to show young children pictures of three blue dogs and one red dog and ask them to identify which one is different.)

Even though the research was carefully structured, the researchers admit that they are far from convinced that supplements can boost intelligence. One reason is that, while the ordinary diet of all the children appeared to be normal and adequate without supplements, it is possible that marginal deficiencies of one or another nutrient may have gone undetected. And since it is well established that a diet deficient in nutrients can hinder both intellectual and physical growth, such deficiencies may have been the reason nonverbal intelligence improved once supplements were given. As the researchers emphasized, much more work must be done in this area before anyone should seriously think that giving supplements to children will make them smarter.

Q. Do sweets and fatty foods increase the possibility that a teenager will have acne?

A. Scientists have found no evidence of a direct link between diet and adolescent acne. The notion originated with the premise that because adolescent acne is caused by an excess of oil in the skin, a diet that contained less fat would reduce this oil. But the oil in the skin is stimulated by the hormones, not French fries. (The rare exception is when there is a clear-cut case of food allergy.)

Acne occurs when follicles under the skin become clogged with oil. Bacteria under the skin feed on the oil and release toxins that spill out onto the skin's surface. The end result: a pimple. Fortunately, treating pimples that crop up on the face, back, or other skin surfaces has been made easier by the recent development of a wide array of effective medications. Some of these new drugs are vitamin A derivatives—that is, compounds that are similar in structure to vitamin A. However, vitamin A itself will not "cure" acne and, in fact, can cause damage to the liver if taken in doses that far exceed the amounts people are likely to consume from foods alone. Only the medications prescribed by a dermatologist will do the trick.

Q. Is there a vitamin that prevents gray hair?

A. While it's true that a deficiency of the B vitamin pantothenic acid causes gray hair in some laboratory animals, humans will not be spared the ravages of time by loading up on supplements containing this nutrient.

Understanding the Health Link

Q. Since cigarette smokers use 100 calories fewer a day than nonsmokers, won't people who quit smoking gain weight?

A. In 1988, the surgeon general reported that a preoccupation with gaining weight plays a major role in influencing whether people start, continue, and even resume smoking after quitting. Apparently, young women are particularly apt to develop a nicotine dependency while trying to lose weight.

Smokers who quit usually gain an average of seven pounds—so the weight gain could not be called an unhealthful one. In fact, according to Jack Henningfield, Ph.D., of the Addiction Research Center at the National Institute of Drug Abuse, it is rare for former smokers to gain unhealthful amounts of weight. As Dr. Henningfield noted, "A few pounds of weight is a small price to pay for greatly increasing your chances of a longer, healthier life."

For those who are concerned, some evidence exists that nicotine gum might help minimize weight gain. A group of long-term nicotine-gum chewers monitored by experts at the University of London's Addiction Research Unit gained less weight than smokers who successfully quit without using it. This is not to say that transferring the dependence to nicotine gum is necessarily a good idea. But since chewing gum decreases exposure to nicotine and completely eliminates the harmful tar and carbon monoxide its users would inhale if they continued to rely on cigarettes, it's certainly preferable to smoking and might be a viable option for people who have trouble kicking the habit, either because they fear weight gain or for other reasons. Moreover, most users give up the gum within three to six months.

Q. Will drinking cranberry juice help prevent or cure urinary tract infection?

A. The widely held belief that cranberry juice plays a role in prevention and treatment of urinary tract infection stems from an assumption that it makes urine more acidic. The reasoning is that since the bacteria that cause urinary tract infections are unlikely to flourish in an acid environment, drinking the acid-producing juice helps control the problem. However, cranberry juice's ability to make the urine acidic has not been well established. (Incidentally, straight cranberry juice is too bitter to be palatable. What you'll find at the supermarket is cranberry juice cocktail, a mixture of water, juice, and sugar that contains 147 calories a cup.)

Q. Are some foods more likely to cause heartburn than others?

A. Heartburn, an uncomfortable burning sensation in the chest that can occur when there is too much acid in the stomach, is a symptom of an underlying disorder called gastroesophageal reflux, a condition in which the contents of the stomach (including acid) flow backward into the esophagus. Although there is no proof that foods stimulate reflux, some substances are known to aggravate heartburn. These include coffee, alcohol, and citrus fruits, all of which make the stomach more acidic. Heartburn sufferers should also avoid fatty foods and chocolate, which interfere with contraction of the sphincter that separates the esophagus from the stomach. Other foods, such as spicy dishes, radishes, and cucumbers, may cause trouble for some people, but not for others. Some doctors counsel their heartburn patients not to lie down immediately after meals. That allows gravity to help in reducing the chances of a backflow, or reflux, of stomach contents.

Q. Are there any nutritional substances that can bolster the immune system?

A. Many essential nutrients, including vitamins B-6 and C and the mineral zinc, play a role in regulating the immune system. Researchers at Tufts have found that large doses of vitamin E also enhance immune responsiveness. After giving one group of healthy men and women over 60 years of age a daily supplement containing several times the recommended dietary allowance for that nutrient, and another group a placebo, they found that the immune function of those who took the vitamin was significantly improved after just 30 days. The group taking the placebo had no change in immune function at all.

As provocative as the findings are, they are by no means a signal for everyone to start taking megadose supplements of vitamin E. While the scientists were able to study much about immune function through a variety of specialized tests, they have yet to examine the direct relationship between vitamin E and the incidences of disease, such as cancer. In addition, they have not carried out long-term tests to find out if the effects last more than 30 days.

Q. Is it true that occasional fasting will eliminate toxins from the body?

A. Nearly every religion has encouraged fasting at one time or another, and fasting for a day or two every few weeks probably doesn't do any harm to a healthy person. But the alleged benefit, that the practice somehow "cleans out the system," is questionable. And fasting for more than a few days at a stretch could be quite harmful.

Ironically, although many fasters believe they are eliminating "toxic wastes," chemicals known as ketone bodies begin to accumulate in the bloodstream if they stop eating for too long. Ketone bodies are quite toxic and place a severe burden on the kidneys.

For some people, fasting can cause fatigue, dizziness, low blood pressure, and even depression. Prolonged fasting leads to a loss of protein from muscles and vital organs, as well as a depletion of the essential minerals calcium, phosphorus, sodium, and postassium.

The bottom line is that if your desire to fast is motivated by a desire to be physically healthier, you're probably choosing the wrong course of action.

Appendix A

Weights and Measures

Abbreviations

oz.	=	ounce
g	=	gram
lb.	=	pound
kg	=	kilogram
mg	=	milligram
ug	=	microgram
ml	=	milliliter
qt.	=	quart
tsp.	=	teaspoon
tbsp.	=	tablespoon

Volume

1 liter	=	1.06 quarts
1 gallon	=	3.79 liters
1 quart	=	0.95 liter
1 cup	=	8 fluid ounces
3 teaspoons	=	1 tablespoon
2 tablespoons	=	1 fluid ounce
16 tablespoons	=	1 cup
2 pints	=	1 quart
4 cups	=	1 quart
32 ounces	=	1 quart

Weights

1 ounce	=	28.4 grams
16 ounces	=	1 pound
1 pound	=	454 grams
1 kilogram	=	1,000 grams or 2.2 pounds
1 gram	=	1,000 milligrams
1 milligram	=	1,000 micrograms

Appendix B

Guide to Frozen Foods

A Tufts panel of experts evaluated popular frozen dinners to assess their nutritional value. Although we acknowledge that new products may have emerged since this test was conducted, we encourage you to use this guide to evaluate a healthy frozen meal. Dinners are recommended based on the criteria that they contain

▶ no more than 30 percent of calories in the form of fat

▶ no more than 800 milligrams of sodium

▶ at least 15 grams of protein

▶ no more than 300 calories per serving

▶ a net weight of 9 ounces or more

We have also supplied a list of side dishes that complement the frozen entrees and help achieve a more complete balance by adding missing amounts of vitamins A and C, along with fiber, a component that few frozen dinners contain in any appreciable amount.

Key

Dinners in the Recommended category may be somewhat higher in fat, sodium or calories than the Highly Recommended meals—or, they may be lower in protein.

+ FAT	= Somewhat high in fat
− PRO	= Somewhat low in protein
+ CAL	= Somewhat high in calories
+ SOD	= Somewhat high in sodium
Add . . .	= The numbers refer to the complementary *Nutritious Side Dishes* listed on pages 297–298 after the frozen foods

HIGHLY RECOMMENDED

Armour Dinner Classics

Chicken Hawaiian	Add 38, 44, or 47
Sirloin Roast with mushroom gravy	Add 17, 21, or 48

Armour Dinner Classics Lite

Baby Bay Shrimp in sherried cream sauce	Add 29, 39, or 45
Chicken Marsala	Add 19, 29, or 45
Chicken Breast in tomato and mushroom sauce	Add 11, 13, or 48
Chicken Burgundy	Add 16, 21, or 39
Chicken Cacciatore	Add 2, 27, or 33
Chicken Oriental	Add 7, 31, or 36
Seafood with natural herbs	Add 26 or 36
Steak Diane in seasoned sauce	Add 19, 22, or 48
Sweet & Sour Chicken	Add 14, 16, or 19

Benihana Oriental Lites

Beef and Mushrooms in sauce	Add 24, 29, or 36
Chicken in sauce	Add 24, 31, or 36
Chicken in spicy garlic sauce	Add 16, 24, or 31
Oriental Beef in wine sauce	Add 16, 29, or 36

Blue Star Dining Lites

Cheese Vegetable Lasagna	Add 35, 36, or 43
Chicken Ala King	Add 20, 31, or 49
Chicken Chow Mein	Add 4, 23, or 42
Country Style Chicken	Add 9, 17, or 36
Sauce and Swedish Meatballs	Add 28, 32, or 42
Zucchini Lasagna	Add 13, 24, or 42

Budget Gourmet, Regular Entrees

Pepper Steak in tomato sauce	Add 16, 24, or 41
Pepper Steak with Rice	Add 28, 39, or 44

Budget Gourmet, Slim Selects

Glazed Turkey	Add 7, 22, or 44
Glazed Turkey in honey sauce	Add 9, 16, or 36
Mandarin Chicken	Add 19, 26, or 41
Oriental Beef and Oriental Vegetables	Add 9, 23, or 24

Dining Lites

Beef Teriyaki	Add 16, 27, or 41
Chicken Ala King	Add 18, 22, or 25
Cheese Cannelloni	Add 11, 35, or 49
Chicken with Noodles	Add 3, 5, or 50
Glazed Chicken	Add 1, 7, or 28

Healthy Choice

Breast of Turkey	Add 8, 12, or 38
Chicken Oriental	Add 16, 17, or 49
Chicken Parmigiana	Add 13, 20, or 37
Oriental Pepper Steak	Add 16, 38, or 47
Salisbury Steak	Add 12, 20, or 25
Sirloin Tips	Add 4, 6, or 10
Sole Au Gratin	Add 8, 24, or 39
Sweet & Sour Chicken	Add 12, 24, or 47

Legume

Cannelloni Florentine	Add 14, 26, or 48
Manicotti Florentine	Add 11, 40, or 50
Meatless Pepper Steak	Add 27, 45, or 50

Le Menu Light Style Dinners

Chicken Cacciatore	Add 14, 19, or 21
Chicken Cannelloni	Add 2, 30, or 40
Glazed Chicken Breast	Add 29, 33, or 48
Herb Roasted Chicken	Add 24, 39, or 49
3-Cheese Stuffed Shells	Add 20, 32, or 38
Turkey Divan	Add 16, 24, or 31
Veal Marsala	Add 8, 11, or 15

Mrs. Paul's Light Entrees

Fish Florentine	Add 38, 47, or 49
Shrimp Primavera	Add 1, 19, or 24
Tuna Pasta Casserole	Add 16, 24, or 43

Stouffer's Lean Cuisine

Fillet of Fish Divan	Add 20, 24, or 25
Linguini with clam sauce	Add 1, 20, or 42
Veal Lasagna	Add 19, 24, or 29
Zucchini Lasagna	Add 16, 19, or 45

Stouffer's Right Course

Beef Dijon with Pasta & Vegetables	Add 4, 30, or 50
Beef Ragout with Rice Pilaf	Add 36, 43, or 47
Chicken Italiano with Fettucini & Vegetables	Add 1, 11, or 20
Homestyle Pot Roast	Add 2, 6, or 19

Tyson Gourmet Selection

Chicken A L'Orange	Add 1, 17, or 49

Weight Watchers

Chicken Ala King	Add 16, 20, or 49
Chicken Cacciatore	Add 16, 24, or 31

Fillet of Fish au Gratin	Add 8, 18, or 45
Imperial Chicken and Mushrooms	Add 29, 36, or 42

Pasta Rigati in meat sauce	Add 3, 24, or 36
Spaghetti with meat sauce	Add 24, 29, or 38
Sweet 'n Sour Chicken Tenders	Add 17, 24, or 38

RECOMMENDED

Armour Dinner Classics

BBQ Chicken / + SOD	Add 4, 13, or 34
Sirloin Roast / + SOD	Add 21, 30, 48

Armour Dinner Classics Lite

Baby Bay Shrimp / + SOD	Add 8, 38, or 44
Beef Pepper Steak	Add 5, 40, or 46
Chicken Breast Marsala / + SOD	Add 1, 8, or 17
Chicken Breast with Mushroom & Tomato Sauce / + SOD	Add 8, 13, or 32
Chicken Cacciatore / + SOD	Add 38, 47, or 50
Chicken Oriental / + SOD	Add 14, 41, or 42
Seafood with Natural Herbs / + SOD	Add 12, 24, or 38
Salisbury Steak with mushroom gravy / + FAT	Add 13, 23, or 35
Steak Diane / + SOD	Add 2, 23, or 40

Banquet Family Favorites Dinners

Spaghetti & Meatballs Dinner / − PRO	Add 1, 4, or 18

Benihana Oriental Lites

Chicken Chow Mein	Add 19, 13, or 32
Chicken in Spicy Garlic Sauce / + SOD	Add 15, 34, or 41
Glazed Chicken / + SOD	Add 8, 13, or 32
Shrimp Chow Mein / − PRO	Add 4, 13, or 44
Shrimp and Oriental Vegetables / − PRO	Add 38, 47, or 50
Sweet and Sour Chicken / + CAL	Add 17, 38, or 44

Blue Star Dining Lites

Cheese Cannelloni with tomato sauce / + FAT	Add 23, 29, or 47
Ziti in tomato sauce	Add 3, 30, or 34

Budget Gourmet, Regular Entrees

Chicken Marsala / + CAL	Add 11, 15, or 32
Sweet & Sour Chicken with Rice / + CAL	Add 17, 38, or 44

Budget Gourmet, Three Dish Dinners

Chicken Cacciatore / + FAT	Add 9, 16, or 29
Roast Chicken / + SOD	Add 7, 8, or 17

Scallops & Shrimp Mariner / + CAL	Add 18, 39, or 47
Sliced Turkey Breast	Add 16, 24, or 29
Teriyaki Chicken / + CAL	Add 16, 42, or 50

Budget Gourmet, Slim Selects

Cheese Ravioli / − PRO	Add 4, 24, or 27
Chicken au Gratin / + FAT	Add 17, 20, or 26
Chicken Enchilada Suiza / + SOD	Add 7, 22, or 25
Fettucini with meat sauce / + FAT	Add 2, 19, or 33
French Recipe Chicken / + FAT	Add 31, 34, or 36
Lasagna, with meat sauce / + FAT	Add 2, 29, or 48
Linguini with scallops & clams / + FAT	Add 1, 8, or 17
Oriental Beef / + SOD	Add 16, 38, or 47
Sirloin of Beef in herb sauce / + FAT	Add 13, 16, or 48
Sirloin Salisbury Steak / + SOD	Add 11, 18, or 25

Dining Lites

Chicken Chow Mein / + SOD	Add 17, 24, or 44
Pepper Steak / + SOD	Add 24, 39, or 47
Sauce & Swedish Meatballs / + FAT	Add 8, 17, or 28

Healthy Choice

Chicken & Pasta Divan / + CAL	Add 29, 37, or 40
Shrimp Creole / + CAL	Add 12, 17, or 24

Legume

Classic Lasagne / + FAT	Add 1, 11, or 15
Mexican Enchiladas with tofu / − PRO	Add 14, 42, or 46
Sweet & Sour Tofu with whole wheat noodles / − PRO	Add 2, 16, or 36
Tofu Sesame Ginger Stir-Fry / − PRO	Add 14, 17, or 47
Vegetable Lasagna / − PRO	Add 1, 11, or 18

Le Menu

Sliced Breast of Turkey with Mushroom Gravy / + SOD	Add 21, 23, or 42

(continued)

RECOMMENDED (cont.)

Le Menu Light Style Dinners

Chicken Chow Mein / + SOD	Add 16, 17, or 38
Salisbury Steak / + SOD	Add 8, 24, or 49
Turkey Divan / + SOD	Add 12, 20, or 30

Morton Dinners

Glazed Ham / + CAL	Add 2, 16, or 43
Sliced Beef Dinner / + SOD	Add 3, 6, or 15
Turkey with dressing and gravy	Add 13, 24, or 48

Mrs. Paul's Light Seafood Entrees

Fish au Gratin	Add 10, 15, or 37
Fish and Pasta Florentine / + FAT	Add 9, 19, or 44
Seafood Lasagne / − PRO	Add 7, 22, or 49
Seafood Rotini / − PRO	Add 1, 17, or 44
Shrimp Cajun Style / − PRO	Add 24, 44, or 47
Shrimp & Clams with linguini / − PRO	Add 1, 8, or 39

Stouffer's

Chicken a la King with Rice / + SOD	Add 17, 28, or 44

Stouffer's Lean Cuisine

Beef and Pork Cannelloni with Mornay sauce / + FAT	Add 11, 14, or 26
Beefsteak Ranchero / + SOD	Add 17, 38, or 49
Breast of Chicken Parmesan / + SOD	Add 1, 18, or 47
Cheese Cannelloni with tomato sauce / + FAT	Add 2, 16, or 36
Chicken and Vegetables with vermicelli	Add 4, 8, or 15
Chicken Cacciatore with vermicelli / + FAT	Add 11, 20, or 38
Chicken Chow Mein	Add 2, 16, or 36
Chicken Oriental / + SOD	Add 17, 28, or 38
Filet of Fish Florentine / + FAT	Add 7, 44, or 45
Filet of Fish Jardiniere / + FAT	Add 2, 16, or 36
Herbed Lamb	Add 11, 14, or 26
Lasagna with Meat and Sauce / + SOD	Add 1, 23, or 25
Linguini with Clam Sauce / + SOD	Add 1, 22, or 44
Oriental Scallops	Add 2, 3, or 48
Shrimp & Chicken Cantonese with noodles	Add 6, 13, or 37

Spaghetti with beef and mushroom sauce / + SOD	Add 8, 18, or 24
Szechuan Beef with Noodles and Vegetables / + FAT	Add 5, 16, or 41
Tuna Lasagna with spinach noodles and vegetables / + FAT	Add 22, 36, or 48
Turkey Dijon / + FAT	Add 17, 26, or 29
Veal Primavera with vermicelli / + FAT	Add 7, 18, or 44
Zucchini Lasagna / + SOD	Add 19, 31, or 42

Stouffer's Right Course

Sesame Chicken / + CAL	Add 16, 38, or 49
Shrimp Primavera / − PRO	Add 3, 15, or 42
Vegetarian Chili / − PRO	Add 1, 4, or 45

Swanson's 4-Compartment Dinners

Beef in barbecue sauce / + CAL	Add 4, 17, or 44
Chicken (dark meat) in barbecue sauce / + CAL	Add 16 or 35
Noodles and Chicken in gravy / − PRO	Add 2, 24, or 48
Polynesian Sweet and Sour Chicken / + CAL	Add 7, 24, or 29
Sweet 'n Sour Chicken / + CAL	Add 16, 17, or 41
Swiss Steak with tomato-beef gravy / + CAL	Add 1, 8, or 24

Swanson's Homestyle Recipe Entrees

Chicken Cacciatore / + SOD	Add 4, 18, or 20
Sirloin Tips in Burgundy Sauce / + FAT	Add 8, 18, or 38

Tyson Chicken Entrees

Chicken Cacciatore with pasta primavera / + FAT	Add 2, 16, or 29
Chicken Marsala / + FAT	Add 13, 29, or 36
Chicken Oriental in teriyaki sauce / SOD-OK	Add 7, 24, or 36
Chicken Picatta in lemon-butter sauce / SOD-OK, + FAT	Add 2, 24, or 29
Chicken Mesquite in tangy barbecue sauce / + CAL	Add 16, 27, or 36

Tyson Gourmet Selections

Chicken Oriental / + SOD	Add 18, 38, or 44
Chicken Mesquite / + CAL	Add 13, 19, or 50

Weight Watchers

Broccoli and Cheese Baked Potato / − PRO	Add 21, 33, or 48
Chicken Divan Baked Potato / + SOD	Add 7, 23, or 44
Imperial Chicken / + SOD	Add 16, 17, or 38
Pasta Rigati / + SOD	Add 3, 32, or 36
Seafood Linguini / − PRO	Add 1, 8, or 18

Spaghetti with Meat Sauce / + SOD	Add 10, 13, or 37

Weight Watchers

Stuffed Sole in Newburg Sauce / SOD-OK	Add 16, 24, or 36
Seafood Linguini / − PRO	Add 27, 29, or 48
Baked Cheese Ravioli / + FAT	Add 3, 28, or 43

NUTRITIOUS SIDE DISHES

Round out your frozen meals with the addition of one of these dishes, designed to add the nutrients missing in the corresponding dinners. Each contains from 100 to 200 calories:

1. Spinach salad: 1 cup chopped spinach, ¼ cup sliced mushrooms, ½ wedged tomato, ½ chopped hard-cooked egg, 1 tablespoon walnuts, 1 tablespoon low-calorie Italian dressing; 2 breadsticks.
2. ½ cup steamed red and green cabbage sprinkled with caraway seeds; 1 cup pineapple chunks garnished with maraschino cherry and a sprig of mint.
3. 4 asparagus spears; 1 cup sliced strawberries with a dollop of low-fat lemon or vanilla yogurt.
4. ½ cup each shredded Iceberg and Romaine lettuce and ¼ cup sliced mushrooms sprinkled with wine vinegar and a dash of basil; ½ cup red grapes with 1 ounce wedge of low-fat cheese.
5. 1 cup cooked green beans tossed with ¼ cup water chestnuts and 1 tablespoon toasted, slivered almonds; 1 sliced orange with ½ sliced grapefruit.
6. 1 small ear corn on the cob with 1 teaspoon margarine; 4″ x 8″ watermelon wedge.
7. ½ cup steamed carrots dusted with parsley; 1 kiwifruit sliced into ½ cup water-packed fruit cocktail.
8. 1 cup Romaine lettuce, ½ cup cherry tomato halves tossed with 1 tablespoon low-calorie Italian dressing and sprinkled with 1 tablespoon Parmesan cheese; ¼ cantaloupe.
9. 3 steamed broccoli stalks sprinkled with sesame seeds; ½ cup each canned, drained mandarin oranges and pineapple chunks mixed with ½ cup low-fat yogurt and garnished with a maraschino cherry.
10. ½ cup steamed artichokes drizzled with lemon juice.
11. Caesar salad: 1 cup Romaine letuce, ¼ cup herbed croutons, ½ chopped hard-cooked egg tossed with 1 teaspoon olive oil, 2 teaspoons lemon juice, dash of garlic and 1 tablespoon Parmesan cheese; 1 cup raspberries with a dollop of low-fat lemon vanilla yogurt.
12. Carrot salad: 1 cup shredded carrots, 1 tablespoon each raisins and diet mayonnaise; 1 poppyseed roll.
13. ½ cup each steamed zucchini and cauliflower seasoned with a squirt of lemon juice and sprinkled with dill; 2″-long slice Italian bread.
14. ½ cup low-fat cottage cheese spooned over 2 water-packed peach halves and garnished with chopped walnuts.
15. 2 tomato halves broiled with 1 ounce part-skim mozzarella cheese and seasoned with a dash of garlic and oregano.
16. Oriental salad: ½ cup each shredded Bibb lettuce and fresh spinach leaves, ¼ cup drained mandarin oranges, ¼ cup herbed croutons, 1½ teaspoons each vinegar and olive oil.
17. 1 cup cantaloupe balls in ½ cup low-fat vanilla yogurt, spiced with a dash of cinnamon and nutmeg.
18. ¼ cucumber, 1 tomato, ¼ red onion, sliced and marinated in low-calorie dressing and seasoned with fresh ground pepper; 1 nectarine.
19. Fruit kabob: 4 strawberries, ¼ cup honeydew chunks, ¼ cup pineapple chunks skewered and dipped in ¼ cup low-fat vanilla yogurt mixed with 1 tablespoon slivered almonds and a taste of honey.
20. Spinach and basil salad: 1 cup fresh spinach leaves, ¼ cup fresh basil leaves tossed with 2 teaspoons olive oil, 1 tablespoon pine nuts and garlic powder to taste; 1 plum.

(continued)

NUTRITIOUS SIDE DISHES (cont.)

21. Waldorf salad: 1 chopped apple, 1 tablespoon each raisins, chopped celery, and chopped walnuts moistened with 1 tablespoon diet mayonnaise.
22. 1 cup steamed broccoli with 1 ounce low-fat cheese melted on top; 3 medium apricots.
23. ½ cup each steamed carrots and zucchini seasoned with dill; 1 cup red grapes.
24. 1 cup Iceberg lettuce with ¼ cup each shredded red cabbage and carrots tossed with wine vinegar and tarragon.
25. 1 cup raw cauliflowerettes and ¼ cup grated carrots with ¼ cup plain low-fat yogurt seasoned with dill.
26. 1 cup cooked green beans sprinkled with sesame seeds and a shake of soy sauce; ½ cup fresh strawberries with a dollop of lemon or vanilla yogurt.
27. 1 cup cooked Brussels sprouts stir fried with ¼ cup water chestnuts in 1 teaspoon of vegetable oil; Blueberry parfait: alternate layers of ½ cup each fresh blueberries and low-fat vanilla yogurt and top with a dash of cinnamon and 2 crumbled vanilla wafers.
28. 1 cup cooked spinach with a zest of lemon juice and dash of nutmeg; 1 cup peach slices sprinkled with ginger.
29. 1 cup shredded cabbage mixed with caraway seeds and 1 tablespoon diet mayonnaise; small poppyseed roll.
30. ½ cucumber, 1 tomato sliced into ½ cup low-fat plain yogurt with chives and lemon juice; 1 nectarine.
31. 1 cup cooked cauliflower with ¼ cup each sliced mushrooms and red pepper strips; 1 small whole wheat roll.
32. 1 cup okra marinated in vinegar seasoned with dry mustard, thyme and a few drops of olive oil; 2″ by 7″ wedge honeydew melon.
33. Iceberg lettuce wedge with low-calorie dressing; ½ medium-sized acorn squash baked with 1 teaspoon each margarine and brown sugar.
34. 1 cup shredded red cabbage cooked with ¼ cup each chopped apple and diced onion, as well as wine vinegar and sugar to taste; 1 small hard roll.
35. ½ cup each carrot, green pepper and onion strips sautéed in a teaspoon of vegetable oil and a dash of basil; 1 pear.
36. 2 stalks steamed broccoli sprinkled with pimento; apple baked with cinnamon and a dash of brown sugar.
37. 1 celery stalk stuffed with low-fat cottage cheese and garnished with pimento; 3 prunes.
38. Fruit bowl: ½ cup each cantaloupe and honeydew, 1 sliced kiwifruit and ⅔ cup raspberries with a sprinkle of lemon; 2 gingersnap cookies.
39. 1 cup cooked collard greens with 1 tablespoon Parmesan cheese; 1 slice Pumpernickel bread.
40. 1 peach and ½ cup sliced strawberries in ½ cup water-packed fruit cocktail; small whole wheat roll.
41. Chinese salad: 1 cup Romaine lettuce, ¼ cup canned, drained mandarin oranges and 2 tablespoons slivered toasted almonds with poppyseed dressing.
42. 1 banana sliced with 1 orange (and its juice) and sprinkled with 1 tablespoon raisins.
43. 1 cup steamed cauliflower topped with 1 ounce melted low-fat cheese and 1 tablespoon bread crumbs; 2 apricots.
44. 3 stalks steamed asparagus; 1 persimmon.
45. Baked potato covered with spinach and 1 tablespoon Parmesan cheese.
46. ½ cup corn with chopped red and green peppers seasoned with chili powder; 1 cup red grapes.
47. Garden salad: 1 cup red leaf lettuce, ¼ sliced cucumber, ¼ wedged tomato, and ¼ cup grated carrot with 1 tablespoon low-calorie dressing (optional: 2 chopped, marinated artichoke hearts).
48. 1 apple baked with margarine, dash of brown sugar, raisins, walnuts, and ¼ cup orange juice.
49. Raw julienne carrots, yellow and green zuchini, red pepper, dipped in plain, low-fat yogurt with scallions.
50. Fresh fruit mix; 1 sliced peach, ¼ cup each strawberries and blueberries, ½ cup honeydew melon balls.

Appendix C

The Nutrition Hotline

Food, Drug, and Alcohol Abuse

Action on Smoking & Health
2013 H. St. N.W.
Washington D.C. 20006
(202) 659-4310

Nonprofit legal action smoking group; provides general information

Alcohol, Drug Abuse, and Mental Health Administration
Department of Health and Human Services
Parklawn Building, Room 12C–15
5600 Fishers Lane
Rockville, Maryland 20857
(301) 443-3783

Handles inquiries and supplies publications about alcohol, drug, and mental health problems

Alcoholics Anonymous World Services
468 Park Avenue South
New York, New York 10163
(212) 686-1100

Answers inquiries, makes referrals regarding AA groups in 110 countries

Alcohol and Drug Problems Association of North America
444 N. Capitol St., Suite 181
Washington D.C. 20001
(202) 737-4340

Provides information, education, and referrals on drug- and alcohol-related problems

Alcohol Education for Youth
1500 Western Ave.
Albany, New York 12203
(514) 456-3800

Answers inquiries and provides education for the prevention of alcohol abuse among youth

American Anorexia/Bulimia Association, Inc.
133 Cedar Lane
Teaneck, New Jersey 07666
(201) 836-1800

Provides information and support for people with eating disorders and their families

Anorexia Nervosa and Associated Disorders, Inc.
P.O. Box 7
Highland Park, Illinois 60035
(312) 831-3438

Provides information and referrals for treatment of eating disorders

Bulimia, Anorexia Self-Help
6125 Clayton Ave., Suite 215
St. Louis, Missouri 63139
(800) 227-4785

Provides support and information for recovery from eating disorders

Center for the Study of Anorexia and Bulimia
One W. 91st St.
New York, New York 10024
(212) 595-3449

Provides support, information, and services related to the psychotherapeutic treatment of eating disorders

Children of Alcoholics Foundation
540 Madison Ave., 23rd floor
New York, New York 10022
(212) 980-5394

Supplies education and support for children with alcoholic parents

Drug and Alcohol Council
396 Alexander St.
Rochester, New York 14607
(716) 244-3190

Provides preventive education and primary intervention for alcohol and drug cases

National Anorexic Aid Society, Inc.
5796 Karl Road
Columbus, Ohio 43229
(614) 436-1112

Provides education, referrals, and services related to anorexia nervosa

National Clearinghouse for Alcohol Information
P.O. Box 2345
Rockville, Maryland 20852
(301) 468-2600

Supplies information, publications, and referrals related to alcoholism

National Council on Alcoholism
12 W. 21st St.
New York, New York 10010
(212) 206-2770

Provides referrals and information regarding alcoholism and its medical, pyschological, and sociological aspects

National Federation of Parents for Drug-Free
  Youth
8730 Georgia Avenue, Suite 200
Silver Spring, Maryland 20910
(301) 554-5437

Helps concerned parents prevent adolescent drug abuse

Office on Smoking and Health
Centers for Disease Control
Park Bldg., Rm. 1–10
5600 Fishers Lane
Rockville, Maryland 20857
(301) 443-1575

Answers inquiries, makes referrals, and publishes a bulletin related to smoking and health

Students Against Drunk Driving
10812 Ashfield Road
Adelphi, Maryland 20783
(301) 937-7936

Devoted to combatting deaths caused by drunken driving; offers education and information programs, as well as student-parent support

Food Policy, Safety, Labeling, Legislation

Center for Food Safety and Applied Nutrition
Food and Drug Administration
200 C St. S.W., Room 3321
Washington D.C. 20204
(202) 245-1236

Provides information on nutrition, food, food technology, and food additives

Center for Science in the Public Interest
1501 16th St. N.W.
Washington D.C. 20036
(202) 332-9110

Engages in research, education, and advisory services dedicated to improving the American diet

Clean Water Action Project
733 15th St. N.W., Suite 1110
Washington D.C. 20005
(202) 638-1196

Promotes public interest in water safety through national education; provides information and referrals

Food and Drug Administration, Consumer Inquiries
5600 Fishers Lane
Rockville, Maryland 20857
(301) 443-3170

Answers inquiries and supplies publications related to food and drug safety and efficacy

Food Safety and Inspection Service
Information Division
Department of Agriculture
14th St. and Independence Ave. S.W.
Washington D.C. 20250
(202) 447-9113

Takes responsibility for meat and poultry inspection; provides consumer information and gives referrals

Public Voice for Food and Health Policy
1001 Connecticut Ave N.W., Suite 522
Washington D.C. 20036
(202) 659-5930

Acts as a national consumer watchdog organization which monitors food and health agencies and congressional committees charged with protecting public health

Illness and Disease Prevention and Treatment

American Cancer Society
Medical Library
4 West 34th St.
New York, New York 10001
(212) 736-3030

Serves as a clearinghouse for information on cancer research, statistics, and public health

American Diabetes Association
505 8th Ave.
New York, New York 10018
(212) 947-9707

Provides information, education, research, and referrals related to diabetes

American Health Foundation
320 East 43rd St.
New York, New York 10017
(212) 953-1900

Engages in disease-prevention programs and public education and information services

American Heart Association
7320 Greenville Ave.
Dallas, Texas 75231
(214) 750-5300

Answers inquiries, makes referrals, and offers reference services related to heart disease

American Lung Association
1740 Broadway
New York, New York 10019
(212) 245-8000

Engages in preventive efforts regarding lung disease; answers inquiries and provides education materials

Association for Research of Childhood Cancer
3653 Harlem Road
Buffalo, New York 14215
(716) 838-4433

Provides support for parents of children with cancer

Centers for Disease Control
Office of Public Affairs
1600 Clifton Road N.E.
Atlanta, Georgia 30333
(404) 329-3286

Answers public's questions on health-related issues

Citizens for the Treatment of High Blood Pressure
1140 Connecticut Ave. N.W., Suite 606
Washington D.C. 20036
(202) 296-4435

Engages in research and funding for treatment of high blood pressure; provides advisory services and conducts seminars

High Blood Pressure Information Center
2121 Wisconsin Ave. N.W., Suite 410
Washington D.C. 20036
(202) 496-1809

Provides education, references, information and seminars related to high blood pressure

Joslin Diabetes Center
One Joslin Place
Boston, Massachusetts 02215
(617) 732-2400

Provides research, education, and information on adult-onset diabetes

Juvenile Diabetes Foundation
60 Madison Ave.
New York, New York 10010
(800) 223-1138

Provides educational programs and information on adolescent-onset diabetes

Lipid Research Clinic
George Washington University Medical Center
2150 Pennsylvania Ave. N.W.
Washington D.C. 20037
(202) 676-4152

Conducts reseach on blood lipids and lipoproteins and their relationship to coronary heart disease; provides patient services and referrals

National Cancer Institute
NIH Bldg. 31, Room 10A18
Bethesda, Maryland 20892
(301) 496-5583

Provides research, training, and information on all aspects of cancer prevention, detection, and rehabilitation

National Diabetes Information Clearinghouse
Box NDIC
Bethesda, Maryland 20892
(301) 468-2162

Supplies information, publications, and referrals related to diabetes

National Digestive Diseases Information Clearinghouse
Box NNDIC
Bethesda, Maryland 20892
(301) 496-9707

Provides information and nationwide referrals related to illnesses of the digestive tract

National Foundation for Cancer Research
7215 Wisconsin Ave. N.W., Suite 332W
Bethesda, Maryland 20814
(301) 654-1250

Distributes publications, makes referrals, and holds seminars related to cancer research

National Heart, Lung, and Blood Institute
Public Inquiries and Reports Branch
National Institutes of Health
Bethesda, Maryland 20892
(301) 496-4236

Answers inquiries regarding heart, lung, and blood diseases

National Kidney Foundation
2 Park Avenue
New York, New York 10016
(212) 889-2210

Provides education, information, research, and referrals related to kidney disease

Skin Cancer Foundation
475 Park Avenue South
New York, New York 10016
(212) 725-5176

Supplies education, information, and services related to skin cancer

Food Industry Associations

Food Marketing Institute
1750 K St. N.W.
Washington D.C. 20006
(202) 452-8444

Serves as the association of supermarket retailers and wholesalers; answers inquiries and provides research information

Food Processors Institute
1401 New York Ave. N.W., Suite 400
Washington D.C. 20005
(202) 393-0890

Provides information on food processing, labeling, safety, and policy

Grocery Manufacturers of America
1010 Wisconsin Avenue N.W., Suite 800
Washington D.C. 20007
(202) 337-9400

Provides information on the grocery industry, labeling, safety, and food quality

Milk Industry Foundation
888 16th St. N.W., 2nd floor
Washington D.C. 20006
(202) 296-4250

Publishes research on milk and milk products

National Association of Wheat Growers
415 Second St N.E., Suite 300
Washington D.C. 20002
(202) 547-7800

Answers inquiries and distributes publications regarding the wheat industry

National Meat Association
734 15th St. N.W.
Washington D.C. 20005
(202) 347-1000

Represents the meat packing and processing industry; answers inquiries

National Restaurant Association
311 First St. N.W.
Washington D.C. 20001
(202) 638-6100

Provides information related to the food-service industry

Soy Protein Council
1255 23rd St. N.W., Suite 850
Washington D.C. 20037
(202) 467-6610

Represents the food protein industry; provides information about research and government actions

Wheat Flour Institute
600 Maryland Ave. S.W.
Washington D.C. 20024
(202) 484-2200

Provides information on wheat flour, nutrition, and diet

Nutrition and Health Information and Services

American Association of Retired Persons
1900 K St. N.W.
Washington D.C. 20049
(202) 728-4880

Promotes education, welfare, research, and other matters related to the elderly

Beltsville Human Nutrition Research Center
Ag Research Service
U.S. Department of Agriculture
Room 223, Bldg. 308
Beltsville, Maryland 20705
(301) 244-2157

Answers inquiries and makes referrals concerning nutrient requirements and metabolism

Bureau of Health Care Delivery and Assistance
Health Resources and Services Administration
Public Health Service
Parklawn Building, Room G-05
5600 Fishers Lane
Rockville, Maryland 20857
(301) 443-2320

Oversees the provision of health and nutrition services; answers inquiries and supplies information

Community Nutrition Institute
2001 S St. N.W.
Washington D.C. 20009
(202) 462-4700

Answers inquiries, conducts seminars, and distributes publications related to national nutrition concerns

Human Nutrition Information Service
Food and Consumer Services
U.S. Department of Agriculture
6505 Belcrest Road
Hyattsville, Maryland 20782
(301) 436-7725

Studies food and nutrition; answers inquiries

International Association for Medical Assistance to Travelers
736 Center St.
Lewiston, New York 14092
(716) 754-4883

Provides information on sanitary conditions and precautions for travelers around the world

Maternity Center Association
48 East 92nd St.
New York, New York 10028
(212) 369-7300

Provides prenatal education and services

National Health Information Clearinghouse
P.O. Box 1133
Washington D.C. 20013
(800) 336-4797

Provides referrals from a database for over 1,000 health-related organizations

President's Council on Physical Fitness and Sports
450 Fifth St. N.W., Room 7103
Washington D.C. 20001
(202) 272-3421

Engages in development and education regarding national fitness programs

Tufts University Diet and Nutrition Letter
80 Boylston St., Suite 353
Boston, Massachusetts 02116
(617) 482-3530

Publishes a monthly consumer newsletter that reflects current nutrition research and guidelines

Index

Page numbers followed by (c) indicate charts. Page numbers followed by (t) indicate tables.

Page numbers followed by (c) indicate charts. Page numbers followed by (t) indicate tables.

Page numbers followed by (c) indicate charts. Page numbers followed by (t) indicate tables.

DEMCO